RARE AND INTERSTITIAL LUNG DISEASES

Clinical Cases and Real-World Discussions

Editors

Claudio Sorino, MD, PhD
Assistant Professor of Medicine and Human Anatomy
University of Insubria
Varese, Italy;
Associate Medical Director of Respiratory Pathophysiology
Department of Pulmonary and Critical Care Medicine
Sant'Anna Hospital
Como, Italy

Sergio Agati, MD
Director
Department of Pulmonary and Critical Care Medicine
Sant'Anna Hospital
Como, Italy

Associate Editors

Sonye Karen Danoff, MD, PhD
Associate Professor of Medicine
Division of Pulmonary and Critical Care Medicine,
Co-Director
Johns Hopkins Interstitial Lung Disease/Pulmonary Fibrosis Program
Baltimore, Maryland

Nicola Scichilone, MD, PhD
Full Professor of Respiratory Medicine
University of Palermo;
Head of the Division of Respiratory Medicine
Department PROMISE
"Giaccone" University Hospital
Palermo, Italy

Francesco Bonella, MD, PhD
Assistant Professor of Medicine
University of Essen;
Head of the Division for Interstitial and Rare Lung Disease
Ruhrlandklinik
Essen, Germany

Michele Mondoni, MD
Assistant Professor of Respiratory Medicine
University of Milan;
Associate Medical Director of Interventional Pulmonology
Department of Health Sciences
ASST Santi Paolo e Carlo
Milan, Italy

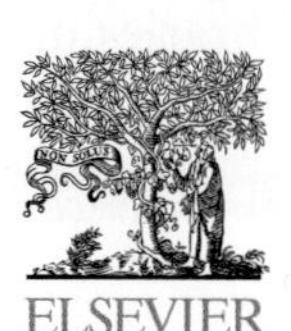

ELSEVIER

Elsevier
1600 John F. Kennedy Blvd.
Ste 1800
Philadelphia, PA 19103-2899

RARE AND INTERSTITIAL LUNG DISEASES:
CLINICAL CASES AND REAL-WORLD DISCUSSIONS ISBN: 978-0-323-93522-7

Senior Content Strategist: Robin Carter/Charlotta Kryhl
Senior Content Development Specialist: Himanshi Chauhan
Publishing Services Manager: Shereen Jameel
Senior Project Manager: Beula Christopher
Senior Book Designer: Renee Duenow

Printed in India

Last digit is the print number: 9 8 7 6 5 4 3 2 1

RARE AND INTERSTITIAL LUNG DISEASES

Clinical Cases and Real-World Discussions

CONTRIBUTORS

Sergio Agati, MD
Director
Department of Pulmonary and Critical Care Medicine
Sant'Anna Hospital
Como, Italy

Fausta Alfano, MD
Respiratory Unit
ASST Santi Paolo e Carlo
Milan, Italy

Arata Azuma, MD, PhD
Professor of Pulmonary Medicine
Department of Pulmonary Medicine and Oncology
Graduate School of Medicine
Nippon Medical School
Tokyo, Japan

Alice Biffi, MD
Respiratory Unit
IRCCS San Gerardo
Monza, Italy

Eda Boerner, MD
Department of Pneumology
Ruhrlandklinik, Universitätsmedizin Essen
Essen, Germany

Francesco Bonella, MD, PhD
Assistant Professor of Medicine
University of Essen;
Head of the Division for Interstitial and Rare Lung Disease
Ruhrlandklinik
Essen, Germany

Stacey-Ann Brown, MD, MPH
Assistant Professor
Department of Pulmonary and Critical Care
Johns Hopkins University
Baltimore, Maryland

Ilaria Campo, PhD
Biologist, Researcher
Pneumology Unit
IRCCS San Matteo Hospital Foundation
Pavia, Italy

Nunzia Cannizzaro, MD
Division of Respiratory Diseases
Paolo Giaccone University Hospital
Palermo, Italy

Stefano Centanni, MD, PhD
Full Professor of Respiratory Medicine
Respiratory Unit
ASST Santi Paolo e Carlo
Department of Health Sciences
Università degli Studi di Milano
Milan, Italy

Daniela Ceriani, MD
Department of Pulmonary and Critical Care Medicine
Sant'Anna Hospital
Como, Italy

Giuseppe Cicchetti, MD, PhD
Advanced Radiology Center
Department of Diagnostic Imaging
Oncological Radiotherapy and Hematology
Fondazione Policlinico Universitario A. Gemelli IRCCS
Rome, Italy

Claudia Cigala, MD
Anatomic Pathology Unit
ASST Santi Paolo e Carlo
Milan, Italy

Angelo Guido Corsico, MD, PhD
Professor of Respiratory Medicine
Department of Internal Medicine and Therapeutics
University of Pavia;
Head of Respiratory Diseases Division
Department of Thoracic and Vascular
IRCCS Policlinico San Matteo Foundation
Pavia, Italy

Vincent Cottin, MD, PhD
Professor of Respiratory Medicine
Claude Bernard University
University of Lyon;
Head
Reference Center for Rare Pulmonary Diseases (OrphaLung)
Louis Pradel Hospital
Hospices Civils de Lyon
Lyon, France

Sonye Karen Danoff, MD, PhD
Associate Professor of Medicine
Division of Pulmonary and Critical Care Medicine,
Co-Director
Johns Hopkins Interstitial Lung Disease/ Pulmonary Fibrosis Program
Baltimore, Maryland

Stefano Elia, MD
Division of Radiology
Esine Hospital
Esine (BS), Italy

Federico Giussani, MD
Pulmonology Unit
Sant'Antonio Abate Hospital
Cantù (CO), Italy

Tomohiro Handa, MD, PhD
Associate Professor
Department of Advanced Medicine for Respiratory Failure
Graduate School of Medicine
Kyoto University
Kyoto, Japan

Lutz-Bernhard Jehn, MD
Clinician Scientist
Interstitial and Rare Lung Disease
Ruhrlandklinik University Hospital
Essen, Germany

Sara Lettieri, MD
Pneumology Unit
IRCCS San Matteo, Hospital Foundation
Pavia, Italy

Roberto Marchese, MD
Division of Pulmonology and Thoracic Surgery
La Maddalena Hospital
Palermo, Italy

Francesca Mariani, MD, PhD
Pneumology Unit
IRCCS San Matteo, Hospital Foundation
Pavia, Italy

Giulio Melone, MD
Department of Pulmonary and Critical Care Medicine
Sant'Anna Hospital
Como, Italy

Riccardo Messina, MD, PhD
Division of Respiratory Medicine
Paolo Giaccone University Hospital
Palermo, Italy

Michele Mondoni, MD
Assistant Professor of Respiratory Medicine
University of Milan;
Associate Medical Director of Interventional Pulmonology
Department of Health Sciences
ASST Santi Paolo e Carlo
Milan, Italy

Stefano Negri, MD
Department of Pulmonary and Critical Care Medicine
Sant'Anna Hospital
Como, Italy

Giovanni Palladini, MD, PhD
Professor
Molecular Medicine
University of Pavia
Pavia, Italy

Sara Piciucchi, MD
Department of Radiology
G.B. Morgagni Hospital/University of Bologna
Forlì, Italy

Davide Piloni, MD, PhD
UOC Pneumologia
IRCCS Policlinico San Matteo Foundation
Pavia, Italy

Silvia Pizzolato, MD
Department of Pulmonary and Critical Care Medicine
Sant'Anna Hospital
Como, Italy

Venerino Poletti, MD
Professor of Medicine
Department of Respiratory Diseases and Allergy
Aarhus University
Aarhus, Denmark;
Department of Medical Specialities-Pulmonology
GB Morgagni Hospital
Bologna, Italy;
University-Forlì-Ravenna Campus
Forlì, Italy

Antje Prasse, MD
Clinical Professor of Pneumology,
Faculty of Medicine,
Director of the Clinic for Pneumology
University Hospital of Basel
Basel, Switzerland

Claudia Ravaglia, MD
Associate Professor
Department of Thoracic Diseases
GB Morgagni - L Pierantoni Hospital
Forlì, Italy

Jannik Ruwisch, MD
Clinician Scientist
Department of Pulmonary Medicine and Infectious Diseases
Hannover Medical School
Lower Saxony, Germany

Ryo Sakamoto, MD
Department of Diagnostic Imaging and Nuclear Medicine
Kyoto University Graduate School of Medicine
Kyoto, Japan

Gianluca Sambataro, MD
Assistant Professor of Rheumatology
Department of Clinical and Experimental Medicine
University of Catania
Internal Medicine Unit, Section of Rheumatology, "Cannizzaro" Hospital
Catania, Italy

Nicola Scichilone, MD, PhD
Full Professor of Respiratory Medicine
University of Palermo;
Head of the Division of Respiratory Medicine
Department PROMISE
"Giaccone" University Hospital
Palermo, Italy

Claudio Sorino, MD, PhD
Assistant Professor of Medicine and Human Anatomy
University of Insubria
Varese, Italy;
Associate Medical Director of Respiratory Pathophysiology
Department of Pulmonary and Critical Care Medicine
Sant'Anna Hospital
Como, Italy

Antonio Spanevello, MD
Full Professor, Respiratory Diseases
Department of Medicine and Surgery
University of Insubria
Varese, Italy

Silvia Terraneo, MD, PhD
Respiratory Unit
ASST Santi Paolo e Carlo
Milan, Italy

Claudio Tirelli, MD
Respiratory Unit
ASST Santi Paolo e Carlo;
Department of Health Sciences
Università degli Studi di Milano
Milan, Italy

Olga Torre, MD
Respiratory Unit
ASST Santi Paolo e Carlo
Milan, Italy

Ada Vancheri, MD
Department of Diseases of the Thorax
Ospedale GB Morgagni
Forlì, Italy

Carlo Vancheri, MD, PhD
Full Professor of Respiratory Medicine
Department of Clinical and Experimental Medicine
University of Catania
University Hospital Policlinico "G. Rodolico - San Marco"
Catania, Italy

Marco Vanetti, MD
Department of Medicine and Surgery
University of Insubria
Varese, Italy

Francesco Varone, MD
UOC Pneumologia
Fondazione Policlinico Universitario "Agostino Gemelli" IRCCS
Roma, Italy

Robert Vassallo, MD
Professor of Medicine,
Associate Chair for Research
Division of Pulmonary and Critical Care Medicine
Mayo Clinic
Rochester, Minnesota

Dina Visca, MD, PhD
Associate Professor
Department of Pneumology
Istituti Clinici Scientifici Maugeri, IRCCS
Tradate, Italy

Akihiko Yoshizawa, MD, PhD
Associate Professor
Department of Diagnostic Pathology
Kyoto University Hospital;
Associate Professor
Center for Anatomical, Pathological, and Forensic Medical Researches
Graduate School of Medicine
Kyoto University
Kyoto, Japan

Martina Zappa, MD, PhD
Department of Medicine and Surgery
University of Insubria
Varese, Italy

FOREWORD

Interstitial lung diseases are rare entities when evaluated individually. Considered altogether, due to their variety (more than 200 pathologies), they constitute a significant part of the clinical activity of physicians dealing with respiratory diseases.

This is an extremely niche area of interest, as it involves not only idiopathic but also autoimmune and rheumatologic pathologies, as well as diseases linked to noxious professional exposures or secondary to the increasingly widespread use of drugs.

To date, we lack a standardized clinical approach that is recognized as effective and efficient in diagnosing most rare respiratory and nonrespiratory diseases, except those few conditions for which a screening process has proven useful. In fact, given their "intrinsic" rarity, loosely recommending second-level tests in all patients with evidence of interstitial lung disease would be inconvenient and uneconomical. Similarly, therapeutic options are in some cases based on a limited number of reported experiences.

However, recent advances such as the availability of antifibrosing drugs have allowed progress in the management of fibrosing lung diseases and raised new research interests.

Given these premises, a surely correct way to improve diagnostic yield and management skills in this field is to increase culture on these pathologies, with an innovative and intelligent approach such as the one proposed by this volume.

I believe it can accompany the working lives of all of us every day and should be placed on the desks of all health care professionals called to diagnose and manage respiratory diseases.

Fabiano Di Marco, MD, PhD
Full Professor of Respiratory Medicine
Department of Health Sciences
University of Milan (Italy);
President
Italian Respiratory Society (SIP-IRS);
Head
Respiratory Disease Unit
Papa Giovanni XXIII Hospital
Bergamo, Italy

PREFACE

The term *interstitial lung diseases* (ILDs), commonly used as a synonym for *diffuse parenchymal lung diseases* (DPLDs), refers to several heterogeneous conditions that affect the lung parenchyma and interstitium. They comprise some rare and ultra-rare disorders.

ILDs can be classified using various criteria, such as acute vs chronic, granulomatous vs non-granulomatous, known vs unknown cause, primary lung disease vs secondary to systemic disease, and related or not to smoking history.

Pulmonary parenchyma includes the main components involved in gas exchange such as respiratory bronchioles and alveoli, whereas lung interstitium indicates the network of extracellular matrix and cells surrounding the bronchoalveolar structures and vessels.

Certain types of ILDs are characterized by inflammation within the interstitial pulmonary space, alveolar septal thickening, fibroblast proliferation, and collagen deposition.

Some disorders frequently affect not only the parenchyma but also the peripheral airways. This is the reason why some airway diseases, such as obliterating bronchiolitis, are also listed under ILDs.

Although the lung circulatory system is not strictly part of the parenchyma or interstitium, vascular disorders are commonly included in the group of ILDs or DPLDs.

The diagnosis of ILDs is often complex and requires a multidisciplinary team that includes the pulmonologist, radiologist, thoracic surgeon, pathologist, and, often, rheumatologist. Moreover, the involvement of general practitioners and nurses is crucial for their management.

Outcomes vary considerably for the different ILDs. Some conditions may undergo spontaneous reversibility or stabilization, whereas many others may evolve toward progressive pulmonary fibrosis (PPF), with consequent impairment of gas exchange and decline in lung function. This leads to breathlessness, diminished exercise tolerance, worsened quality of life, respiratory failure, and early mortality.

Several years ago, the weapons available to treat ILDs were few and, despite many efforts, the results were often disappointing. Yet patients with ILDs passed by our clinics and we were there, trying to do something to help them.

We tried therapies that were not effective. We were not discouraged, we studied, we joined forces through multidisciplinary approaches, we refined the interpretation of imaging, and we reduced the invasiveness of interventional diagnostic procedures.

Knowledge in this area is constantly evolving. The most important progress is the availability of pharmacologic therapies. Antifibrotic drugs have been shown to be effective in counteracting idiopathic pulmonary fibrosis, historically known as one of the worst prognosis ILDs. Moreover, clinical trials have demonstrated that even patients with different forms of progressive fibrosing ILDs can benefit from a treatment effective in slowing functional decline.

We lost many patients; others are struggling, but we are by their side and we will continue to fight with them.

It took longer than expected to complete the project, but this was because many authors spend most of their time caring for people.

We thank Dr. Agazio Francesco Ussia for his contribution to anatomical pathologic issues and Dr. Alessandra Cancellieri for her cytopathologic assistance.

We also thank all the colleagues who work alongside us and those who, unfortunately, are no longer with us.

We hope this book will help increase readers' skills in diagnosing and treating various ILDs, as well as stimulate the interest of many physicians in ILDs.

Claudio Sorino
Sergio Agati

Rare diseases don't exist
until you know them.

CLAUDIO SORINO

CONTENTS

VIDEO CONTENTS

PART I

Fibrosing Interstitial Lung Diseases

CHAPTER 1

Fibrotic Hypersensitivity Pneumonitis After Long-Term Exposure to Household Mold

Alice Biffi ■ Claudio Sorino ■ Silvia Pizzolato ■ Sergio Agati

History of Present Illness

A 58-year-old man presented to the outpatient clinic complaining of cough and shortness of breath during exercise. These symptoms had begun about 1 year earlier and had progressively worsened. Chest radiography, requested by the primary care physician, revealed a reticular interstitial pattern, diffusely involving both lungs (Fig. 1.1). Consequently, he was referred to the pulmonology department.

Past Medical History

The patient was a plumber and a former smoker of 20 cigarettes per day, with a 30-pack-year history of smoking. When asked about potentially harmful exposures, he said he lived in a damp, old house. He had never undergone pulmonary function testing. He took daily medications only for arterial hypertension.

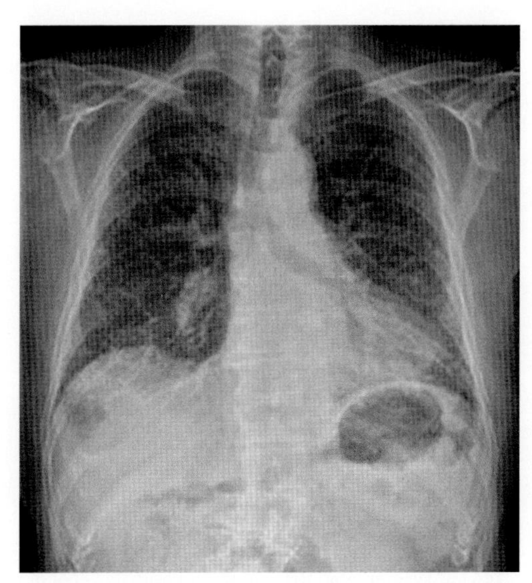

Fig. 1.1 Posteroanterior chest radiograph showing a diffuse reticular interstitial lung pattern, with loss of lung volume.

Physical Examination and Early Clinical Findings

At the time of the visit to the pulmonologist, the patient was in fair general health condition, afebrile, and cooperative. Oxygen saturation measured by pulse oximetry (SpO_2) was 95% on room air but rapidly decreased to 86% when he started to move. Similarly, he had shortness of breath and tachypnea when walking.

On chest examination, there were bilateral fine crackles, especially on pulmonary bases, and bronchiolar squeaks. There was also digital clubbing at the physical examination. He did not complain of joint stiffness or other signs or symptoms of a rheumatological disease.

Discussion Topic 1

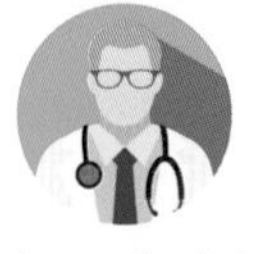

Pulmonologist A

The patient has bilateral fine crackles. They are typical of pulmonary fibrosis.

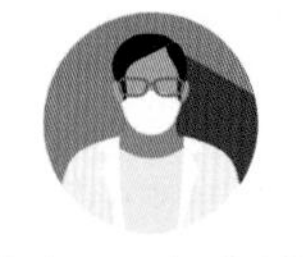

Pulmonologist B

A chest computed tomography (CT) scan will be mandatory to confirm this and evaluate the pattern of fibrosis.

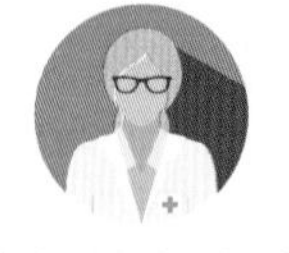

Pulmonologist C

I agree. Meanwhile, let's start performing spirometry and lung diffusion test to evaluate the presence of impaired lung function and gas exchange.

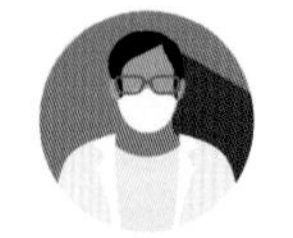

Pulmonologist B

Considering the patient's exposure to molds, searching for specific precipitin IgG should be useful.

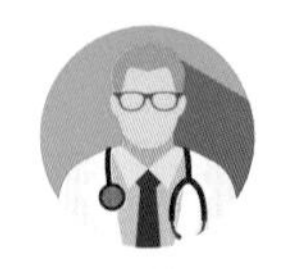

Pulmonologist A

Do you think he may have hypersensitivity pneumonitis (HP)?

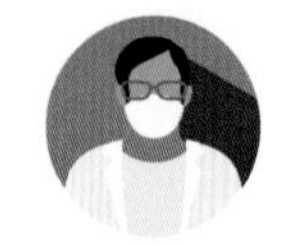

Pulmonologist B

It's only one of the possible differential diagnoses but should be considered, given his exposure.

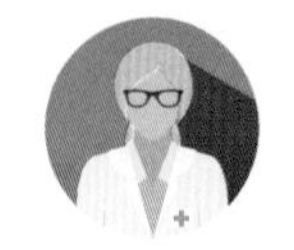

Pulmonologist C

Yes, but keep in mind that precipitin positivity is not in itself diagnostic, and if the precipitins are negative, we can't exclude HP. We should also screen for autoimmune and connective tissue diseases.

Clinical Course

During the visit, the patient underwent pulmonary function tests that showed a restrictive pattern and a significant reduction in the diffusing capacity of the lungs for carbon monoxide (DLCO) (Fig. 1.2).

Autoimmunity tests (antinuclear antibody [ANA], anti-extractable nuclear antigens [ENA], anti-neutrophil cytoplasmic antibodies [ANCA], rheumatoid factor) were negative. A slight

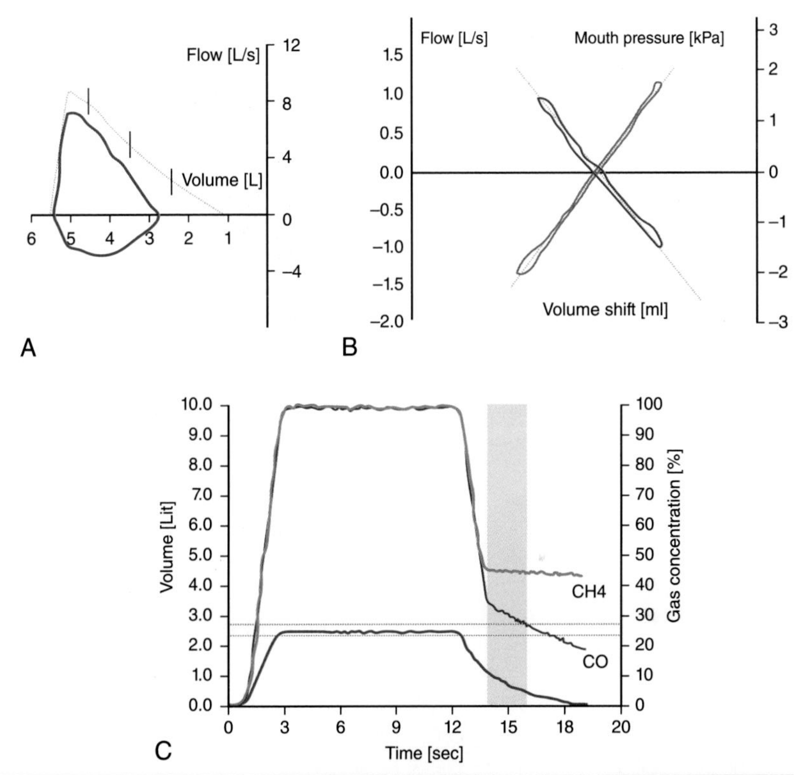

D

ID: ****** ******		Gender: Male		Height: 175 cm
Age: 58 years		Race: Caucasian		Weight: 80 kg
	Observed	Predicted	LLN	% Observed/Predicted
FEV_1 (Lit)	2.16	3.51	2.89	62
FVC (Lit)	2.49	4.27	3.75	58
FEV_1/FVC	0.82	0.79	0.67	103
Raw (TkPa*s/L)	0.35	0.30	—	118
RV (Lit)	1.16	1.99	1.25	59
TLC (Lit)	3.82	6.51	5.47	59
DLCO (mL/min/mmHg)	3.93	9.89	6.72	40

Fig. 1.2 Pulmonary function test results. (A) Flow-volume curve; (B) plethysmography; (C) diffusing capacity; (D) measured parameters. A normal FEV_1/VC ratio with a reduction of both FEV_1 and VC below the LLN suggests a restrictive pattern. The reduction of TLC and RV below the LLN confirms lung restriction. FEV_1, forced expiratory volume in 1 second; LLN, lower limit of normal; FVC, forced vital capacity; RV, residual volume; TLC, total lung capacity. DLCO, diffusing capacity of the lungs for carbon monoxide.

increase in nonspecific markers of inflammation was found erythrocyte sedimentation rate [ESR] 34.5 mm/hr (normal values for men aged 51–85 < 20 mm/hr) and C-reactive protein [CRP] 21.2 mg/L (normal values < 10 mg/L).

Searching for specific precipitin IgG was done, and a slight increase in IgG for pigeon droppings and *Aspergillus fumigatus* was found.

High-resolution computed tomography (HRCT) of the chest revealed bilateral reticular opacities with distortion of the pulmonary parenchyma, traction bronchiolectasis, honeycombing in the medium lung fields, and small areas of ground-glass opacities. Radiological changes in the lung parenchyma were relatively base-sparing but had no clear base-to-apex gradient (Fig. 1.3).

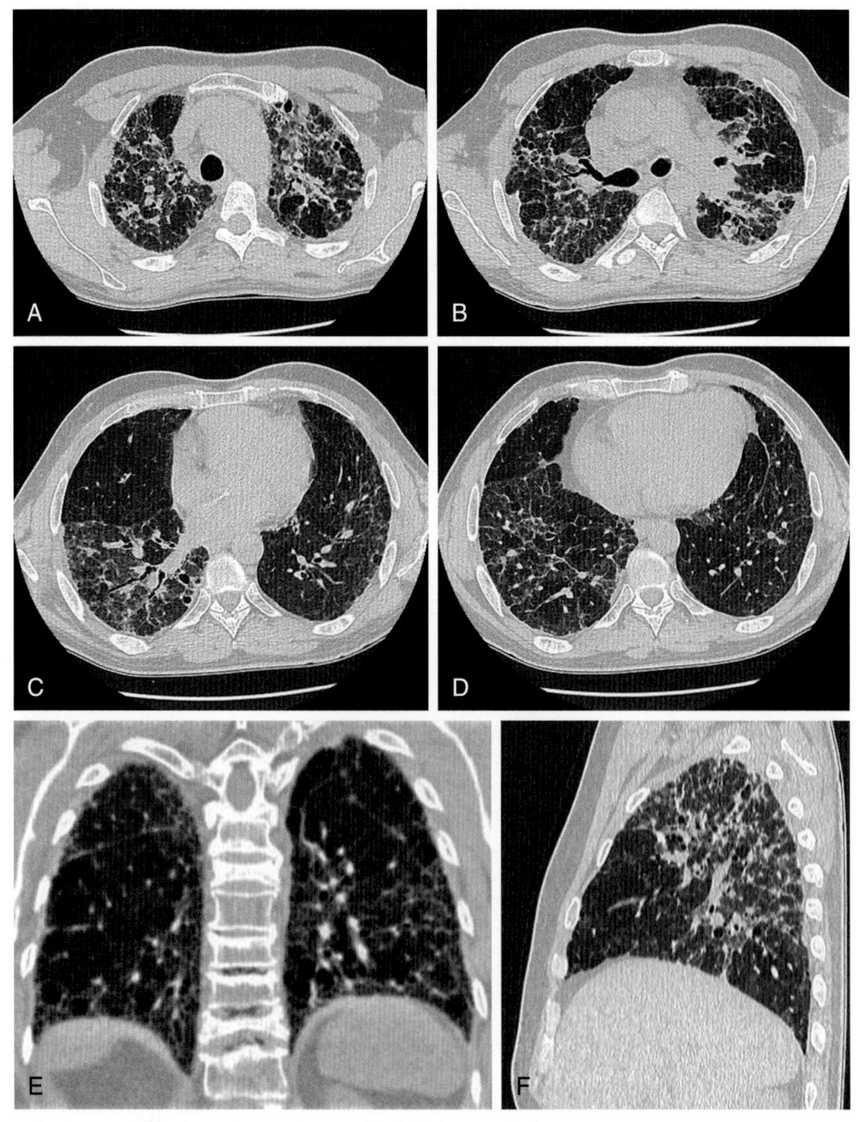

Fig. 1.3 Axial (A–D), coronal (E), and sagittal (F) HRCT scans of the chest with lung window setting showing bilateral reticular alterations, traction bronchiolectasis, honeycombing in the medium lung fields, and small areas of ground-glass opacities.

Discussion Topic 2

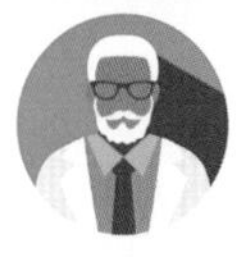

Radiologist

The chest CT pattern isn't exhaustive. There are signs of fibrosis, scarce areas of ground glass, and some subpleural honeycombing. There's no clear basal-apical gradient.

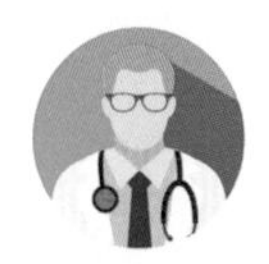

Pulmonologist A

We can only infer that the patient has a fibrosing interstitial lung disease (ILD).

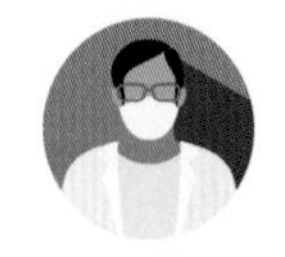

Pulmonologist B

Could we consider this pattern as indeterminate for usual interstitial pneumonia (UIP)?

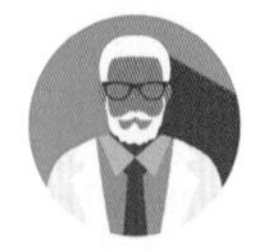

Radiologist

It could be. It does not meet UIP or probable UIP criteria.

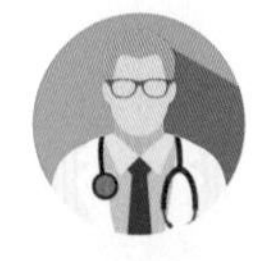

Pulmonologist A

About one-third of atypical HRCT features conceal an underlying histopathological pattern of UIP.

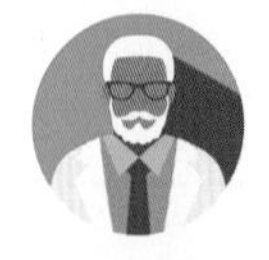

Radiologist

If there was evidence of fibrosing ILD and contextual signs of small airway disease, a diagnosis of fibrotic HP would have been very likely.

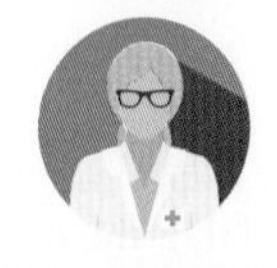

Pulmonologist C

What are the HRCT features of small airway disease?

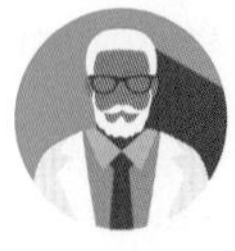

Radiologist

They are ill-defined centrilobular nodules, ground glass, mosaic attenuation, air trapping, and the so-called "three-density pattern," which is a combination of areas of normal lung parenchyma, areas of ground-glass attenuation, and areas of mosaic attenuation or hyperlucency. It was formerly known as the "headcheese sign" and indicates the association of ILD and airway obstruction. In my opinion, mosaic attenuation is one of the most important findings for the diagnosis of fibrotic HP. HRCT acquisition at end-expiration is useful for better identifying this feature.

Continued on following page

Discussion Topic 2 (Continued)

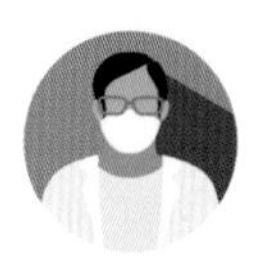

Pulmonologist B

What about the presence of precipitins IgG for pigeon droppings and Aspergillus fumigatus in a patient with possible mold exposure?

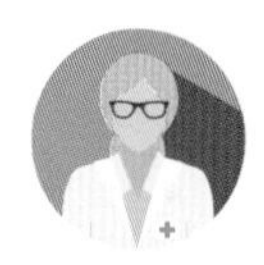

Pulmonologist C

The precipitins have a controversial diagnostic value for the lack of specificity in HP. The tests cannot differentiate between sensitization and disease.
We need other information to discriminate HP from other ILDs, in particular, idiopathic pulmonary fibrosis (IPF).

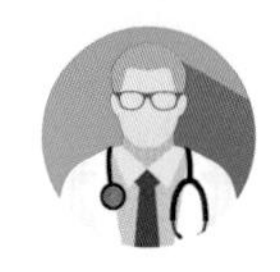

Pulmonologist A

We could perform bronchoscopy with bronchoalveolar lavage (BAL).
A significant lymphocytosis would reinforce the suspicion of HP diagnosis.

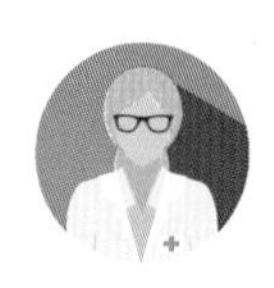

Pulmonologist C

I only partially agree. Lymphocytosis in BAL fluid is common in nonfibrotic forms, that is, what we called acute and subacute HP in the past. Guidelines suggest a 30% threshold of lymphocytes to distinguish HP from non-HP ILD.
However, BAL fluid differential cell count is usually not altered in fibrotic HP, which is a chronic and often progressive form. Even the CD4:CD8 ratio, which is often altered in nonfibrotic forms, may remain preserved in the fibrotic form.

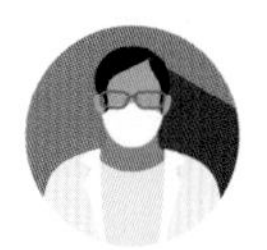

Pulmonologist B

If BAL isn't exhaustive, I'm afraid a surgical lung biopsy will be needed for the diagnosis.

BAL was done. Total cells were 200.000/mL with neutrophils 5%, macrophages 88%, and lymphocytes 5% of total cells.

Because neither chest HRCT scan nor BAL was conclusive in distinguishing idiopathic pulmonary fibrosis (IPF) from HP, after a multidisciplinary team meeting (MDD), the patient was offered a pulmonary biopsy in video-assisted thoracic surgery (VATS).

The histological examination on the lung biopsy showed fibrosis predominantly centrilobular and bridged between different lobule centers. Honeycombing and centrilobular microgranuloma were also reported (Fig. 1.4).

The case was discussed again during an MDD with radiologists, pulmonologists, and pathologists. Considering the suspected exposure to mold, the HRCT pattern, and the histological findings, a diagnosis of fibrotic HP was made.

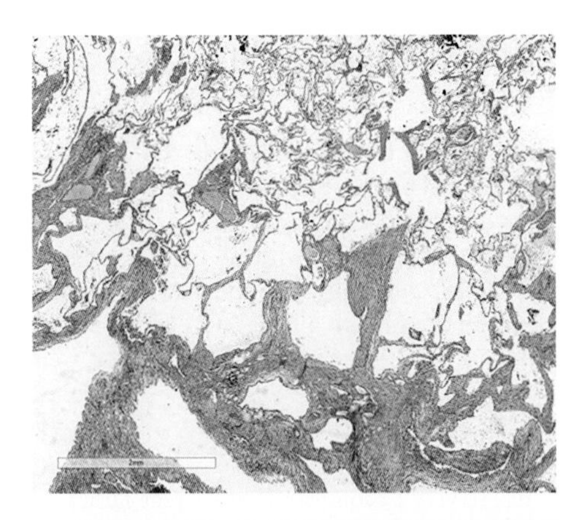

Fig. 1.4 Histology of lung biopsy showing areas of centrilobular fibrosis, microgranulomas, and cystic spaces lined with bronchiolar epithelium and fibrotic wall (honeycombing).

Discussion Topic 3

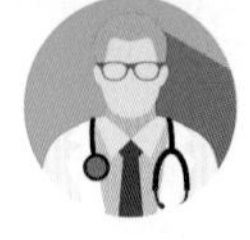

Pulmonologist A

We have a clinical suspicion of HP, but imaging is not conclusive. What information does the histology of lung biopsy samples give us?

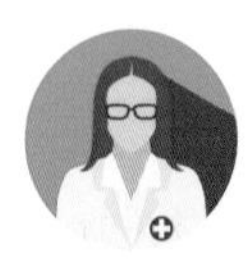

Pathologist

It suggests fibrotic HP. According to international guidelines, a typical fibrotic HP pathological pattern has three features: (1) airway-centered fibrosis with or without widespread peribronchiolar metaplasia and bridging fibrosis, (2) fibrosing interstitial pneumonia (e.g., UIP or nonspecific interstitial pneumonia [NSIP] pattern), and (3) poorly formed granulomas.
Sometimes, histological UIP pattern in HP is hardly differentiated from UIP pattern in IPF; only the careful search for residues of noncaseating microgranulomas and/or the persistence of mononuclear inflammation can confirm the diagnosis.

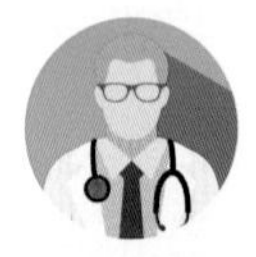

Pulmonologist A

Given the diagnosis of HP, the patient's symptoms and the lung function impairment, we can do a trial of steroids and recommend him to clean the house from mold.

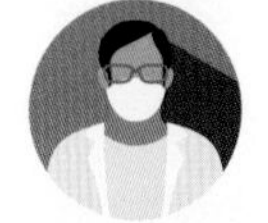

Pulmonologist B

We can also add an immunosuppressive drug if the clinical and functional improvement after steroid treatment is insufficient.

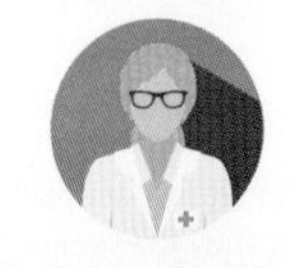

Pulmonologist C

Unfortunately, many patients with fibrotic HP do not respond to steroid or immunosuppressive drugs. They tend to have a behavior similar to patients with IPF, with a poor prognosis.

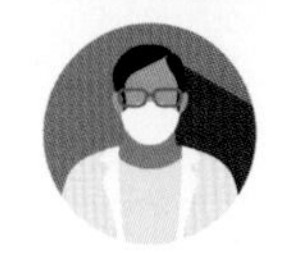

Pulmonologist B

Remember that the patient is young, with few comorbidities, and could be eligible for lung transplantation if the disease progresses.

Recommended Therapy and Further Indications at Discharge

The patient was recommended to avoid antigen exposure and to take prednisone at a dosage of 1 mg/kg per day. After 6 months, pulmonary function tests showed a further reduction in pulmonary volumes, whereas HRCT chest scan demonstrated an increase in fibrosis.

A trial with an immunosuppressive drug (azathioprine) was done, with no improvement of any pulmonary function parameters and progressive clinical worsening with the need for supplemental oxygen even at rest, so the drug was stopped after 8 months.

Follow-Up and Outcomes

One year after the diagnosis, the patient had more dyspnea and decreased exercise tolerance, documented by a 50-m reduction in the 6-minute-walk test (6MWT) compared with 1 year earlier.

Moreover, pulmonary function tests showed a forced vital capacity (FVC) decline of 8%. A new echocardiogram ruled out an increase in pulmonary pressure. In the meanwhile, antifibrotic drug use was approved for patients with pulmonary fibrosis other than IPF with a progressive course, grouped under the name of progressive pulmonary fibrosis (PPF). Thus, nintedanib 150 mg twice daily was started, and the patient was followed in the outpatient clinic.

In the following 3 months, FVC remained stable. However, considering the need for oxygen supplement, the low value of DLCO, and the patient's age, he was referred for evaluation for lung transplantation.

Focus On

New Classification of HP and Diagnosis of Fibrotic HP

Historically, HP was classified as acute, subacute, or chronic, based on the duration of symptoms. However, this classification is now considered to have poor clinical utility, as the presence of fibrosis is the critical determinant of prognosis.

Recently, two guidelines on the diagnosis of HP were published, by the American Thoracic Society/Japanese Respiratory Society/Asociación Latinoamericana de Tórax (ATS/JRS/ALAT) and by the American College of Chest Physicians (CHEST). They propose to categorize patients as having nonfibrotic HP (purely inflammatory) or fibrotic HP (mixed inflammatory and fibrotic or purely fibrotic).

Fibrotic HP should always be considered in the differential diagnosis in patients presenting with fibrotic ILD.

The diagnosis of fibrotic HP is particularly challenging, given the absence of an identifiable exposure in up to 50% of patients.

Based on the CHEST guidelines, a confident diagnosis of HP can be made in patients who have an identified exposure and a typical HP pattern on HRCT scan. According to the ATS/JRS/ALAT guidelines, a confident diagnosis of HP also requires evidence of BAL lymphocytosis.

For patients with suspicion of fibrotic HP who do not fulfill the criteria listed above, transbronchial lung cryobiopsy or surgical lung biopsy may be considered.

Focus On

Radiological Pattern of Fibrotic HP

HRCT chest scan of patients with fibrotic HP is usually characterized by bilateral reticular alterations with distortion of the pulmonary parenchyma and traction bronchiolectasis. Honeycombing may be present in $> 50\%$ of cases.

Unlike IPF, patients with fibrotic HP have fibrosis and honeycombing mainly in the middle and upper pulmonary lobes.

Focus On (Continued)

Radiological Pattern of Fibrotic HP

Together with parenchymal distortion, there may be ground-glass opacity, ill-defined centrilobular nodules, and mosaic attenuation, typical of the nonfibrotic form of the disease.

The mosaic attenuation pattern is caused by air trapping and occurs as patches of hypodensities (darker areas) within the lung parenchyma. They correspond to areas where vessels are reduced in number and caliber due to hypoxic vasoconstriction, which is believed in turn to be secondary to bronchiolitis and local alveolar hypoventilation. These alterations are more evident on expiratory CT scans.

The combination of areas of normal parenchyma, ground-glass opacity, and mosaic attenuation (or areas of hyperlucency) can give what is called "three-density pattern."

Other signs that can be found on HRCT of the chest are:

- Emphysema, found in almost 20% of nonsmoking patients, particularly in cases of "farmer's lung"
- Mediastinal lymphadenopathies
- Thin-walled cysts often associated with ground-glass opacity

The most recent international guidelines for the diagnosis of HP (ATS/JRS/ALAT and CHEST guidelines) differentiate two HRCT patterns for nonfibrotic HP (typical and compatible) and the following two patterns for fibrotic HP:

1. Typical fibrotic HP pattern, which is characterized by lung fibrosis with middle lung predominance and relatively spared lower lung zones (or with random distribution) and at least one abnormality that is indicative of small airway disease (e.g., ill-defined centrilobular nodules and/or ground glass, mosaic attenuation, three-density pattern, and air trapping).
2. Compatible-with-fibrotic HP pattern, which may be characterized by several patterns and distribution of interstitial fibrosis different from that of the typical HP pattern (e.g., predominantly peripheral or basal reticulation, honeycombing with/without traction bronchiectasis), and concurrent abnormalities indicative of small airway disease.

Focus On

Therapeutic Options for Fibrotic HP

Identifying and eliminating the exposure to the causative agent is the first step in the management of patients with HP. Persistent exposure to a pathogenic noxa correlates with a worse prognosis and a more rapid decline in lung function. There are no clear guidelines for the treatment of HP; thus, the choice of therapy is based on observational data and expert advice. There is one randomized trial, carried out on patients with "farmer's lung" in which the effectiveness of an 8-week course of steroid therapy was compared with placebo. A faster improvement in lung function was observed in the steroid group compared with the placebo group, but after 12 months, there were no significant differences between the two groups.

Although not tested in randomized controlled trials, it is still common practice in HP to use immunosuppressive drugs.

Concerns have been raised over the chronic use of immunosuppression in patients with fibrotic HP given the harmful effects of prednisone plus azathioprine observed in patients with IPF.

Another important problem is the definition of response to treatment; it is debated whether to consider as a response also a stabilization of the pulmonary disease. The decision to continue the drugs in these cases should always be weighed against side effects.

Recently, a phase III randomized placebo-controlled clinical trial (INBUILD study) showed that nintedanib (an intracellular tyrosine kinase inhibitor used in IPF patients) was effective in reducing the annual rate of FVC decline compared with placebo in patients with progressive fibrosing ILD other than IPF (including HP).

The RELIEF study investigated the effects of pirfenidone (another antifibrotic drug available for IPF) in patients with progressive pulmonary fibrosis other than IPF. The study was prematurely terminated due to low recruitment but demonstrated a smaller decline in FVC% predicted over 48 weeks in patients who received pirfenidone compared with placebo.

Lung transplantation should be considered in selected patients with HP who are not responsive to other therapies, despite the possibility of HP recurrence on the transplanted lung.

LEARNING POINTS

- Typical fibrotic HP pattern on chest HRCT scan includes lung fibrosis with relative sparing of the bases and at least one sign of small airway disease (e.g., centrilobular nodules, mosaic attenuation, or air trapping).
- Mosaic attenuation has a high diagnostic value for HP, particularly in pulmonary parenchymal zones without evident fibrosis.
- Multidisciplinary discussion is crucial to diagnosing fibrotic HP and selecting patients for invasive investigation.
- BAL fluid lymphocyte cellular analysis and, in selected patients, transbronchial lung cryobiopsy or surgical lung biopsy may be useful in suspected HP when clinical and imaging do not lead to a reliable diagnosis.
- Identifying and eliminating the antigen exposure is the first step in the management of patients with HP.
- A causative agent is not identified in 30% to 50% of HP cases evaluated at ILD referral centers.
- Current treatment of fibrotic HP includes glucocorticoids, immunosuppressants, and antifibrotic (in progressive fibrosing ILD), but optimal therapeutic options should be better evaluated.

Further Reading

Behr J, Prasse A, Kreuter M. Pirfenidone in patients with progressive fibrotic interstitial lung diseases other than idiopathic pulmonary fibrosis (RELIEF): a double-blind, randomised, placebo-controlled, phase 2b trial. *Lancet Resp Med.* 2021;9:476–486.

Chandra D, Cherian SV. Hypersensitivity pneumonitis. [Updated 2021 Jul 15]. In: *StatPearls* [Internet]. Treasure Island, FL: StatPearls Publishing; 2022 Jan. Available at: https://www.ncbi.nlm.nih.gov/books/NBK499918/.

Costabel U, Miyazaki Y, Pardo A, et al. Hypersensitivity pneumonitis. *Nat Rev Dis Primers.* 2020;6(1):65.

Dias OM, Baldi BG, Pennati F, et al. Computed tomography in hypersensitivity pneumonitis: main findings, differential diagnosis and pitfalls. *Exp Rev Respir Med.* 2018;12(1):5-13.

Efared B, Ebang-Atsame G, Rabiou S, et al. The diagnostic value of the bronchoalveolar lavage in interstitial lung diseases. *J Negat Results Biomed.* 2017;16(1):4. Published 2017 Mar 1.

Fernández Pérez ER, Travis WD, Lynch DA, et al. Executive summary diagnosis and evaluation of hypersensitivity pneumonitis: CHEST guideline and expert panel report. *Chest.* 2021;160:595-615.

Flaherty KR, Wells AU, Cottin V, et al; INBUILD Trial Investigators. Nintedanib in progressive fibrosing interstitial lung diseases. *N Engl J Med.* 2019;381(18):1718-1727.

Hamblin M, Prosch H, Vašáková M. Diagnosis, course and management of hypersensitivity pneumonitis. *Eur Respir Rev.* 2022;31:210169.

Patolia S, Tamae Kakazu M, Chami HA, et al. Bronchoalveolar lavage lymphocytes in the diagnosis of hypersensitivity pneumonitis among patients with interstitial lung disease. *Ann Am Thorac Soc.* 2020;17(11):1455-1467.

Raghu G, Remy-Jardin M, Richeldi L, et al. Idiopathic pulmonary fibrosis (an update) and progressive pulmonary fibrosis in adults: an official ATS/ERS/JRS/ALAT clinical practice guideline. *Am J Respir Crit Care Med.* 2022;205(9):e18-e47.

Raghu G, Remy-Jardin M, Ryerson CJ, et al. Diagnosis of hypersensitivity pneumonitis in adults. an official ATS/JRS/ALAT clinical practice guideline. *Am J Respir Crit Care Med.* 2020;202(3):e36-e69.

CHAPTER 2

Idiopathic Pulmonary Fibrosis With a Typical Usual Interstitial Pneumonia Pattern on Chest High-Resolution Computed Tomography

Ada Vancheri ■ Claudia Ravaglia ■ Sara Piciucchi ■ Claudio Sorino ■ Venerino Poletti

History of Present Illness

A 65-year-old man has been complaining of exertional dyspnea and dry cough for 2 years. During this period, he was treated with oral steroids, inhaled bronchodilators, and antibiotics without any improvement. He was initially identified as having a chronic obstructive pulmonary disease (COPD). Due to the clinical worsening, a chest radiograph was performed, which showed a basal reticular interstitial lung pattern (Fig. 2.1). Therefore, the patient was referred to a pulmonologist.

Past Medical History

The patient was a former smoker (40 pack-years) and a retired office worker, without significant occupational or environmental exposure to other noxious particles or gases. He had no family history of respiratory diseases. The only comorbidities were high blood pressure and type 2 diabetes mellitus for which he assumed antihypertensive therapy (valsartan) and oral hypoglycemic agents (glimepiride and metformin).

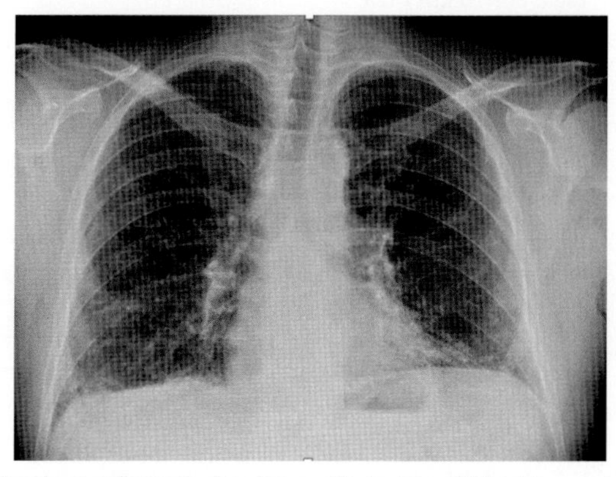

Fig 2.1 Posteroanterior chest radiograph showing a reticular interstitial pattern mainly in the lower zones.

Physical Examination and Early Clinical Findings

At the physical examination, bilateral Velcro sounds were present in the lower fields of the lungs. Peripheral oxygen saturation (SpO_2) was 95% at rest in room air. The patient had no skin alterations, neither xerostomia nor xerophthalmia, no Raynaud phenomenon, nor other signs of connective tissue diseases (CTDs).

Discussion Topic 1

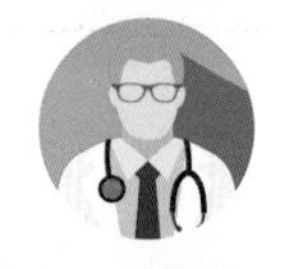

Pulmonologist A

The patient has Velcro sounds in the lower pulmonary fields. They are very specific for fibrosing interstitial lung diseases (ILDs).

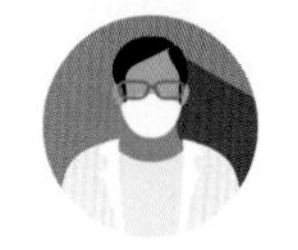

Pulmonologist B

This is consistent with radiological findings: chest radiograph shows an interstitial pattern. We need to perform a high-resolution computed tomography (HRCT) scan of the lungs.

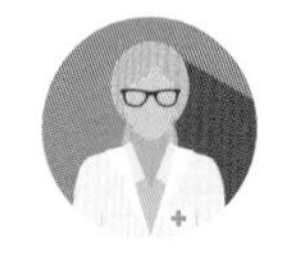

Pulmonologist C

We need pulmonary function tests, too. I would also be curious to see those performed previously, as a diagnosis of COPD had been made.

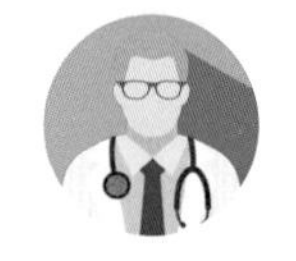

Pulmonologist A

The patient has a significant smoking history and is in the typical range of age of idiopathic pulmonary fibrosis (IPF).

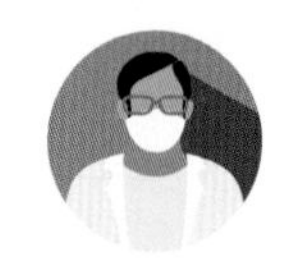

Pulmonologist B

I didn't find symptoms or signs suggestive of CTDs, which are a relevant cause of secondary ILD.

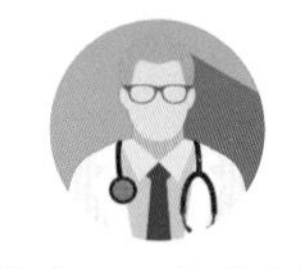

Pulmonologist A

I believe an autoimmunity screening and a rheumatological evaluation should be performed anyway.

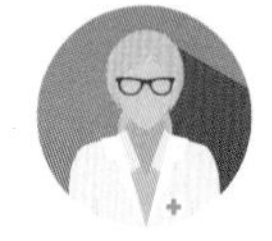

Pulmonologist C

We should also measure serum precipitins, which may raise the suspicion of hypersensitivity pneumonitis (HP). It is the third most common ILD, after IPF and CTD-related ILD, and patients are often unaware of environmental contact with organic antigens.

Clinical Course

The presence, at the lower lobes of the lungs, of bilateral Velcro sounds, very specific for ILDs, suggested to the pulmonologists to deepen the diagnostic process by performing an HRCT of the lungs. This showed the typical radiological findings of a UIP pattern: peripheral reticulations, traction bronchiectasis, and honeycombing with a basal predominance (Fig. 2.2; Fig. 2.3).

Pulmonary function tests (Fig 2.4) revealed a restrictive lung pattern and a moderate reduction in diffusion capacity for carbon monoxide (DLCO).

Antinuclear antibodies (ANAs), extractable nuclear antigen (ENA) screening, rheumatoid factor (RF), anti-cyclic citrullinated peptide antibodies (anti-CCP), and the myositis panel were all negative. A rheumatological evaluation confirmed the absence of physical signs attributable to an underlying CTD. Specific serum IgG antibodies to various avian proteins, bacterial compounds, or molds (precipitins) resulted to be negative. The case was discussed by a dedicated multidisciplinary team (MDT) involving pulmonologists, radiologists, and rheumatologists.

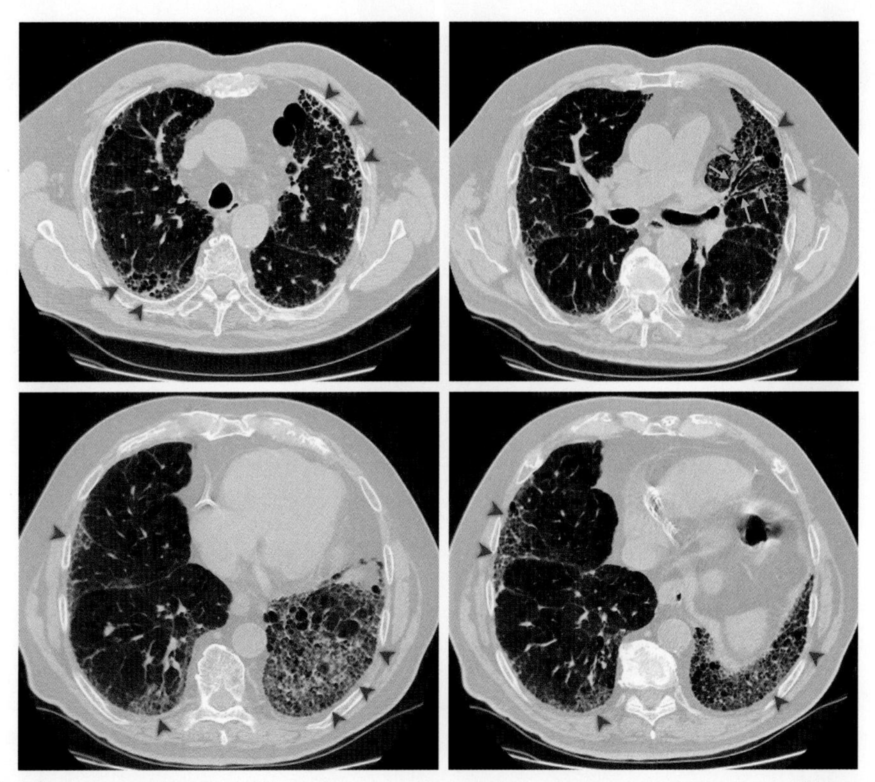

Fig 2.2 High-resolution chest CT scan (lung parenchyma window, transverse view) showing a UIP pattern with peripheral and basal honeycombing (red arrowheads) and traction bronchiectasis (yellow arrows).

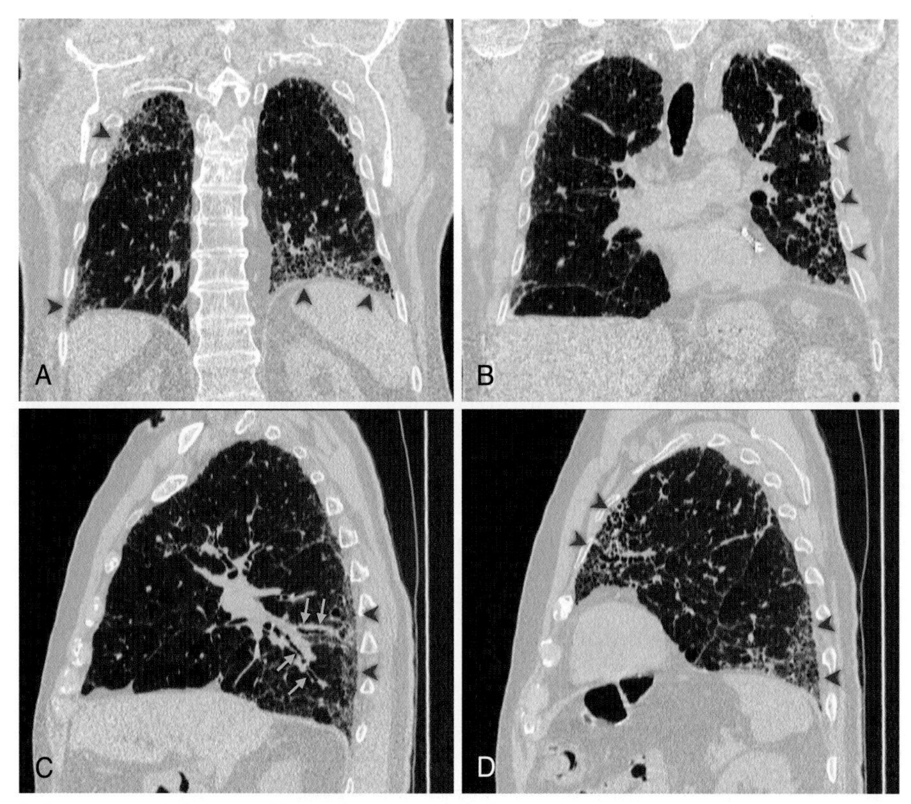

Fig 2.3 High-resolution chest CT scan (lung parenchyma window), in the coronal (A, B) and sagittal (C, D) views showing reticulations, traction bronchiectasis (yellow arrows), and honeycombing (red arrowheads) with a peripheral and basal distribution typical of the UIP pattern.

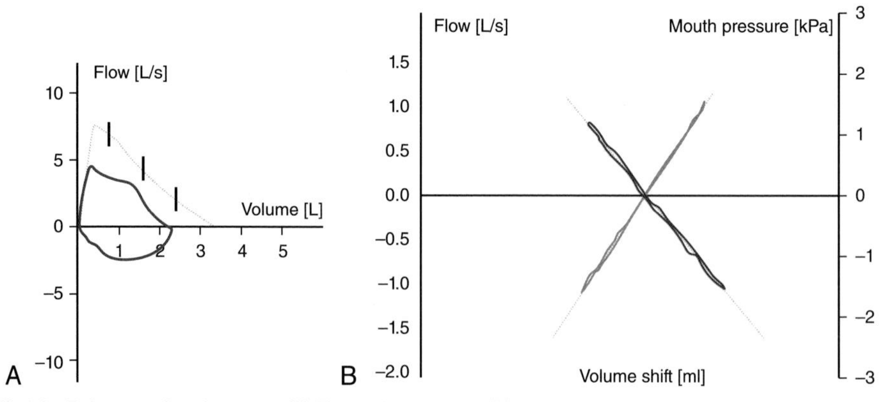

Fig 2.4 Pulmonary function tests. (A) Flow-volume curve; (B) body plethysmography;

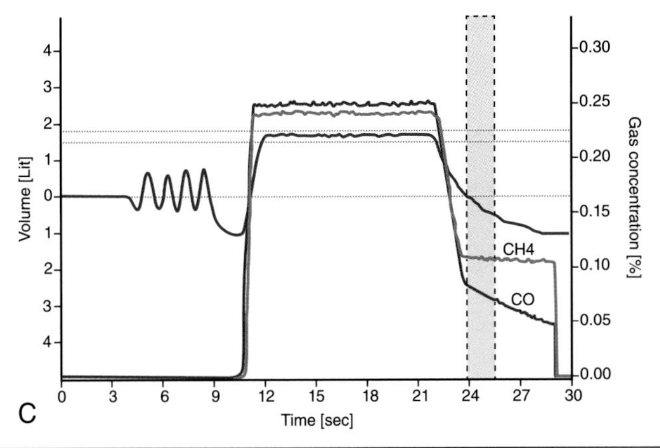

D

ID: ****** ******		Gender: Male		Height: 160 cm
Age: 65 years		**Race: Caucasian**		**Weight: 68 kg**
	Observed	**Predicted**	**LLN**	**% Observed/Predicted**
FEV_1 (Lit)	2.04	2.47	1.82	82.6
FVC (Lit)	2.44	3.23	2.53	87.9
FEV_1/FVC	83.6	77.7	64.2	107
Raw (TkPa*s/L)	0.35	0.30	0.30	116
RV (Lit)	1.45	1.90	1.15	76.1
TLC (Lit)	4.12	5.45	4.33	75.6
DLCO (mL/min/mmHg)	11.3	22.2	21.8	51.0

Fig 2.4, cont'd (C) lung diffusion test; (D) measured parameters. There is a restrictive pattern, with a preserved FEV_1/FVC ratio and a reduction in all lung volumes. Moderate impairment in the diffusing capacity of the lungs is also evident. FEV_1, forced expiratory volume in 1 second; LLN, lower limit of normal; FVC, forced vital capacity; RV, residual volume; TLC, total lung capacity. DLCO, diffusing capacity of the lungs for carbon monoxide.

Discussion Topic 2

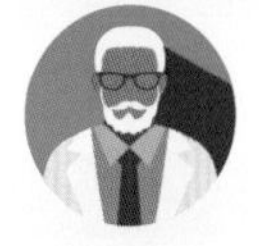

Radiologist

A radiological UIP pattern is evident: subpleural reticulations, honeycombing, and traction bronchiectasis.

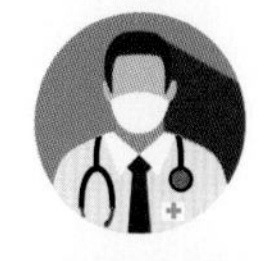

Rheumatologist

Autoimmunity is negative and no symptoms or signs of CTDs are present. Similarly, no serum precipitins were detected.

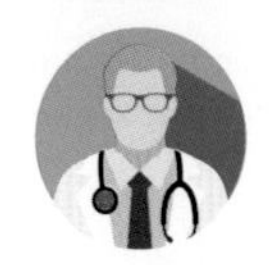

Pulmonologist A

Do you think that a surgical lung biopsy or cryobiopsy will be necessary?

Continued on following page

Discussion Topic 2 (Continued)

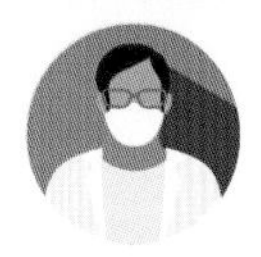

Pulmonologist B

Not in this case; we have all the elements to diagnose IPF. I believe that the cellular analysis of the bronchoalveolar lavage fluid does not provide additional useful information either.

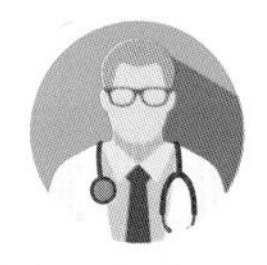

Pulmonologist A

We should perform echocardiography with an estimation of pulmonary pressures.

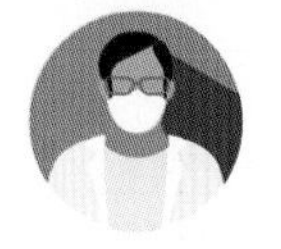

Pulmonologist B

I will also schedule a 6-minute walk test and nocturnal pulse oximetry to see if the patient has a latent respiratory failure.

Based on the available clinical and laboratory data, the MDT ascribed the UIP radiological pattern observed in this patient to IPF as no findings suggestive of another diagnosis were found.

At the 6-minute walk test (6MWT), the patient covered a distance of 350 m (67% predicted). He experienced severe dyspnea and had a significant oxygen desaturation after just 2 minutes (lowest SpO_2 = 86%, mean SpO_2 = 90.6%).

The patient also underwent overnight pulse oximetry, which showed nocturnal hypoxemia with a mean SpO_2 of 89.8% and a small number of desaturations per hour of sleep (oxygen desaturation index [ODI] was 34.6). Overall, the patient spent 29.4% of the night with $SpO_2 < 90\%$. The lowest value of SpO_2 was 81%.

Echocardiography revealed mild mitral and tricuspid regurgitation with preserved systolic function and no significant increase in pulmonary artery pressure.

Discussion Topic 3

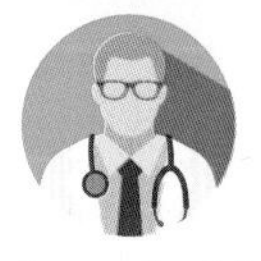

Pulmonologist A

We should offer the patient antifibrotic therapy.

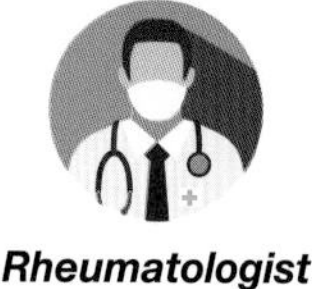

Rheumatologist

Both nintedanib and pirfenidone are effective in reducing the decline in lung function of patients with IPF. How do you decide which one is most appropriate for the patient?

Discussion Topic 3 (Continued)

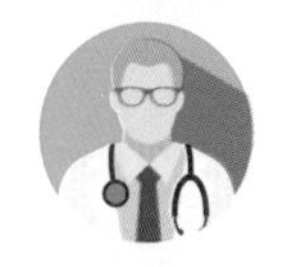

Pulmonologist A

First, you should ensure that there are no contraindications. Subsequently, I usually inform the patient about the possible side effects of each drug and I share the decision with him/her.

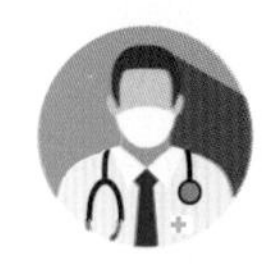

Rheumatologist

How well are these drugs tolerated?

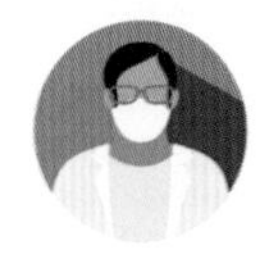

Pulmonologist B

They have a reasonable long-term tolerability profile. The main adverse effects of both pirfenidone and nintedanib are gastrointestinal and hepatic. Patients may develop abdominal distention or pain, nausea, vomiting, diarrhea, gastroesophageal reflux disease, weight loss, and anorexia. Moreover, patients treated with pirfenidone often develop a photosensitivity skin rash.

Recommended Therapy and Further Indications

When the diagnosis of IPF was made, the pulmonologist explained to the patient the opportunity to start an antifibrotic therapy. The patient accepted this advice. The physicians did not find drug interaction or other comorbidities that can preclude nintedanib or pirfenidone prescription. Therefore, they shared this important decision with the patient and explained the possible side effects of such drugs and their frequency. During the discussion, the patient expressed concern about photosensitivity, which occurs in about one out of three patients during treatment with pirfenidone. Conversely, he didn't care about diarrhea, which is more common when taking nintedanib. Thus, nintedanib 150 mg, 1 pill after breakfast and 1 pill after dinner was started. Monthly laboratory tests (complete blood count, direct and total bilirubin, transaminase, γ-glutamyl transpeptidase, and serum creatinine) were scheduled.

Unfortunately, the drug intake was temporarily stopped for a significant alteration of transaminases after about 3 months. The pulmonologists waited for normalization of these parameters and started again with a lower dosage of the same drug, nintedanib 100 mg twice daily. Oxygen supplement during sleep and effort was recommended. Further echocardiography was scheduled to assess the presence of arterial hypertension.

Follow-Up and Outcomes

After approximately 1 year of follow-up, symptoms were relatively stable, as well as lung volumes and diffusion capacity. In detail, the forced vital capacity was 73% predicted, and DLCO was 50% predicted. The new chest HRCT revealed no signs of radiological progression. The extent of reticulation and honeycombing was approximately the same. No ground-glass opacities or other alterations that might suggest acute exacerbation emerged. The mean pulmonary arterial pressure estimated by echocardiography was near the upper limit of normal (25 mmHg).

Focus on

Overview of Idiopathic Pulmonary Fibrosis

Idiopathic pulmonary fibrosis (IPF) is a rare disease characterized by exhaustion of alveolar stem cells, acquisition of senescent associated secretory phenotype (SASP) by these cells, and afterward aberrant activation of different pathways (e.g., *Wnt, Hedgehog*). These pathogenetic steps determine the appearance of a profibrotic microenvironment of the affected lung parenchyma with subsequent proliferation of fibroblasts and deposition of extracellular matrix and collagen. When then aberrant signals reach the bronchiolar compartment, a dysplastic proliferation of basaloid bronchiolar cells takes place with pulmonary fibrosis and honeycomb changes. This causes a progressive and relentless loss of lung function and alterations of gas exchanges, which lead to respiratory failure.

Patients with IPF are usually older than 50 years, with a peak of frequency around 65 years. Both incidence and prevalence are reported to be steadily increasing. The disease affects males more often than females. Smoking and metal or wood dust inhalation are recognized as risk factors. Other conditions associated with IPF include gastroesophageal reflux, chronic viral infections such as Epstein-Barr virus or hepatitis C, and a family history of ILD. IPF is limited to the lung and occurs without constitutional or other symptoms that suggest a multisystem disease.

Despite recent advances, the prognosis is poor, with a median survival of 2–3 years without treatment. Succeeding an early diagnosis is fundamental in order to treat the disease at its beginning, when lung fibrosis is not yet at an advanced stage. In particular, the antifibrotic therapy is based either on pirfenidone or nintedanib. Both reduce by about 50% the decline of lung function expressed as forced vital capacity. The choice between them is based on age, functional lung tests, concomitant therapy, possible side effects, and patient lifestyle. Adverse events may occur, and dosing modification of antifibrotic therapy might be necessary, especially in the initial phase of treatment. Collaboration between the pulmonologist and the general practitioner is essential, and supportive care should be provided to the patient and family, including psychological support for managing symptoms such as anxiety, anger, sadness, and fear. Patients should also receive information and education about supplemental oxygen, disease progression and prognosis, drug treatments, and end-of-life planning.

Focus on

Imaging of IPF

HRCT of the chest is the most important tool for the identification of interstitial lung diseases (ILDs). It allows the study of lung parenchyma thanks to the thin-section CT scanning and the high number of acquisitions. The most common radiological pattern of IPF is the usual interstitial pneumonia (UIP) pattern, associated with a worse prognosis.

The radiologic UIP pattern is characterized by three elements:

1. Honeycombing (a series of cystic airspace stacked with well-defined walls just sited beneath the pleura; the cysts are typically 3-10 mm in diameter but can be as large as 2.5 cm).
2. Traction bronchiectasis (bronchial/bronchiolar dilatation of the lumen).
3. Subpleural and basal predominance of reticulation and honeycombing.

Honeycombing must be distinguished from traction bronchiectasis, paraseptal emphysema, and airspace enlargement with fibrosis (AEF). Honeycombing with a basal and peripheral predominance is an essential HRCT criterion for the typical ("definite") UIP pattern. Subpleural and basal-predominant reticulation and traction bronchiectasis/bronchiolectasis without honeycombing should be regarded as "probable UIP." Ground-glass opacification may be present in both UIP and probable UIP, but it is not a prevalent feature. Other radiological characteristics that may be present in IPF are the asymmetrical distribution of fibrosis, dendriform pulmonary ossification, and mediastinal lymphadenopathy.

The diagnostic approaches for UIP and probable UIP patterns on HRCT are similar, and if no other causes of ILD are detected (e.g., CTD, hypersensitivity pneumonia, asbestosis, etc.), the sole radiological pattern usually allows making a diagnosis of IPF without need for histologic confirmation.

Focus on

Monitoring and Follow-Up of IPF Patients

The follow-up of IPF is fundamental and includes the evaluation of three elements: symptoms, lung function, and radiological appearance. A medical visit and pulmonary function tests (PFTs) are recommended every 3 to 6 months.

Worsening of dyspnea and reduction of exercise tolerance are the main clinical indicators of disease progression.

An absolute decline in FVC $\geq$ 5% predicted or a reduction in DLCO (corrected for Hb levels) $\geq$10% predicted within 1 year of follow-up may suggest a disease progression. Although the rate of FVC decline is directly related to the progression of the disease and mortality, different factors can affect this value. For example, the presence of emphysema increases lung compliance balancing the opposite effect of fibrosis and leading to higher-than-expected FVC values. Similarly, DLCO may be altered by concomitant clinical problems, such as emphysema, pulmonary hypertension, and anemia.

HRCT of the lungs should be performed every year after the diagnosis of IPF. It allows for identifying a radiological progression, defined as an increased extent of reticulations, traction bronchiectasis, or honeycomb cysts. Transverse, coronal, and sagittal HRCT sections of the initial and follow-up CT examinations should be compared side by side. Moreover, chest HRCT is also useful to detect lung cancer, as the prevalence of this fearsome event in patients with IPF is much higher.

The identification of IPF progression remains challenging. Therefore, multidisciplinary expertise is needed to differentiate it from other events such as heart failure, bacterial superinfections, or acute exacerbation of IPF.

LEARNING POINTS

1. IPF is a progressive disease that requires early diagnosis and treatment.
2. The collaboration of different specialists (i.e., pulmonologist, radiologist, rheumatologist, and pathologist) is essential to improve the accuracy of the diagnosis of IPF.
3. For patients with ILD of apparently unknown cause and HRCT pattern of UIP, the diagnosis of IPF does not require cellular analysis of the BAL fluid nor lung biopsy.
4. Pirfenidone and nintedanib are approved and recommended antifibrotic drugs for patients with IPF. In referral centers, patients can also benefit from inclusion in clinical trials.
5. Treatment of IPF can slow down the disease progression by reducing the decline in lung function, although gastrointestinal side effects are frequent.
6. PFTs, DLCO, and 6MWT, associated with HRCT, are important tools for the follow-up of patients with IPF

Further Reading

Chilosi M, Carloni A, Rossi A, Poletti V. Premature lung aging and cellular senescence in the pathogenesis of idiopathic pulmonary fibrosis and COPD/emphysema. *Transl Res*. 2013;162:156-173.

Kinoshita T, Goto T. Molecular mechanisms of pulmonary fibrogenesis and its progression to lung cancer: a review. *Int J Mol Sci*. 2019;20(6):1461.

Lynch DA, Sverzellati N, Travis WD, et al. Diagnostic criteria for idiopathic pulmonary fibrosis: a Fleischner Society White Paper. *Lancet Respir Med*. 2018;6(2):138-153.

Nathan SD, Wanger J, Zibrak JD, et al. Using forced vital capacity (FVC) in the clinic to monitor patients with idiopathic pulmonary fibrosis (IPF): pros and cons. *Exp Rev Respir Med*. 2021;15:175-181.

Noble PW, Albera C, Bradford WZ, et al. Pirfenidone in patients with idiopathic pulmonary fibrosis (CAPACITY): two randomised trials. *Lancet*. 2011;377(9779):1760-1769.

Raghu G, Remy-Jardin M, Richeldi L, et al. Idiopathic pulmonary fibrosis (an update) and progressive pulmonary fibrosis in adults an official ATS/ERS/JRS/ALAT Clinical Practice Guideline. *Am J Respir Crit Care Med.* 2022;205(9):e18-e47.

Renzoni EA, Poletti V, Mackintosh JA. Disease pathology in fibrotic interstitial lung disease: is it all about usual interstitial pneumonia? *Lancet.* 2021;398:1437-1449.

Richeldi L, Du Bois RM, Raghu G, et al. Efficacy and safety of nintedanib in idiopathic pulmonary fibrosis. *N Engl J Med.* 2014;370:2071-2082.

Sorino C, Liou TG, Pistelli R. Overview of the pulmonary function tests. In: *Diagnostic Evaluation of the Respiratory System.* 1st ed. Jaypee Brothers Medical Publishers (P) Ltd; 2017:63-68.

Spagnolo P, Kropski JA, Jones MG, et al. Idiopathic pulmonary fibrosis: disease mechanisms and drug development. *Pharmacol Ther.* 2021;222:107798.

Wolters PJ, Collard HR, Jones KD. Pathogenesis of idiopathic pulmonary fibrosis. *Annu Rev Pathol.* 2014; 9:157-179.

CHAPTER 3

Idiopathic Pulmonary Fibrosis in a Smoker With Indeterminate Usual Interstitial Pneumonia Pattern on High-Resolution Computed Tomography

Fausta Alfano ■ Claudio Tirelli ■ Claudio Sorino ■ Stefano Centanni ■ Michele Mondoni

History of Present Illness

A 73-year-old Caucasian man was referred to the respiratory unit complaining of worsening exertional dyspnea and productive cough, lasting for about 4 months.

Following an acute bronchitis, the primary care physician heard fine crackles on chest auscultation. He requested a chest radiography, which showed bilateral basal interstitial thickening.

Past Medical History

The patient, a retired policeman, was a former smoker with a 30-pack-year smoking history, without referred exposure to noxious inhalants.

He had hypertension and type 2 diabetes. He had developed Bell's palsy at the age of 30.

He took daily medications for hypertension (ramipril) and diabetes (metformin). His family history was negative for respiratory disease or connective tissue diseases.

Two years earlier, the patient had undergone a chest computed tomography (CT) scan, requested by the primary care physician following repeated acute bronchitis. It had revealed bibasilar subtle ground-glass opacities with fine reticulations (Fig. 3.1), and a subsequent pulmonary consultation had been requested. Following a complete clinical recovery after antibiotic therapy, the patient did not undergo any other medical examination.

Physical Examination and Early Clinical Findings

At the outpatient pulmonology visit, the patient was afebrile, alert, and cooperative. He had no peripheral edemas, whereas digital clubbing was evident. Chest auscultation confirmed inspiratory crackles in both lower lung fields. Cardiac and abdominal examinations were normal. Oxygen saturation measured by pulse oximetry (SpO_2) was 95% on room air, respiratory rate was 22 breaths/min, heart rate was 70 beats/min, and blood pressure was 130/80 mmHg.

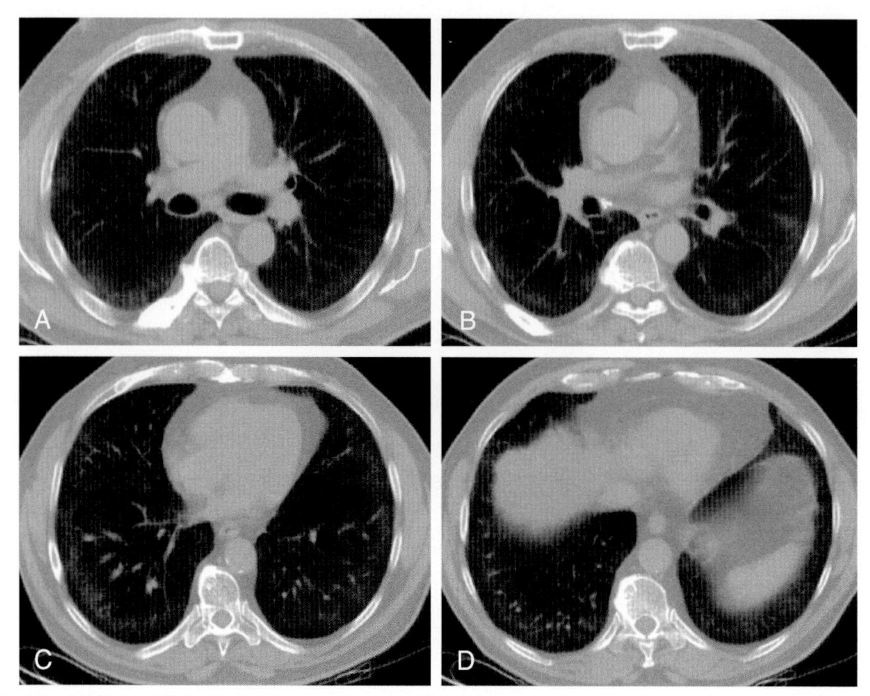

Fig. 3.1 Axial chest CT scan (lung parenchyma window) performed 2 years before the current presentation, showing subtle ground-glass opacities and fine reticulations at the lung bases.

Discussion Topic 1

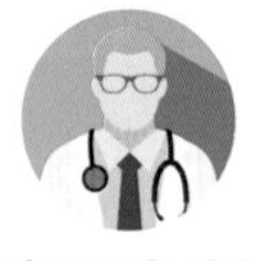

Pulmonologist A

Did you also hear the fine crackles on chest auscultation?

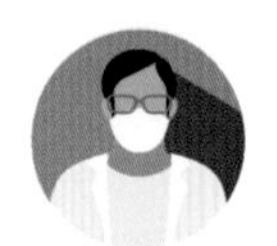

Pulmonologist B

Yes. And the patient also has nail clubbing. Both suggest that he may have idiopathic pulmonary fibrosis (IPF).

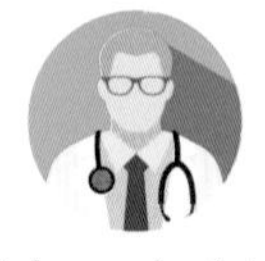

Pulmonologist A

A new chest CT scan will be needed. We should also consider other possible interstitial lung diseases (ILDs).

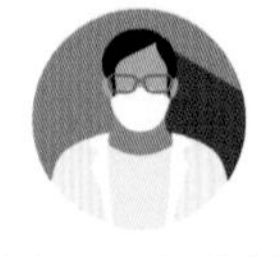

Pulmonologist B

I'll ask for autoantibodies associated with connective tissue diseases.

Discussion Topic 1 (Continued)

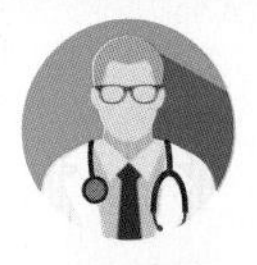

Pulmonologist A

Can we do everything on an outpatient basis?

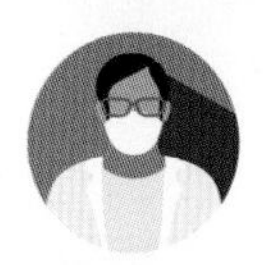

Pulmonologist B

I think so, I will work to get the chest CT scan quickly and organize the blood draw.

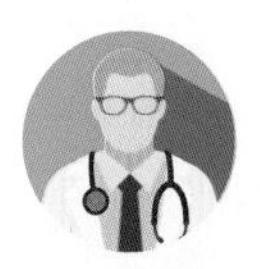

Pulmonologist A

He should also undergo pulmonary function tests, arterial blood gas analysis, and a 6-minute-walk test (6MWT).

Pulmonary function tests demonstrated a moderate restrictive pattern with a forced expiratory volume in 1 second (FEV_1) of 79% of the predicted value, forced vital capacity (FVC) of 68% of predicted, FEV_1/FVC ratio (Tiffenau-Pinelli index) of 116%, and total lung capacity (TLC) of 67% of predicted. Diffusing capacity of the lungs for carbon monoxide (DLCO) was moderately reduced (51% of the predicted value). A slight reduction in the distance covered at the 6MWT was found (400 m, equal to 74% of predicted) but without significant oxygen desaturation (average SpO_2 92.5%, minimum SpO_2 91%).

Clinical Course

A new high-resolution CT (HRCT) scan of the chest was immediately obtained. It revealed the presence of peripheral interstitial thickenings and ground-glass opacities, with basal predominance. No honeycombing was detected. Notably, a subpleural sparing was present (Fig. 3.2).

A complete autoimmunity serological screening was required to rule out the presence of an underlying connective tissue disease. Antinuclear antibodies (ANAs), extractable nuclear antigen (ENA) antibodies, anti-citrulline antibodies, anti-synthetase antibodies, and rheumatoid factor were all negative.

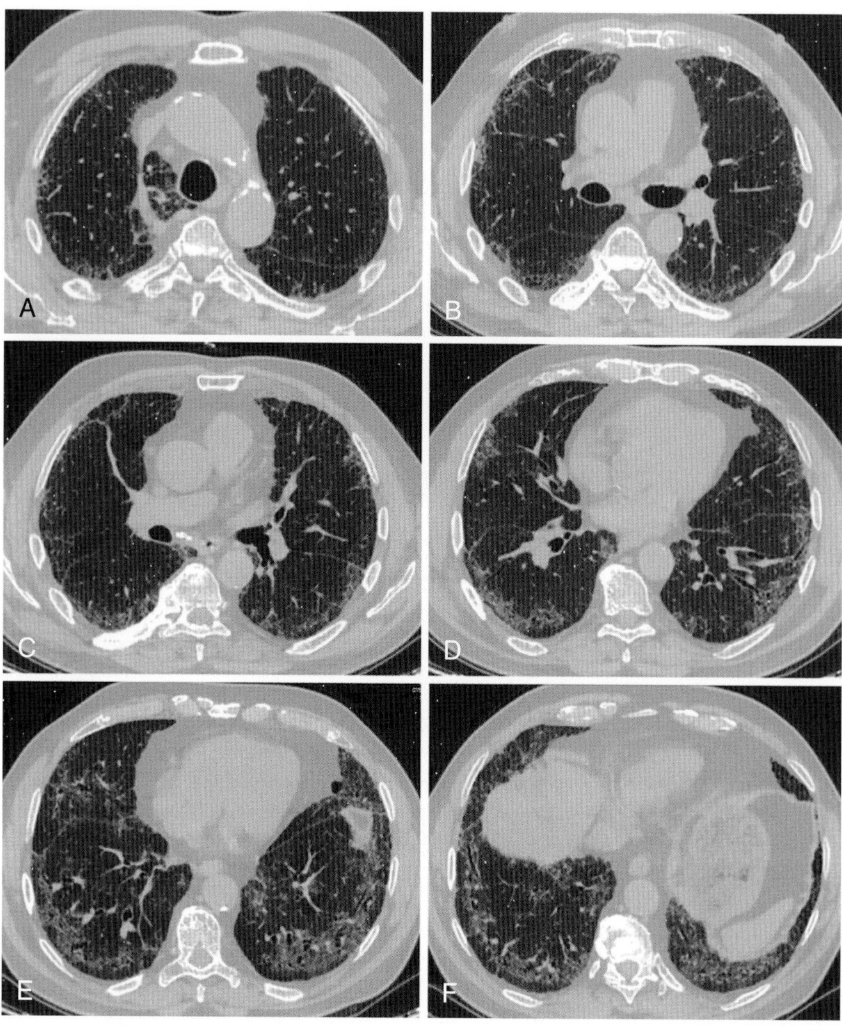

Fig 3.2 Axial HRCT of the chest (lung parenchyma window) showing disease progression with interstitial thickening and ground-glass opacities, mostly located in the periphery of the lungs with basal predominance and with subpleural sparing.

Discussion Topic 2

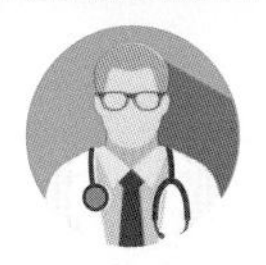

Pulmonologist A

Our patient has signs of lung fibrosis with a radiologic pattern indeterminate for usual interstitial pneumonia (UIP). A bronchoscopy with bronchoalveolar lavage (BAL) should be scheduled.

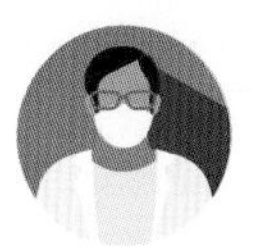

Pulmonologist B

Are you sure we need it? BAL cellular analysis is not useful to diagnose IPF. Perhaps a transbronchial biopsy (TBB) of the lung could be more effective for diagnosis.

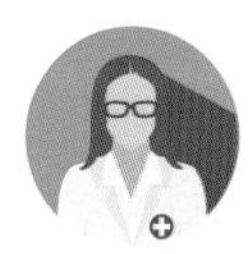

Pathologist

No cellular pattern is specific for IPF, and TBB does not provide adequate specimens for the pathological diagnosis of UIP.

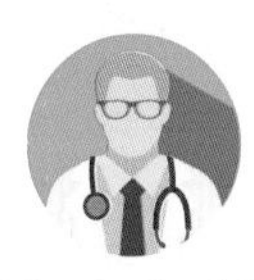

Pulmonologist A

BAL will certainly not provide a definite diagnosis of IPF. However, in the presence of a newly detected ILD of unknown cause without a UIP or probable UIP pattern, BAL cellular analysis may be useful to rule out alternative diagnoses, such as sarcoidosis, eosinophilic pneumonia, hypersensitivity pneumonitis, malignancies, and infections.
Don't worry; BAL is usually well tolerated with a very low rate of complications. Instead, considering the risk/benefit ratio, I would avoid TBB.

The patient underwent a bronchoscopic examination, which showed no inspection abnormalities. Bronchoalveolar lavage (BAL) cytological analysis revealed 90% macrophages, 5% lymphocytes, 1% eosinophils, and 3% neutrophils.

A multidisciplinary discussion (MDD) was then scheduled, in the presence of pulmonologists, thoracic radiologists, a rheumatologist, and a pathologist. On the basis of the clinical case to be discussed, a thoracic surgeon was also invited.

Discussion Topic 3

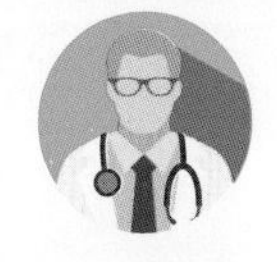

Pulmonologist A

We have a 73-year-old former smoker with a newly detected ILD of unknown origin. There is evidence of clinical worsening and radiological progression through two CT scans approximately 24 months apart.

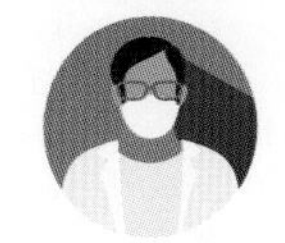

Pulmonologist B

He is clinically suspected of having idiopathic pulmonary fibrosis (IPF). However, HRCT chest findings are indeterminate for UIP, and BAL findings don't suggest any other differential diagnosis.

Continued on following page

Discussion Topic 3 (Continued)

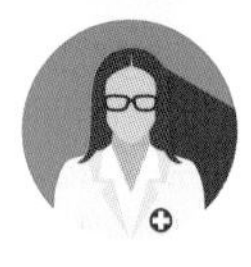

Pathologist

A lung biopsy is recommended by international guidelines. By combining the CT pattern with histopathological findings, we may obtain a definite diagnosis.

Thoracic Surgeon

Surgical lung biopsy provides samples from multiple lobes; the surgical technique most frequently performed in this context is video-assisted thoracic surgery (VATS).

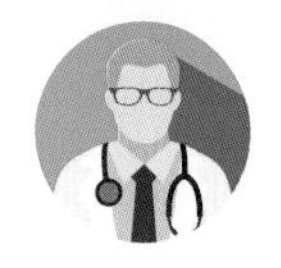

Pulmonologist A

Surgical lung biopsy is associated with a non-negligible rate of complications. In particular, acute exacerbation of IPF should be considered.

Thoracic Surgeon

Awake-VATS may reduce the complications related to endotracheal intubation and mechanical ventilation. It is usually well tolerated. Several studies showed that it results in low morbidity and mortality, excellent diagnostic yield, short hospital stays, and lower costs.

The MDD suggested a surgical lung biopsy for an etiological diagnosis. A biopsy during awake-VATS was proposed to the patient. Surgical biopsy samples were obtained from multiple lobes (upper right lobe, middle and lower right lobe). Histopathology revealed dense fibrosis with architectural distortion, patchy fibrosis, honeycombing, and fibroblast foci. No ancillary findings suggestive of an alternative diagnosis were present. The findings were consistent with a histologic UIP pattern (Fig. 3.3).

No complications were recorded during and immediately after surgery, and the patient was discharged after a few days.

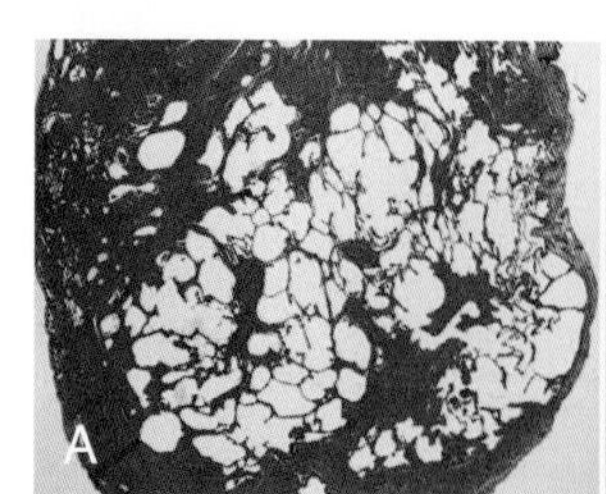

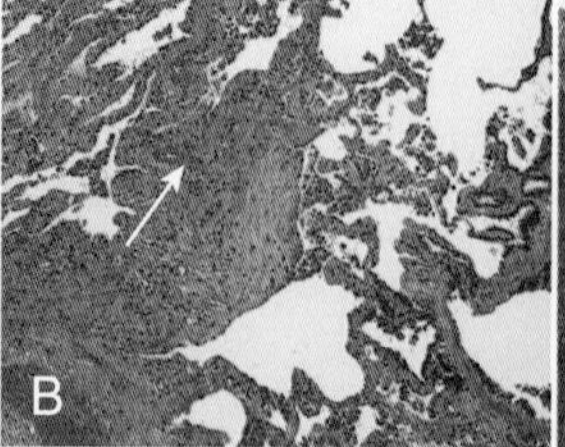

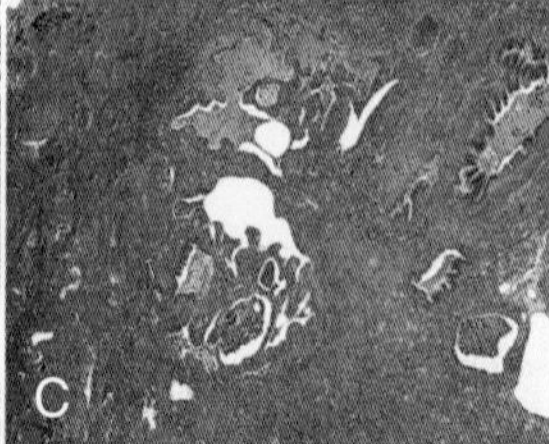

Fig. 3.3 Histopathological evaluation (hematoxylin-eosin staining) of surgical biopsy. (A) Low-magnification photomicrograph showing subpleural patchy fibrosis. (B) Higher-magnification photomicrograph showing fibroblast foci (arrow). (C) Low-magnification photomicrograph showing fibroblast foci and honeycombing.

Discussion Topic 4

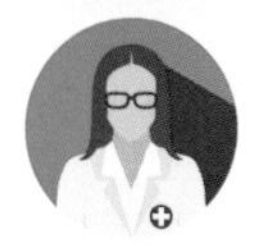

Pathologist

I carefully examined the lung biopsy samples and can affirm that it is a histological UIP. There is an advanced fibrosis with architectural distortion, honeycombing, and fibroblast foci at the interface between the advanced fibrosis and regions of uninvolved lung parenchyma.

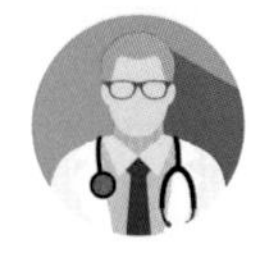

Pulmonologist A

The presence of honeycomb change and fibroblast foci alone is not sufficient to establish the diagnosis of UIP/IPF.

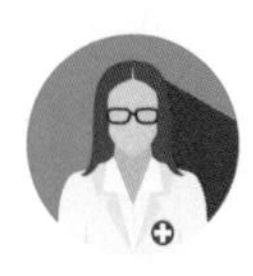

Pathologist

True, but they are important diagnostic findings. The distribution of fibrosis is particularly important because in UIP/IPF, it begins at the periphery of the lobules and works its way toward the centrilobular regions. This results in peripheral "rings" or "donuts" of fibrosis in the subpleural and paraseptal regions of the lobules. The fibrosis should be patchy with areas of advanced fibrosis alternating with nonfibrotic lung parenchyma. Often, the demarcation between the advanced fibrosis and nonfibrotic lung is very clear.

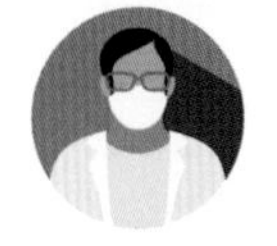

Pulmonologist B

Didn't find airway-centered changes, organizing pneumonia, or other histological features to suggest an alternative etiology?

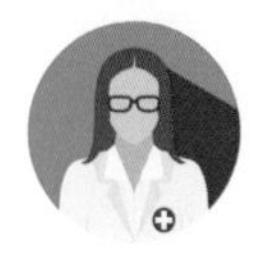

Pathologist

Certainly not. This is crucial in saying that it is UIP/IPF. In particular, there were no prominent airway-centered changes, granulomas, areas of interstitial inflammation lacking associated fibrosis, prominent lymphoid hyperplasia including secondary germinal centers, marked chronic fibrous pleuritis, hyaline membranes, and organizing pneumonia.

Recommended Therapy and Further Indication

The patient immediately started antifibrotic therapy with pirfenidone. No major adverse events were described during treatment, except for moderate dyspepsia and weight loss. Moreover, the patient showed a depressed mood. Nutritional and psychological support was successfully introduced.

Follow-up and Outcomes

The patient was followed for 2 years after the diagnosis. Worsening in lung function and symptoms was recorded. He developed respiratory failure, initially on exertion and later at rest; thus, supplemental oxygen was provided.

The patient was then admitted to the pulmonology unit for acute bronchitis. At the chest CT scan, no new pulmonary infiltrates suspected for an acute exacerbation of IPF were detected.

However, a further worsening of the respiratory failure required high-flow oxygen supplementation. A patent foramen ovale (PFO) was diagnosed with transthoracic and transesophageal echocardiography, and its percutaneous closure was attempted with the aim of reducing hypoxemia due to right-to-left shunt. However, no clinical improvement was obtained, respiratory failure further worsened, and the patient died 3 months later.

Focus on

Velcro Crackles and ILD

Crackles are discontinuous, short explosive noises, considered to be produced by the sudden opening of abnormally closed small airways.

They are best detected during slow, deep inspirations and are often referred to as crepitations in the UK and as rales in the United States.

Fine crackles are softer, shorter in duration, and higher in pitch than coarse crackles. They resemble the sound produced by rubbing strands of hair together in front of the ear or by pulling apart strips of Velcro.

Fine crackles at auscultation are easily recognized by clinicians and are heard in about 60% of patients with IPF. They appear early in the course of IPF, usually in the basal areas of the lungs, where the pulmonary abnormalities begin. As the disease progresses, they can also extend to the upper zones.

The presence of crackles, together with dyspnea or gas exchange abnormalities, may indicate ILD even with a normal chest radiograph.

They are not specific for IPF: they are found in 20% of patients with sarcoidosis and in the majority of patients with idiopathic nonspecific interstitial pneumonia, ILD associated with connective tissue disease, and asbestosis.

Velcro crackles may occasionally be heard in healthy individuals, especially if elderly, or in patients with chronic obstructive pulmonary disease or bronchiectasis.

Focus on

Multidisciplinary Discussion in the Diagnosis of IPF

In patients with newly detected ILD of unknown cause who are clinically suspect of having IPF, recent studies and international guidelines suggest M-D for diagnostic decision-making.

A pulmonologist, a radiologist, and a pathologist are the most frequently involved physicians in multidisciplinary teams. Further input from a rheumatologist and a thoracic surgeon often is useful.

MDD is deemed particularly useful in case of CT pattern different from UIP or probable UIP or in case of discordant clinical, radiological, and histopathological findings. It increases interobserver agreement and diagnostic confidence and can help to avoid unnecessary testing (e.g., lung biopsy).

No specific recommendations exist on how to conduct an MDD. However, face-to-face or voice-to-voice interactions are suggested in case of formal clinical reports with discordance between experts in different disciplines.

Focus on

Awake-VATS in the Diagnosis of IPF/ILD

VATS under general anesthesia is the most frequent surgical technique used for the histopathological diagnosis of ILD. Despite a high diagnostic accuracy, the rate of complications related to the technique is not negligible. Prolonged air leaks, pneumonia, and acute exacerbation of interstitial pneumonia, which can lead to respiratory failure, prolonged hospitalization, and death, have been described after surgical biopsies performed with general anesthesia and mechanical ventilation.

The inflammatory response to surgical intervention (i.e., the exposure to high oxygen concentration), the effect of positive-pressure ventilation, and the overdistention of the lung related to the use of general anesthesia with one-lung ventilation (barotrauma) are potential triggering factors of exacerbation.

Focus on (Continued)

Awake-VATS in the Diagnosis of IPF/ILD

Awake lung biopsy is performed under spontaneous breathing, with regional anesthesia and conscious sedation.

Several regional anesthesia techniques have been described: serratus anterior plane block, thoracic epidural analgesia, selective intercostal block, and thoracic paravertebral blockade.

Recent uncontrolled studies reported excellent outcomes with such a technique. Awake-VATS appears to significantly reduce the rate of postoperative complications, intensive care unit admission, reinterventions, and mortality compared with intubated surgery, with a similar diagnostic yield.

LEARNING POINTS

- Fine crackles at lung auscultation should prompt a thorough diagnostic process for ILD as they are a frequent early sign of IPF.
- In patients with suspected IPF, a lung biopsy is recommended in the absence of a UIP or probable UIP pattern at the chest HRCT, particularly if expertise on transbronchial cryobiopsy is not available.
- Complications of surgical lung biopsy (SLB) with endotracheal intubation include pneumonia, prolonged hospital stay, prolonged air leak, and acute exacerbation of ILD.
- Nutritional support may be useful in patients with IPF with weight loss and gastrointestinal adverse events related to antifibrotic therapy.
- Awake-VATS has a diagnostic yield comparable to SLB, is well tolerated, and may reduce the risk of acute exacerbation related to general anesthesia, endotracheal intubation, and mechanical ventilation.
- In patients with newly detected ILD of unknown cause who are clinically suspected of having IPF, a multidisciplinary discussion is recommended for diagnostic decision-making.

Further Reading

Faverio P, Fumagalli A, Conti S, et al. Nutritional assessment in idiopathic pulmonary fibrosis: a prospective multicentre study. *ERJ Open Res.* 2022;8(1):00443-2021.

Faverio P, Fumagalli A, Conti S, et al. Sarcopenia in idiopathic pulmonary fibrosis: a prospective study exploring prevalence, associated factors and diagnostic approach. *Respir Res.* 2022;23:228.

Flaherty KR, King Jr TE, Raghu G, et al. Idiopathic interstitial pneumonia: what is the effect of a multidisciplinary approach to diagnosis? *Am J Respir Crit Care Med.* 2004;170(8):904-910.

Pompeo E, Rogliani P, Atinkaya C, et al; ESTS Awake Thoracic Surgery Working Group. Nonintubated surgical biopsy of undetermined interstitial lung disease: a multicentre outcome analysis. *Interact Cardiovasc Thorac Surg.* 2019;28(5):744-750.

Pompeo E, Rogliani P, Cristino B, et al. Awake thoracoscopic biopsy of interstitial lung disease. *Ann Thorac Surg.* 2013;95(2):44.

Raghu G, Remy-Jardin M, Myers JL, et al; American Thoracic Society, European Respiratory Society, Japanese Respiratory Society, and Latin American Thoracic Society. Diagnosis of idiopathic pulmonary fibrosis; an official ATS/ERS/JRS/ALAT clinical practice guideline. *Am J Respir Crit Care Med.* 2018;198(5):e44-e68.

Raghu G, Remy-Jardin M, Richeldi L, et al. Idiopathic pulmonary fibrosis (an update) and progressive pulmonary fibrosis in adults: an official ATS/ERS/JRS/ALAT clinical practice guideline. *Am J Respir Crit Care Med.* 2022;205(9):e18-e47.

Richeldi L, Launders N, Martinez F, et al. The characterisation of interstitial lung disease multidisciplinary team meetings: a global study. *ERJ Open Res.* 2019;5(2):00209-2018.

Rossi G, Spagnolo P, Wuyts WA, et al. Pathologic comparison of conventional video-assisted thoracic surgical (VATS) biopsy versus non-intubated/"awake" biopsy in fibrosing interstitial lung diseases. *Respir Med.* 2022;195:106777.

Smith ML. The histologic diagnosis of usual interstitial pneumonia of idiopathic pulmonary fibrosis. Where we are and where we need to go. *Mod Pathol.* 2022;35(suppl 1):8-14.

Walsh SLF, Maher TM, Kolb M, et al; IPF Project Consortium. Diagnostic accuracy of a clinical diagnosis of idiopathic pulmonary fibrosis: an international case-cohort study. *Eur Respir J.* 2017;50(2):1700936.

CHAPTER 4

Interstitial Lung Abnormalities Evolving to Histologically Proven Nonspecific Interstitial Pneumonia

Ada Vancheri ■ Claudio Sorino ■ Sergio Agati ■ Venerino Poletti

History of Present Illness

A 59-year-old woman underwent an abdominal computed tomography (CT) scan for suspected acute gallstones cholecystitis.

Imaging included the lower lung zones, where reticular alterations were incidentally found. Thus, she was referred to the pulmonology clinic.

Past Medical History

The patient was a warehouse worker without any occupational exposure. She had never smoked cigarettes or had bird exposure. No family members had respiratory diseases. About 10 years earlier, she underwent a hysterectomy because of uterine fibroma. She was not taking any medication on a regular basis.

Physical Examination and Early Clinical Findings

At the pulmonology evaluation, the patient was alert and cooperative and just complained of shortness of breath during intense efforts like climbing stairs. She had no cough or chest pain. Her oxygen saturation at the pulse oximeter (SpO_2) was 96% while she was at rest in room air, with a respiratory rate of 15 breaths/min. Blood pressure was 125/80 mmHg, and heart rate was 70 bpm.

The physical examination revealed Velcro sounds at the lower pulmonary fields that endorsed the suspicion of interstitial lung disease. She had no clubbing, no hand joint deformities, and no peripheral edema.

Clinical Course

Pulmonary function tests (PFTs) showed normal lung volumes with forced vital capacity (FVC) 96.3% predicted. Lung diffusion was slightly reduced (diffusing capacity of the lungs for carbon monoxide [DLCO] 78.8% predicted) although still within the lower limits of normal (LLN). A chest high-resolution CT (HRCT) scan confirmed the presence of interstitial lung abnormalities (ILAs) with a few bilateral ground-glass opacities and reticulation, mainly in the peripheral zones and lower lobes (Fig 4.1).

The patient admitted sporadic arthralgias, but usually only after heavy work. At a rheumatological evaluation, there were no current signs of connective tissue disease (CTD), whereas the autoimmunity panel was negative except for low titer (1:40) antinuclear antibodies (ANAs).

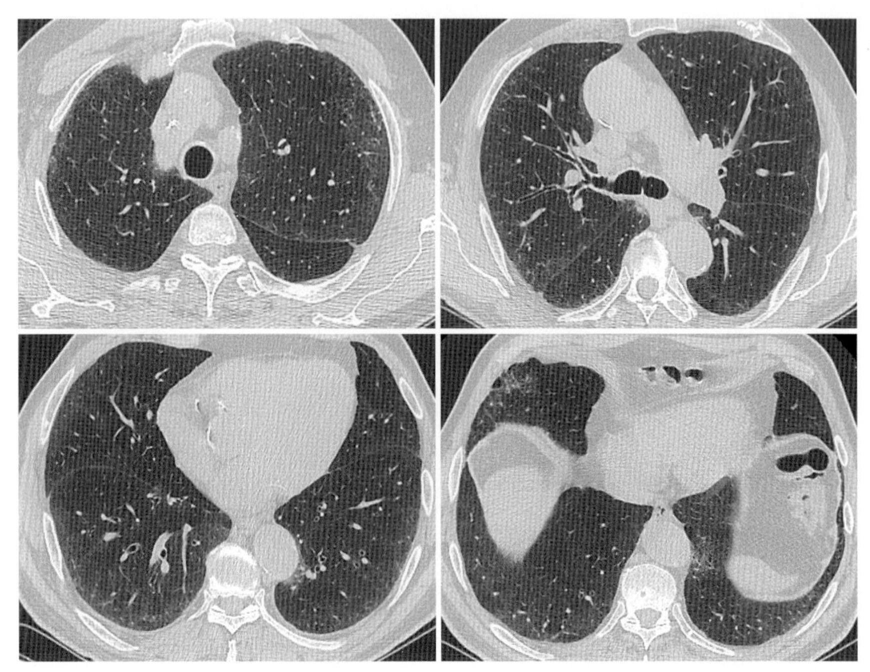

Fig. 4.1 High-resolution CT (HRCT) scan of the chest showing mainly subpleural nonfibrotic interstitial lung abnormalities (ILAs).

Discussion Topic 1

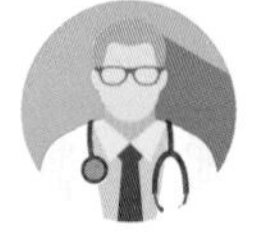

Pulmonologist A

Velcro sounds have high sensitivity for pulmonary interstitial changes. Chest HRCT scan confirmed the presence of ground-glass opacities and subpleural reticulation.

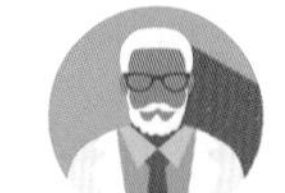

Radiologist

These are just nuanced interstitial lung abnormalities incidentally encountered. It is not easy to understand what the underlying process is.

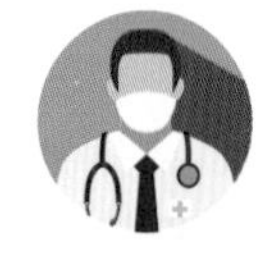

Rheumatologist

Autoimmunity is almost negative and no symptoms or signs of CTD are present, except for sporadic joint pain.

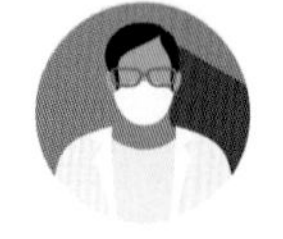

Pulmonologist B

However, we should monitor the patient. ILAs progress within 5 years in at least half of patients.

Discussion Topic 1 (Continued)

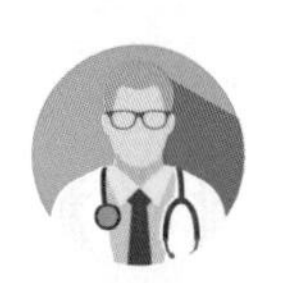

Pulmonologist A

What if it was the onset of an interstitial lung disease (ILD) that could benefit from antifibrotic treatment?

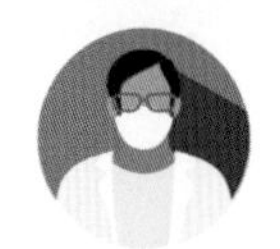

Pulmonologist B

Thinking about idiopatic pulmonary fibrosis (IPF)?

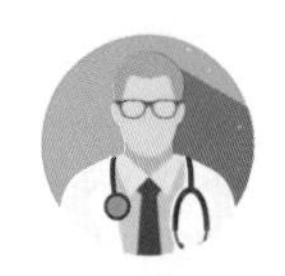

Pulmonologist A

Yes, it would require early therapy to slow the evolution of lung damage and the deterioration of respiratory function. A lung cryobiopsy would be useful for this.

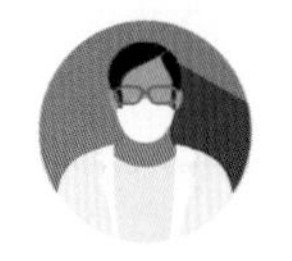

Pulmonologist B

Pulmonary function test (PFT) results are normal, and the patient currently has no respiratory symptoms. Perhaps a follow-up would be sufficient to evaluate whether the clinical and/or radiological picture evolves.

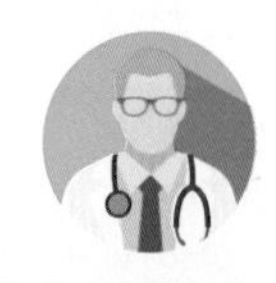

Pulmonologist A

How about a bronchoscopy with bronchoalveolar lavage (BAL)? Could it provide useful information?

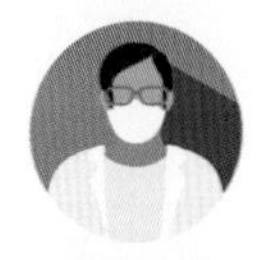

Pulmonologist B

Alone, the BAL cytological analysis has a limited value in distinguishing the different ILDs. It plays a significant role when the clinical and radiological features raise suspicion of some specific forms of ILD, such as sarcoidosis, hypersensitivity pneumonitis, or eosinophilic pneumonia. However, this is not the case.

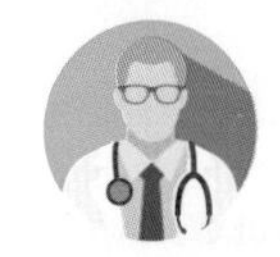

Pulmonologist A

We should explain to the patient the potential benefits and risks of lung cryobiopsy and those of follow-up so that she can consciously choose between the two possibilities.

At a first multidisciplinary evaluation, the specialists agreed on the diagnosis of ILAs, and the patient was informed about the current difficulty in establishing whether she had a disease that would progress to pulmonary fibrosis. She refused cryobiopsy as she was afraid of adverse events and she felt fine. Clinical, radiological, and functional follow-up was scheduled, with PFTs every 6 months and chest HRCT scan every 12 months.

In the following 3 years, the patient reported a progressive reduction of exercise tolerance with dyspnea when walking on flat ground.

Contextually, a deterioration in lung volumes and gas exchanges was observed (Fig. 4.2): FVC decreased to 88.5%, then to 84.2%, and finally to 77.1% of predicted; DLCO reduced to 68.8%, then to 61.2%, and finally to 48.5% of predicted.

At the 3-year follow-up, the patient covered a normal distance (420 m) at a 6-minute walk test (6MWT), although she experienced significant breathlessness and had a slight oxygen desaturation (mean SpO_2 94.2%, lowest SpO_2 88%).

Imaging also showed a worsened ILD with a greater extension of both the reticulation and the areas of hyperdensity with ground-glass pattern (Fig. 4.3).

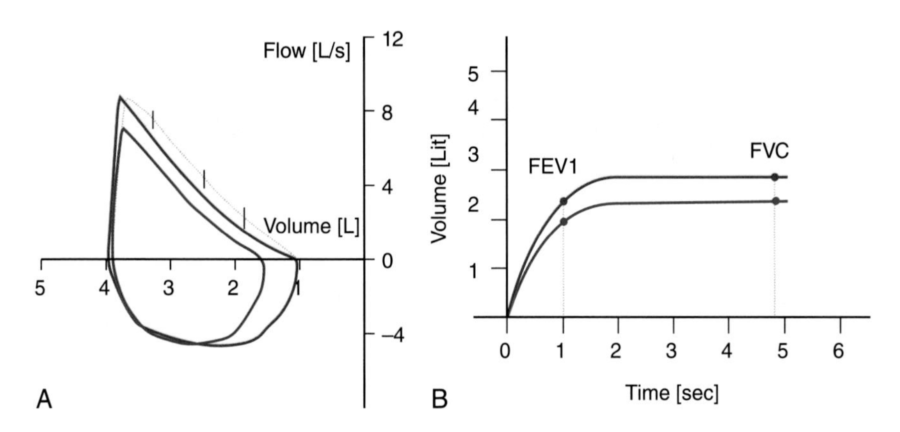

C

Gender: Female	Race: Caucasian			Height: 159 cm		Weight: 74 Kg		
	Age: 59 years					Age: 62 years		
	Observed	Predicted	Z-Score	LLN	% Predicted	Observed	Predicted	% Predicted
FEV_1 (Lit)	2.34	2.41	–0.201	1.89	97.1	1.92	2.36	81.5
FVC (Lit)	2.93	3.04	–0.249	2.31	96.3	2.30	2.98	77.1
FEV_1/FVC	0.80	0.80	0.031	0.68	100.2	0.83	0.79	105.1
FEF 25–75 (Lit/sec)	2.13	2.16	–0.040	1.09	98.6	1.93	2.16	89.3
RV (Lit)	1.50	1.62	–0.275	0.98	92.6	1.23	1.66	74.1
TLC (Lit)	4.76	4.87	–0.192	3.94	97.7	3.44	4.85	70.9
DLCO (mL/min/ mmHg)	15.1	19.1	–1487	14.7	78.8	9.2	18.9	48.5

Fig. 4.2 Comparison of pulmonary function tests at the first observation (red lines) and 3 years later (blue lines). The development of lung restriction and impairment of lung diffusion is evident. (A) Flow-volume curve. (B) Volume-time curve. (C) Measured parameters. FEV_1, forced expiratory volume in 1 second; LLN, lower limit of normal; FVC, forced vital capacity; RV, residual volume; TLC, total lung capacity. DLCO, diffusing capacity of the lungs for carbon monoxide.

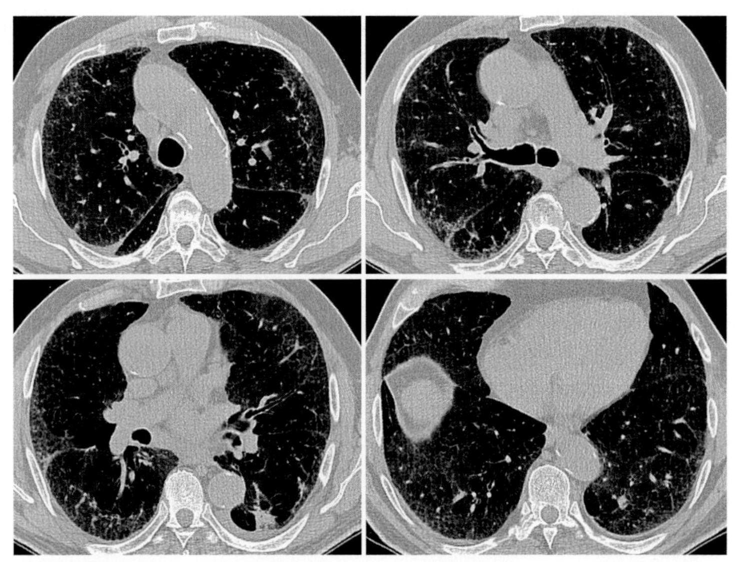

Fig. 4.3 HRCT of the chest showing a progression of the interstitial findings with a greater extension of subpleural reticulation and ground-glass opacities.

Discussion Topic 2

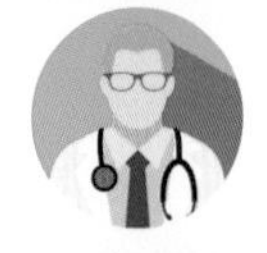

Pulmonologist A

The patient complains of increasing respiratory symptoms. It has been about 3 years since abnormalities were first detected on CT scan of the chest.

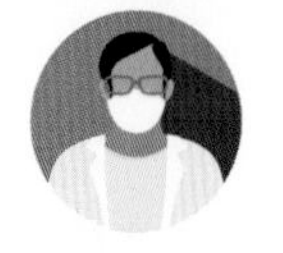

Pulmonologist B

Both PFTs and imaging show worsening findings: total lung capacity decreased by more than 1 Liter, and a greater extension of the interstitial pattern is evident.

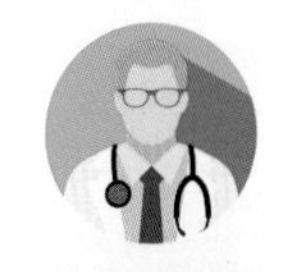

Pulmonologist A

Moreover, the 6MWT revealed oxyhemoglobin desaturation on exercise.

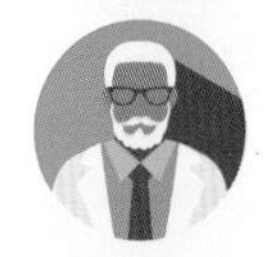

Radiologist

Since the patient is now symptomatic, I would no longer define her radiological findings as ILAs but rather as actual ILD, with a radiological picture of nonspecific interstitial pneumonia (NSIP).

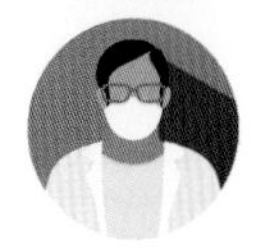

Pulmonologist B

We need to reach a diagnosis. Lung cryobiopsy should be proposed again.

After a new multidisciplinary discussion, the execution of transbronchial cryobiopsy was proposed again to determine the ILD pattern.

The patient accepted and underwent transbronchial cryobiopsy as an outpatient procedure.

Blood tests confirmed that she had normal platelet counts, international normalized ratio (INR), and liver and kidney function. She received deep sedation using propofol and remifentanil and was intubated with a rigid tracheoscope. After a bronchoalveolar lavage with 150 mL of saline in the lateral segment of the middle lobe, transbronchial cryobiopsies at about 1 cm from the pleura were obtained using a 1.7 mm probe. The freezing time was 8 seconds for each biopsy. Two biopsy samples from two different sites of the middle lobe were obtained to improve diagnostic yield.

The procedure was complicated by iatrogenic pneumothorax requiring hospitalization, placement of a small-bore chest tube, and oxygen supplement. A lung expansion was promptly obtained. Drainage was maintained in the pleural space for 3 days. When there was no evidence of air leaks, the chest tube was closed for 24 hours and finally removed after a chest radiograph confirmed that pneumothorax had not recurred (Figs. 4.4, 4.5, 4.6).

BAL cellular profile showed a slight lymphocytosis (macrophages 79%; lymphocytes 16%; neutrophils 5%). The culture for common pathogens was negative as well as microscopy for alcohol/acid-fast bacilli and rRNA-PCR for Mycobacterium tuberculosis complex.

The histological pattern of the lung biopsy was cellular NSIP (Fig 4.7).

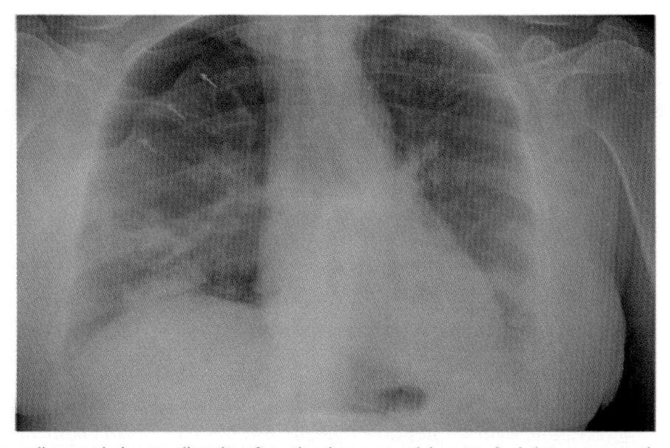

Fig 4.4 Chest radiograph immediately after the lung cryobiopsy. A right pneumothorax is evident.

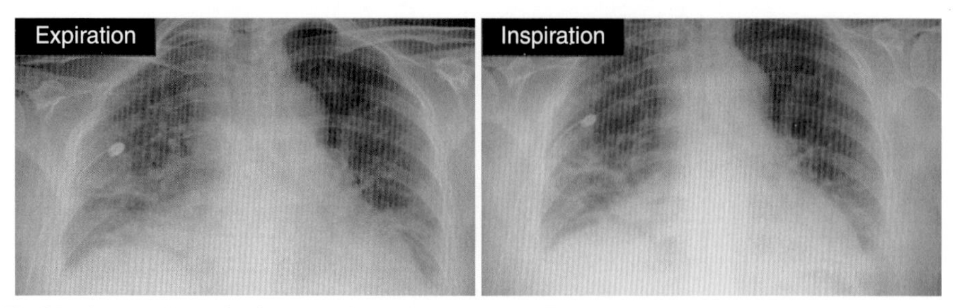

Fig. 4.5 Chest radiograph after right chest tube placement. The lung is expanded on both inspiration and expiration.

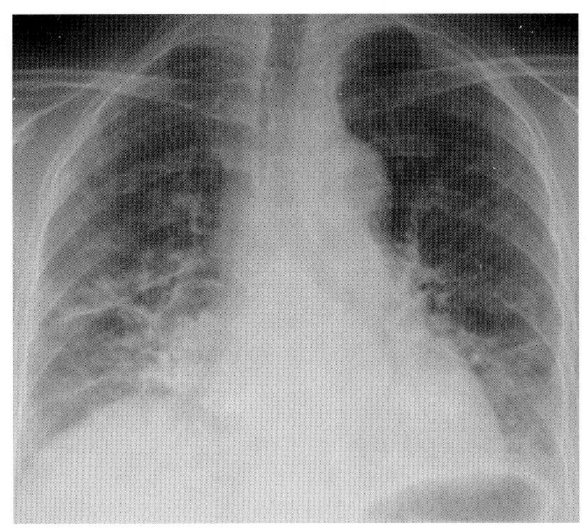

Fig 4.6 Chest radiograph after right chest tube removal showing absence of right pneumothorax.

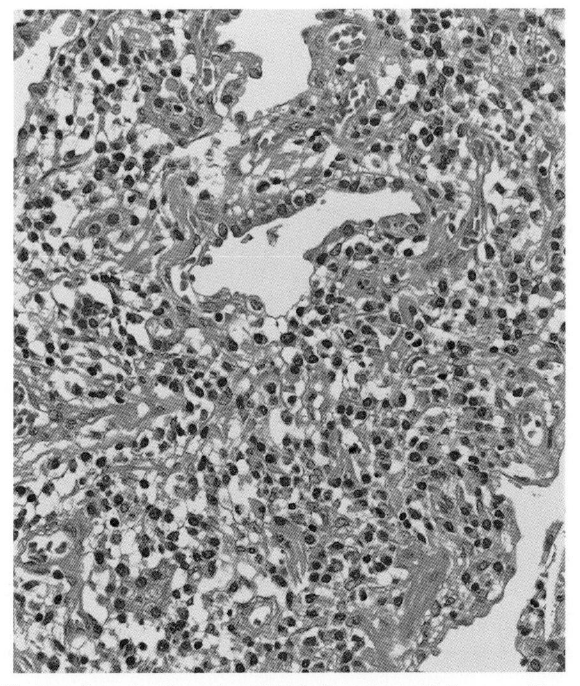

Fig 4.7 Histological findings (hematoxylin-eosin staining) of transbronchial lung cryobiopsy showing a cellular NSIP with diffuse and uniform inflammation and lymphoplasmacytic infiltration of the alveolar walls.

Discussion Topic 3

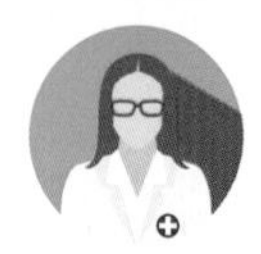

Pathologist

In the histological sample, there are elements to diagnose ILD with cellular NSIP pattern. Unlike the fibrotic form, which has thickening and scarring of lung tissue, here we have mainly inflammation of the cells of the interstitium.

Most importantly, histology excluded findings of acute lung injury, including hyaline membranes, granulomas, organism or viral inclusions, dominant airway disease or organizing pneumonia, eosinophils, and coarse fibrosis.

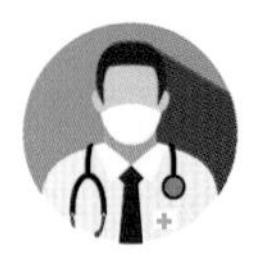

Rheumatologist

The autoimmunity panel showed just ANA 1:160, and the patient has no signs or symptoms of CTD.

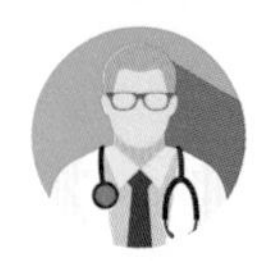

Pulmonologist A

We have no alternative but to say that it's idiopathic NSIP.

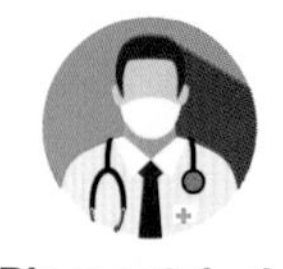

Rheumatologist

The idiopathic form of NSIP is rare. Most cases of idiopathic NSIP appear to be an early manifestation of undifferentiated CTD.

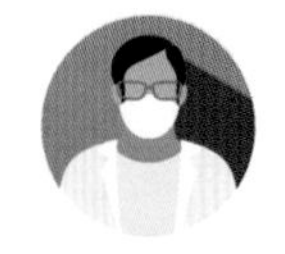

Pulmonologist B

We should offer therapy based on currently available clinical information.

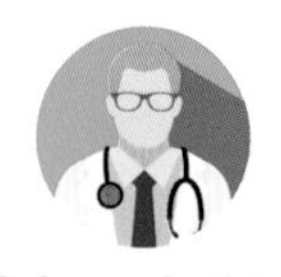

Pulmonologist A

Patients with the cellular type of NSIP often respond well to treatment with oral corticosteroids.

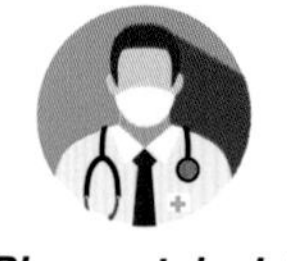

Rheumatologist

However, patients who don't respond to corticosteroid therapy may require additional treatment with immunosuppressants.

Recommended Therapy and Further Indications

Again, after a multidisciplinary discussion among pulmonologists, pathologists, rheumatologists, and radiologists, the diagnosis of idiopathic NSIP was made. Oral prednisone was started at the dosage of 35 mg per day (about 0.5 mg/kg/day).

After a few months, the patient reported xerophthalmia and arthralgias, so the pulmonologist decided to carry out further investigations. The autoimmunity panel was repeated and showed a homogeneous ANA staining pattern (1:1280), and extractable nuclear antigen (ENA) screening was positive for anti-SSA Ro60 (211 KUi/L). At a new rheumatological evaluation, a Schirmer test confirmed the presence of a sicca syndrome. At that point, a diagnosis of pulmonary fibrosis with NSIP pattern due to Sjögren syndrome was made. Considering that the lung cryobiopsy had shown a cellular pattern, mycophenolate mofetil was added with an initial dosage of 500 mg bid.

Follow-Up and Outcomes

In the following months, the patient obtained a progressive improvement in dyspnea. Mycophenolate mofetil was titrated to 1000 mg bid and prednisone tapered to 5 mg/day in about 12 weeks.

PFTs and 6MWT at 6 and 12 months showed slight progressive improvement.

A chest CT scan performed 1 year after the initiation of therapy revealed a marked reduction in diffuse ground-glass opacities. No intercurrent infections occurred.

Focus On

Interstitial Lung Abnormalities: Clinical Significance, and Differential Diagnosis

Interstitial lung abnormalities (ILAs) are incidental radiological findings affecting > 5% of any lung zone at complete or partial chest CT scan where interstitial lung disease (ILD) was not previously suspected. The most frequent radiological alterations are ground-glass opacities, reticulation, traction bronchiectasis or bronchiolectasis, and honeycombing.

Studies suggest that ILAs progress over 5 years in > 50% of individuals and are associated with worsened respiratory symptoms, exercise capacity, lung function, and mortality.

Abnormalities identified during screening for ILD in high-risk groups (e.g., those with CTD or familial ILD) are considered subclinical or preclinical ILD and not ILAs because they are not incidental.

Similarly, abnormalities found in subjects with respiratory symptoms, clinical signs, or functional impairment are usually considered mild ILD rather than just ILAs.

Entities that should be distinguished from ILAs include gravity-dependent atelectasis, which occurs in the dependent portions of the lungs due to a combination of reduced alveolar volume and increased perfusion. They are commonly seen in the posterior lung bases on CT, particularly in elderly individuals, and disappear in prone CT of the chest.

Centrilobular nodules are no longer included in the definition of ILAs as they are a typical, usually nonprogressive manifestation of smoking-related respiratory bronchiolitis.

Other non-ILA findings include apical caps or pleuroparenchymal fibroelastosis-like lesions, focal paraspinal fibrosis in close contact with spine osteophytes, interstitial edema, and findings of aspiration such as patchy ground-glass and tree-in-bud opacities.

The risk factors to develop ILAs are older age, tobacco smoke or other inhalation exposures, and genetic predisposition.

ILAs should be categorized as nonsubpleural, subpleural without fibrosis, and subpleural with fibrosis. The subpleural distribution or the presence of fibrosis is associated with an increased frequency of progression.

The existing evidence is insufficient to determine a definitive management plan or timing for the follow-up of ILAs. Reasonably, it can be useful to visit the patient and perform PFTs at 3 and 12 months, whereas chest HRCT can be performed after 12 to 24 months unless there is previous clinical deterioration. Fig 4.8 shows the algorithm proposed by the Fleischner Society, based on the available literature and consensus clinical opinion.

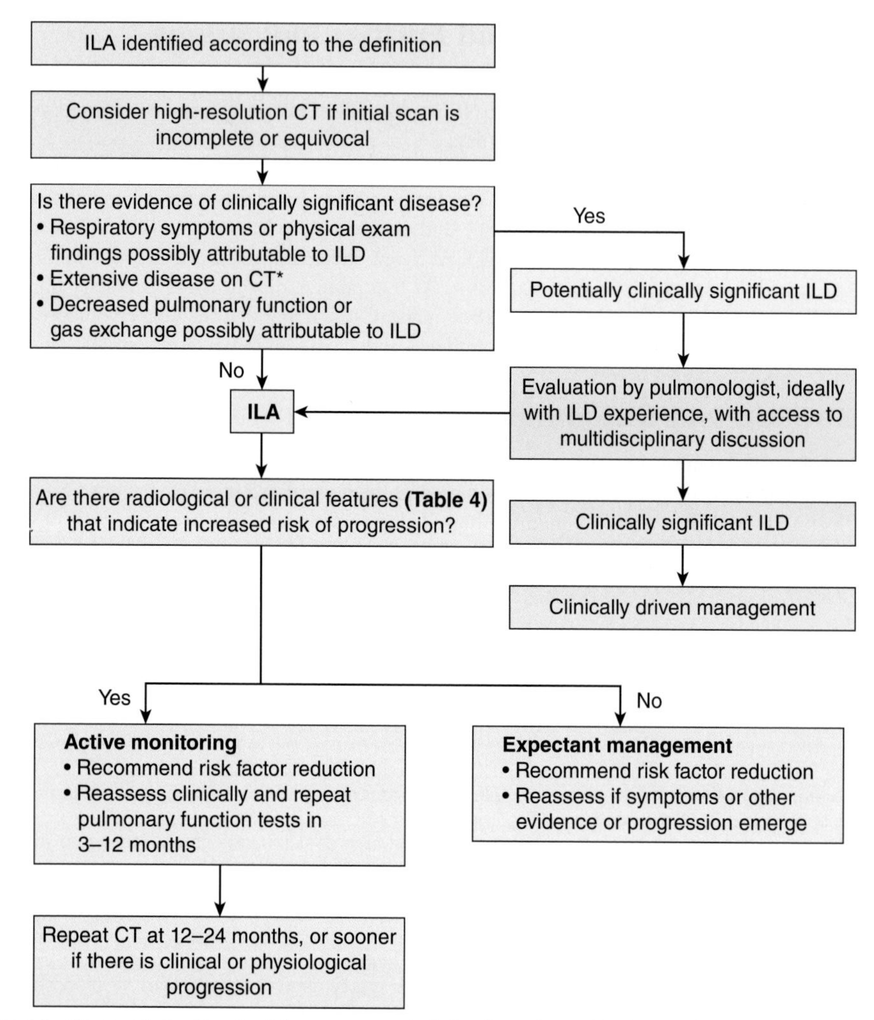

Fig. 4.8 Proposed algorithm for ILAs management. Action items for radiologists are in blue, action items for treating physicians or pulmonologists are in green, and action items for ILD expert pulmonologists are in pink. * Nontrivial abnormalities present in three or more lung zones (above bottom of aortic arch, between aortic arch and top of inferior pulmonary vein, and below inferior pulmonary vein).
[Adapted from Hatabu H, Hunninghake GM, Richeldi L, et al. Interstitial lung abnormalities detected incidentally on CT: a position paper from the Fleischner Society. *Lancet Respir Med*. 2020;8(7):726-737.]

Focus On

Role of Transbronchial Cryobiopsy in ILD

Histopathological evaluation is often required to obtain a diagnosis of interstitial lung disease (ILD) when clinical, laboratory, and radiological data are inconclusive. Surgical lung biopsy (SLB) has long been considered the gold standard, although it is associated with significant complications. In-hospital mortality in elective SLB is estimated to be around 2% and significantly higher in nonelective procedures.

Transbronchial lung cryobiopsy (TBLC) is increasingly recognized as a potential alternative to SLB, especially for patients who are clinically unfit to undergo SLB.

Focus On (Continued)

Role of Transbronchial Cryobiopsy in ILD

The diagnostic yield of TBLC is likely to be somewhat lower than SLB, whereas indirect comparisons suggest lower mortality, shorter hospitalization stay, and lower associated costs in TBLC compared to SLB. In ILDs, subpleural biopsies are suggested, even if they have an increased risk of pneumothorax, while biopsies obtained in the most central areas increase the bleeding risk.

A systematic review suggests that adverse effects occur in 23.1% of patients undergoing TBLC. The incidence of pneumothorax is 9.4%; that of moderate-severe bleeding is 14.2%. Overall adverse event rates of TBLC and SLB are difficult to compare because populations and definitions of complications varied across studies and because pneumothorax is not considered a complication for SLB since all patients require chest tube drainage after the procedure.

The treatment of iatrogenic pneumothorax depends on its entity. In most cases, rest is sufficient to recover, whereas in other cases, the placement of a chest tube is needed. The use of a prophylactic bronchial blocker can lead to improved management of bleeding. The reduction in serious adverse events outweighs the reduced diagnostic yield of TBLC. However, this is recommended only in centers experienced in performing TBLC with competent operators able to safely apply sedation, promptly manage complications, and ensure airway protection.

TBLC is not commonly used for the diagnosis of ILD-CTD, but occasionally it can be performed if the radiological pattern is not clear and if histopathological information is expected to change management.

Focus On

Overview of NSIP Diagnosis, Prognosis, and Treatment

Nonspecific interstitial pneumonia (NSIP) is one class of idiopathic interstitial pneumonia (IIP) that lacks the histopathological features of the other subtypes of IIP. It occurs with a homogeneous appearance of interstitial lung fibrosis and inflammation, typically bilateral and with a certain predisposition for the lower lobes.

The most common features on chest CT scans are ground-glass opacities, fine reticulations, pulmonary volume loss, and traction bronchiectasis. Subpleural sparing, when present, has a high specificity for NSIP.

NSIP can be idiopathic (iNSIP), secondary to connective tissue disease (CTD, mainly systemic sclerosis, polymyositis/dermatomyositis, rheumatoid arthritis, and Sjögren syndrome), induced by drugs (e.g., amiodarone, methotrexate, nitrofurantoin, chemotherapeutic agents, and statin), or associated with HIV infection and with hypersensitivity pneumonitis.

Differential diagnoses include other idiopathic interstitial pneumonia, hypersensitivity pneumonitis, and IgG4-related systemic disease.

Two major radiological and histological NSIP profiles have been described: the "cellular" (or "inflammatory") and the "fibrotic" type. The first is characterized by prominent lymphocytic inflammation on biopsy and bronchoalveolar lavage (BAL), a mixed NSIP/organizing pneumonia HRCT pattern, and a better response to corticosteroid and immunosuppressive treatment. Fibrotic NSIP shows high fibrotic background on biopsy and no lymphocytosis on BAL. It mainly occurs with reticulations and traction bronchiectasis on HRCT and has a worse survival rate than the cellular form.

Nonetheless, fibrotic NSIP should be distinguished from UIP/idiopathic pulmonary fibrosis (IPF) as the former has a significantly better prognosis and possible response to steroid therapy. Overall, five-year survival is about 40% for patients with IPF/UIP and 90% for those with NSIP and a fibrotic component.

Treatment of NSIP depends on the cause and severity of the disease. For patients with mild symptoms and minimal impairment on PFTs, a close follow-up to detect possible disease progression can be scheduled. Patients with iNSIP who have moderate to severe symptoms, significant impairment in lung volumes, and diffuse changes on chest HRCT may receive systemic corticosteroids. Prednisone 0.5–1 mg/kg/day, up to a maximum dose of 60 mg/day, is one of the most commonly starting doses. For those who respond/stabilize with this treatment, the prednisone should be gradually tapered over 6 to 9 months to a dosage of 5–10 mg/day with the goal of discontinuing therapy after 1 year.

In the case of a poor tolerance or response to treatment after 3 to 6 months, a further immunosuppressive agent like azathioprine or mycophenolate may be considered.

Continued on following page

Focus On (Continued)

Overview of NSIP Diagnosis, Prognosis, and Treatment

Pulse methylprednisolone at a dosage of 1000 mg/day for 3 days, followed by systemic prednisone, may be administrated to hospitalized patients with severe NSIP and acute respiratory failure.

In cases of secondary NSIP, treatment should be focused on the underlying cause (e.g., removal from the exposure for drug-induced NSIP, systemic corticosteroid or immunosuppressant agents for CTD-related NSIP, and antiretroviral therapy for HIV infection). A standardized protocol for drug dosage or duration in CTD-NSIP does not exist. As for iNSIP, prednisone is usually started at 0.5–1 mg/kg/day, and the association with other drugs can be useful to obtain steroids sparing and improve survival chances. The disease-modifying antirheumatic drugs (DMARDs) act on the immune system; the most used are methotrexate, mycophenolate mofetil, azathioprine, and cyclophosphamide. Other drugs are under evaluation, such as biological therapies, in particular rituximab, a chimeric anti-CD20 autoantibody that acts against B cells.

Follow-up with PFTs and chest CT scan is crucial to evaluate the treatment response and even to detect a progressive phenotype that may benefit from antifibrotic therapy.

Pneumocystis jirovecii pneumonia prophylaxis with low-dose trimethoprim/sulfamethoxazole should be offered to patients receiving high-dose prednisone for prolonged periods (≥ 0.6 mg/kg/day or 30 mg/day for ≥ 4 weeks) or those on multiple immunosuppressive agents, as this opportunistic respiratory infection may be severe and worsen lung function.

LEARNING POINTS

- Interstitial lung abnormalities (ILAs) are generally incidental radiological findings of potential ILD without respiratory symptoms.
- Nonspecific interstitial pneumonia (NSIP) is the second most common pattern of ILD, usually characterized by bilateral ground-glass opacities, reticulations, pulmonary volume loss, traction bronchiectasis, and subpleural sparing.
- NSIP can, rarely, be an idiopathic entity or secondary to connective tissue diseases (CTDs), drug exposure, hypersensitivity pneumonitis (HP), and HIV infection.
- Surgical biopsy or transbronchial cryobiopsy can identify a prevalent cellular or fibrosing pattern of NSIP and distinguish it from UIP/IPF.
- Cellular NSIP is characterized by inflammatory interstitial infiltrates and has a better treatment response and overall prognosis than fibrosing NSIP.
- Therapeutic strategies of NSIP are based on corticosteroid/immunosuppressant agents or antifibrotic drugs.

Further Reading

Abdelghani R, Thakore S, Kaphle U, et al. Radial endobronchial ultrasound-guided transbronchial cryobiopsy. *J Bronchology Interv Pulmonol.* 2019;26(4):245-249.

Berardicurti O, Marino A, Genovali I, et al. Interstitial lung disease and pulmonary damage in primary Sjögren's syndrome: a systematic review and meta-analysis. *J Clin Med.* 2023;12(7):2586.

Hata A, Schiebler ML, Lynch DA, Hatabu H. Interstitial lung abnormalities: state of the art. *Radiology.* 2021;301(1):19-34.

Hatabu H, Hunninghake GM, Richeldi L, et al. Interstitial lung abnormalities detected incidentally on CT: a position paper from the Fleischner Society. *Lancet Respir Med.* 2020;8(7):726-737.

Hino T, Lee KS, Yoo H, et al. Interstitial lung abnormality (ILA) and nonspecific interstitial pneumonia (NSIP). *Eur J Radiol Open.* 2021;8:100336.

Korevaar DA, Colella S, Fally M, et al. European Respiratory Society guidelines on transbronchial lung cryobiopsy in the diagnosis of interstitial lung diseases. *Eur Respir J.* 2022;60(5):2200425.

Luppi F, Sebastiani M, Silva M, et al. Interstitial lung disease in Sjögren's syndrome: a clinical review. *Clin Exp Rheumatol.* 2020;38(suppl 126):291-300.

Maldonado F, Danoff SK, Wells AU, et al. Transbronchial cryobiopsy for the diagnosis of interstitial lung diseases: CHEST guideline and expert panel report. *Chest.* 2020;157(4):1030-1042.

Yoo H, Hino T, Hwang J, et al. Connective tissue disease-related interstitial lung disease (CTD-ILD) and interstitial lung abnormality (ILA): evolving concept of CT findings, pathology and management. *Eur J Radiol Open.* 2022;9:100419.

PART II

Smoking-Associated Interstitial Lung Diseases

CHAPTER 5

Respiratory Bronchiolitis-Interstitial Lung Disease

Francesco Varone ■ Claudio Sorino ■ Giuseppe Cicchetti

History of Present Illness

A 61-year-old Caucasian man presented to the pulmonology outpatient clinic due to shortness of breath during exercise and nocturnal dyspnea. These symptoms had begun a few months earlier. He also had a cough with sputum almost every morning. However, he said that the cough did not bother him and considered it a normal consequence of cigarette smoking. A chest radiograph, prescribed by the general practitioner, showed a widespread reduced transparency of the lung fields with a slight reticulonodular pattern.

Past Medical History

The patient was a retired bricklayer, current smoker of about 20 cigarettes a day, with a 47-pack-year history of smoking. He reported previous exposure to concrete dust. He denied exposure to organic agents such as birds and feathers nor to asbestos fibers. His family history was negative for pulmonary illness. He had no history of drug abuse, weight loss, or anorexia. He reported a transient ischemic attack a few years earlier. Since then, he was prescribed oral clopidogrel 75 mg once daily. On that occasion, he underwent a high-resolution computed tomography (HRCT) of the chest. However, this was not available at the time of the first pulmonology visit.

Physical Examination and Early Clinical Findings

At the time of the visit to the pulmonologist, the patient was afebrile (body temperature 36.7° C [98.06 °F]), alert, and cooperative. His body mass index was normal. Oxygen saturation measured by pulse oximeter (SpO_2) was 95% on room air, heart rate was 85 beats/min, and blood pressure was 130/90 mm Hg.

Physical examination revealed inspiratory crackles on both lung bases. Moreover, a moderate increase in the convexity of the nail fold (finger clubbing) was noticed. He had no skin pallor, peripheral edema, or jugular vein distention. The patient denied Raynaud phenomenon, arthralgias, myalgias, sicca syndrome, or other symptoms suggesting a connective tissue disease. He admitted to having some daytime sleepiness since dyspnea disturbed his night rest.

Discussion Topic

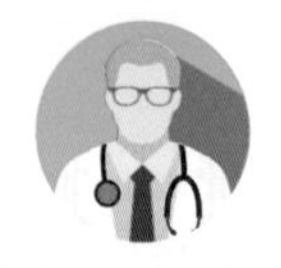

Pulmonologist A

The findings on thoracic auscultation and the strong history of smoking suggest a pulmonary cause of the shortness of breath.

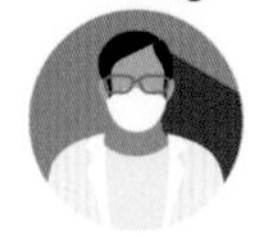

Pulmonologist B

We need to evaluate pulmonary function with spirometry and diffusion capacity of the lung for carbon monoxide (DLCO).

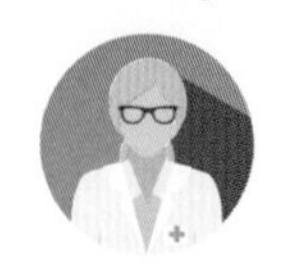

Pulmonologist C

Velcro crackles suggest an interstitial lung disease (ILD) and should be further investigated with an HRCT of the chest.

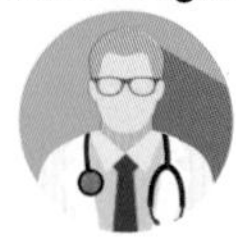

Pulmonologist A

I agree. The patient was also exposed to cement dust, which can contain several substances harmful to the lungs such as crystalline silica.

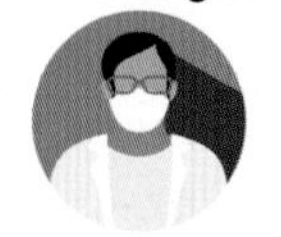

Pulmonologist B

Moreover, the presence of finger clubbing also raises suspicion of idiopathic pulmonary fibrosis (IPF) or lung cancer.

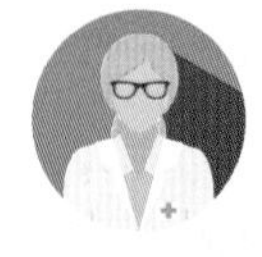

Pulmonologist C

Ok, we will plan a diagnostic workup considering COPD, occupational lung diseases, pulmonary fibrosis and even lung cancer as possible differential diagnoses.

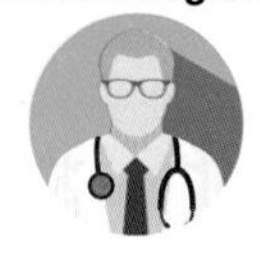

Pulmonologist A

Finger clubbing may also indicate a hypoxemia during sleep or exertion. We should schedule a 6-minute walk test (6MWT) and an overnight pulse oximetry test.

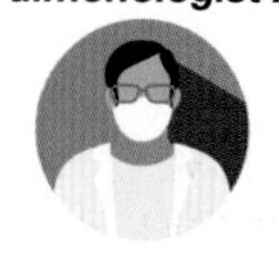

Pulmonologist B

The patient does not appear to have clinical signs of heart failure, but I would also recommend a cardiological evaluation with electrocardiogram and echocardiogram.

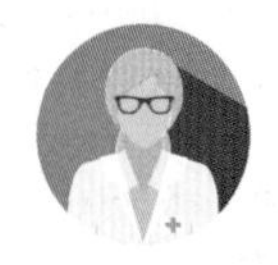

Pulmonologist C

A complete laboratory panel and autoantibodies could also be useful. Anyway, we should encourage smoking cessation.

Clinical Course

The patient underwent pulmonary function tests that showed lung volumes within normal limits but with a slowing in the terminal portion of the spirogram (mid-flows) suggestive of an obstruction in small airways: forced expiratory volume in 1 second (FEV_1)/forced vital capacity (FVC) ratio was 71.5%, FEV_1 was 90% predicted, FVC 94% predicted, forced mid-expiratory flow ($FEF_{25-75\%}$) 51% predicted, total lung capacity (TLC) 88% predicted, residual volume (RV) 96% predicted. A moderate reduction in the diffusion lung capacity was present (DLCO 60% predicted). The six-minute walk test (6MWT) on room air showed a normal walking distance without oxygen desaturation during exercise. At the overnight pulse oximetry test, oxygen levels were quite low but just sufficient (mean SpO_2 90.7%, > 88% for 99% of the time) and without fluctuations suggestive for sleep apnea. Blood tests showed no anemia nor polyglobulia, normal electrolytes, renal and hepatic function, and markers of inflammation. Testing for antinuclear antibodies (ANA), extractable nuclear antigen antibodies (ENA), and anti-neutrophil cytoplasmic antibodies (ANCA) were negative. The electrocardiogram and echocardiogram did not reveal signs of heart failure nor increase in pulmonary arterial pressure. The Mantoux tuberculin skin test (TST) was negative at 72 hours.

The HRCT of the chest (Fig. 5.1) demonstrated a diffuse extensive bilateral parenchymal involvement, with multiple poorly defined centrilobular nodules, confluent ground-glass opacities, and some low attenuation areas. Abnormalities were slightly predominant in the subpleural regions of the upper-mid lung zones. Fine reticulation was evident in the subpleural lung parenchyma without traction bronchiectasis or bronchiolectases and any other signs of coarse fibrosis. The apical region of both lungs showed multiple clustered cysts of variable size, with regular thickened wall (<2 mm), compatible with *airspace enlargement with fibrosis* (AEF). Lung volumes appeared preserved. Diffuse bronchial wall thickening was also evident. The case was discussed by the interstitial lung diseases (ILD) multidisciplinary team.

Discussion Topic

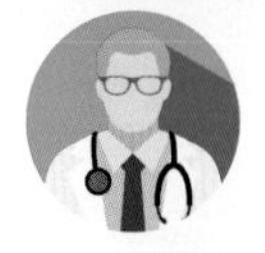

Pulmonologist A

Our patient is a heavy smoker exposed to cement dust. Lung flows and volumes are within normal limits and do not allow the diagnosis of COPD. However, the DLCO is slightly reduced.

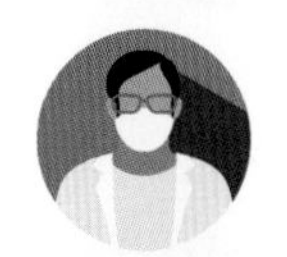

Pulmonologist B

Chest HRCT scan showed multiple poorly-defined nodules and ground glass opacities (GGOs). The abnormalities are inconsistent with a UIP pattern, do you agree?

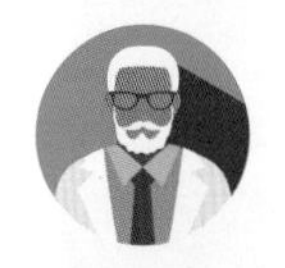

Radiologist A

Yes, I do. There is minimal reticulation, traction bronchiectasis is almost absent, and there is no evidence of honeycombing or volume loss. This is clearly not a UIP pattern, so I would rule out a diagnosis of IPF.

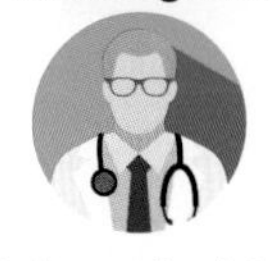

Pulmonologist A

Laboratory results showed no abnormalities, in particular nothing to suggest connective tissue disease. Given his work, an occupational lung disease should be taken into account.

Continued on following page

Discussion Topic (Continued)

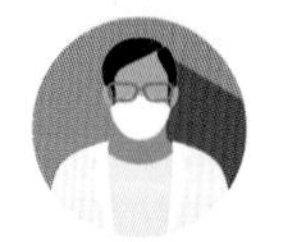

Pulmonologist B

In my opinion, the lack of pleural plaques or perilymphatic nodules, architectural distortion and nodal enlargement/calcifications makes occupational disease unlikely.

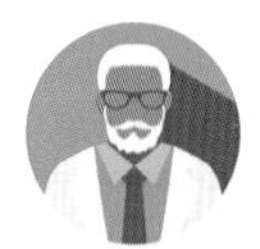

Radiologist A

Ill-defined micronodules and confluent GGOs, with mild mid-upper predominance, may also be present in hypersensitivity pneumonitis (HP), so a differential diagnosis should also be made with it.

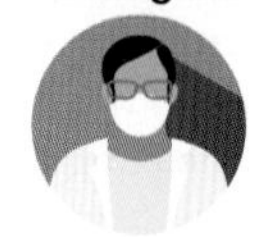

Pulmonologist B

HP is rare in smokers. Additionally, the multiple thin-walled cysts in the upper lobes suggest airspace enlargement with fibrosis (AEF). Together with some paraseptal emphysema, it makes smoking-related diseases more likely.

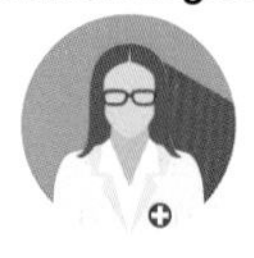

Pathologist

I recommend performing a bronchoscopy with bronchoalveolar lavage (BAL). If this demonstrates the absence of lymphocytosis, we can definitively rule out HP.

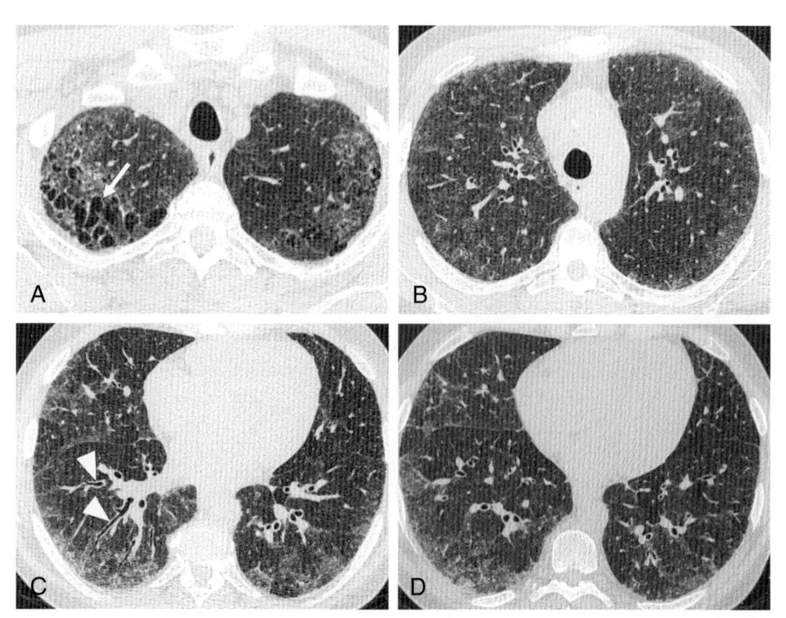

Fig. 5.1 (A-D) Chest HRCT axial images in the lung parenchymal window, demonstrating bilateral multiple poorly defined centrilobular nodules and confluent ground-glass areas, prevalent in the subpleural zones. Fine reticulation is also present in both lungs, without honeycombing. Multiple clustered cysts of variable size, with slightly thickened wall, were evident in the pulmonary apexes (mainly in the right one), consistent with air-space enlargement with fibrosis (AEF) (arrow in A). Note the diffuse marked bronchial wall thickening, especially evident in the lower lobes (arrowheads in C).

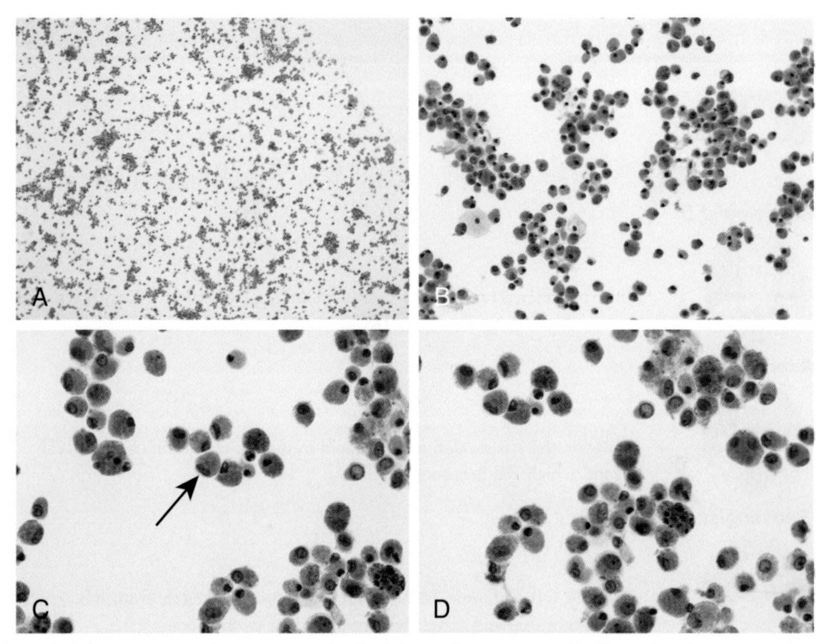

Fig. 5.2 (A-D) Microscope slide smears of BAL fluid at different magnifications showing predominance of alveolar macrophages (as in normal individuals) but with brownish-pigmented macrophages (arrow in C).

The patient underwent outpatient bronchoscopy under mild sedation (midazolam 5 mg intravenous) and local anesthesia (topical lidocaine). On endoscopic evaluation, some areas of anthracosis were observed bilaterally in the bronchial mucosa. There were no alterations of bronchial patency or lesions suspicious of malignancy. A BAL was performed in the middle lobe with the instillation of 150 ml of saline solution (5 aliquots of 30 ml). BAL fluid differential cell count showed the presence of 91% macrophages, most of which characteristically exhibited brown pigments due to high exposure to cigarette smoke (Fig. 5.2) BAL fluid culture was negative, no acid-fast bacilli (AFB) were identified, and cytological examination did not find any cells with malignant atypia.

Discussion Topic

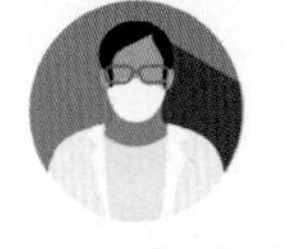

Pulmonologist B

On differential cell counts of BAL fluid, more than 90% of the elements were brownish-pigmented macrophages. This finding is compatible with the diagnosis of smoking-related ILD.

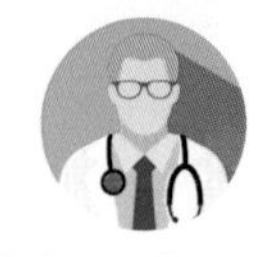

Pulmonologist A

I believe the most likely diagnosis is respiratory bronchiolitis-interstitial lung disease (RB-ILD).

Continued on following page

Discussion Topic (Continued)

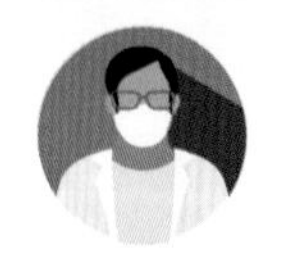

Pulmonologist B

How do you distinguish simple RB from RB-ILD?

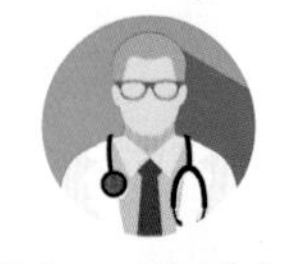

Pulmonologist A

Some consider them to be two similar smoking-related ILDs, with RB-ILD usually showing more severe HRCT and histological abnormalities than RB.

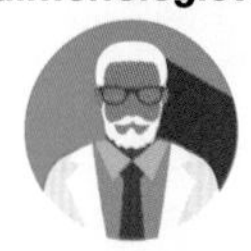

Radiologist

However, there is no defined threshold in disease extent on chest HRCT beyond which RB becomes RB-ILD.

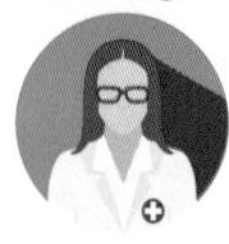

Pathologist

Similarly, RB-ILD may be histologically indistinguishable from RB, which is a very common, and often incidental, finding in smokers.

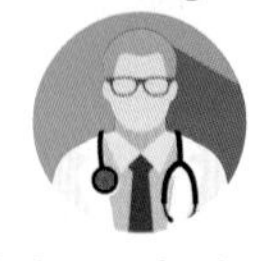

Pulmonologist A

This is true. Actually, the presence of symptoms such as progressive dyspnea and chronic cough often helps differentiate RB-ILD from RB. Furthermore, the presence of RB-ILD is suggested by the finding of inspiratory crackles, heard in more than half of patients.

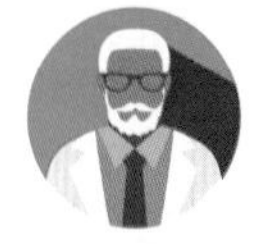

Radiologist

Desquamative interstitial pneumonia (DIP) is another possible smoking-related ILD. In our patient, it is less likely due to the absence of lower lung predominance and cystic changes.

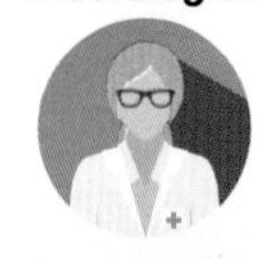

Pulmonologist C

The boundaries between RB-ILD and DIP are also blurred. In daily practice, the distinction can be difficult. Follow-up may further help clarify as RB-ILD usually does not progress to pulmonary fibrosis.

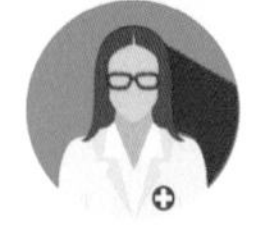

Pathologist

Histology can sometimes differentiate RB-ILD and DIP since in the former the macrophages are confined to the centrilobular area, while in DIP they involve the lobule more diffusely. Furthermore, interstitial fibrosis, lymphoid follicles, giant cells, and eosinophils are more frequent in DIP than in RB-ILD.

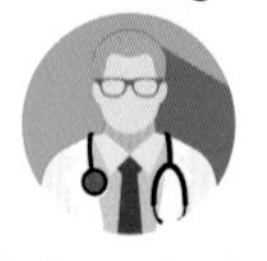

Pulmonologist

So do you think we need histology?

Discussion Topic (Continued)

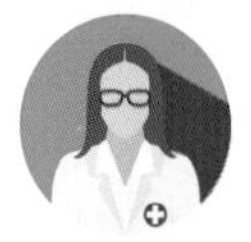

Pathologist

I think it's not necessary at this time. When clinical, functional and radiological features strongly support a diagnosis of RB-ILD, lung biopsy can be avoided and re-evaluation can be planned after a period of smoking cessation. If the patient has no improvement after quitting smoking or even if symptoms and imaging worsen, we may reconsider the need for a lung biopsy.

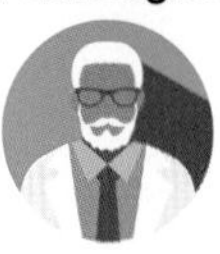

Radiologist

We should definitely look at the previous chest HRCT, to evaluate if the disease is stable or progressive.

Finally, the patient was able to provide the doctors with the previous HRCT scan of the chest (Fig. 5.3), which showed the presence of similar diffuse parenchymal abnormalities, particularly the poorly defined centrilobular nodules and ground-glass opacities, with upper-mid lung predominance, as well as the AEF in the upper lobes and the diffuse bronchial wall thickening. However, the comparison between the two examinations showed a clear progression of lung abnormalities at follow-up images, with an increase in the extent of involved areas and evidence of fine reticulation (Fig. 5.4).

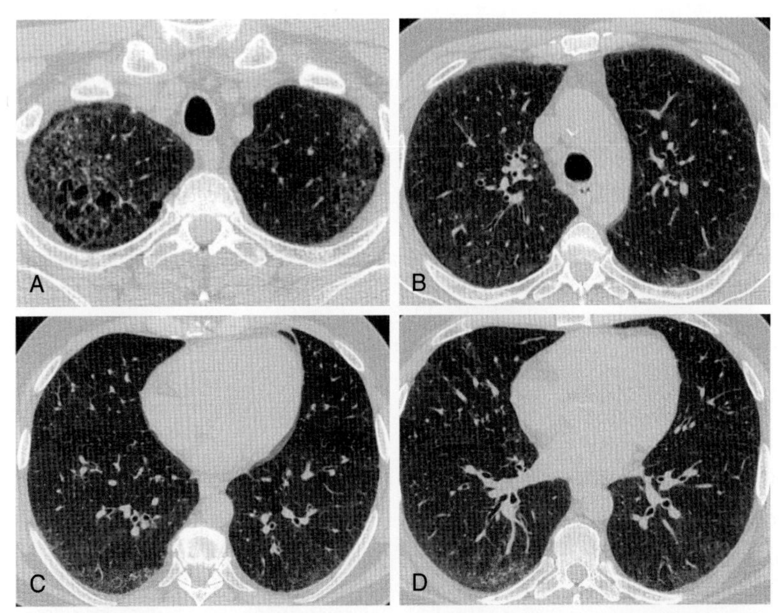

Fig. 5.3 (A-D) HRCT axial images with parenchymal lung window setting performed 4 years before the current clinical evaluation. There are diffuse bilateral parenchymal abnormalities similar to those shown in Fig. 5.1, in particular multiple poorly defined centrilobular nodules and confluent ground-glass areas, prevalent in the subpleural and dorsal regions, but with a lesser extent, some sparing of the lower lobes and almost absent reticulation. The airspace enlargement with fibrosis (AEF) was already present in the apical zones (A, B).

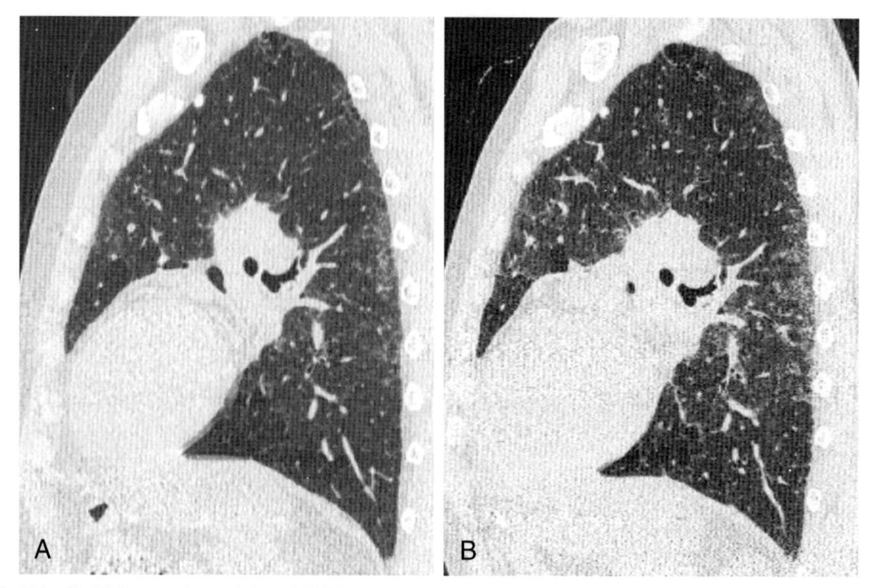

Fig. 5.4 (A-B) Comparison of chest HRCT images in sagittal reconstruction (lung window setting) performed 4 years before (A) and at the current presentation (B). A progression of the parenchymal abnormalities, slightly prevalent in the mid-lung zones, is evident. Lung volume is preserved.

Recommended Therapy and Further Indications

The patient was advised to immediately quit smoking. Apart from this, no pharmacological therapy was prescribed except mucolytics when necessary to manage mucus hypersecretion. Doctors scheduled a strict follow-up with lung function tests and HRCT of the chest in order to detect eventual disease progression.

Follow-up and Outcomes

The patient made up his mind to quit smoking and he succeeded without medical or pharmacological help. He has been actively followed by the ILD outpatient clinic. After 2 years, the main functional parameters, in particular FEV_1, FVC, and DLCO, remained quite stable. Similarly, symptoms remained stable over time. The patient was advised to continue abstaining from smoking and to receive flu and pneumococcal vaccinations.

Focus on

Overview and management of RB-ILD

Respiratory bronchiolitis (RB) is a common inflammatory reaction of respiratory bronchioles that occurs predominantly in long-term active smokers. First described in 1974 by Niewoehner and coworkers, it is characterized by the presence of clusters of pigmented alveolar macrophages within respiratory bronchioles and surrounding airspaces. The majority of patients with RB are asymptomatic, but a small portion of smokers with RB may develop a clinically significant interstitial lung disease, which is termed RB-ILD. The main symptoms of RB-ILD are cough and dyspnea. Pulmonary function tests (PFTs) may show an obstructive, restrictive, or a mixed obstructive–restrictive pattern. DLCO is usually decreased.

Focus on (Continued)

Radiological appearance of RB-ILD

Clubbing in RB-ILD is uncommon but possible. It may result from chronic hypoxemia, and when present, it raises suspicion of IPF or lung cancer.

Prolonged survival is common in RB-ILD patients. Smoking cessation is considered the most important measure in the management of RB-ILD. Usually, quitting smoking leads to significant improvement in symptoms and lung function tests. Some case-reports suggest that oral corticosteroids could be an option for RB-ILD. However, steroid treatment is not usually prescribed in these patients, given the lack of well-designed clinical trials exploring this issue.

Focus on

Radiological appearance of RB-ILD

On chest HRCT, RB consists of multiple ill-defined ground-glass centrilobular micronodules as well as patchy multifocal ground-glass opacities (GGOs). RB-ILD shows similar abnormalities but usually more extensive, represented by low attenuation centrilobular micronodules, GGOs, as well as mild subpleural reticulation, bronchial wall thickening, and lobular areas of air-trapping—which are better depicted on expiratory images. These findings mainly involve the upper lung zones and are generally associated with emphysema (usually not extensive). In some cases, peribronchovascular reticular changes with traction bronchiectasis can be seen, reflecting an airway-centered interstitial fibrosis.

Although not specific, chest X-ray may reveal subtle reticulonodular interstitial pattern.

In some cases, HRCT reveals multiple clustered cysts of variable size, with visible and occasionally thick walls, predominantly located in the upper lobes or in the posterior upper and middle portions of the lower lobes, in the subpleural areas, without abutting the pleura. These findings are referred to as airspace enlargement with fibrosis (AEF) or smoking-related interstitial fibrosis (SRIF), and may coexist with RB-ILD features. Indeed, they can be expression of multiple patterns of smoking-related injury, sometimes with overlapping features, which can be gathered under the term of *smoking-related lung injury*.

Partial regression of centrilobular micronodules and GGOs can occur in patients at follow-up, after smoking cessation. The degree of improvement of the RB-ILD abnormalities on HRCT may depend on the duration of smoking cessation and on the amount of inflammation and fibrosis. On the contrary, Remy-Jardin and coworkers reported that centrilobular micronodules, GGOs, and emphysema can increase in extent in persistent smokers over long follow-up periods.

Focus on

Differential diagnosis of RB-ILD

Given the presence in RB-ILD of upper lobe predominant centrilobular nodules, GGOs, and some degrees of air trapping, hypersensitivity pneumonitis (HP) may be considered among the differential diagnosis for RB-ILD. However, HP patients are usually nonsmokers and cigarette smoking is considered somewhat protective against HP. Therefore, smoking history and/or presence of emphysema are important clues that may help in distinguishing among the two entities. Moreover, the diagnosis of RB-ILD is supported when BAL fluid analysis shows pigmented macrophages and absence of lymphocytosis.

Compared to desquamative interstitial pneumonia (DIP), GGOs in RB-ILD are less extensive and more poorly defined; also, parenchymal abnormalities tend to predominate in the upper lung zones, compared to the mid-lower lung predominance of DIP, which may also demonstrate evidence of small cysts within the GGOs. Nevertheless, the two entities may overlap and even coexist in the same patient. It should be kept in mind that DIP is usually a more clinically aggressive disease compared to RB-ILD.

If RB-ILD is associated with AEF/SRIF changes on HRCT, the presence of confluent thick-walled cysts may resemble honeycombing, and therefore a UIP pattern. Nonetheless, the differential diagnosis with UIP is usually straightforward, due to poor evidence of peripheral traction bronchiectasis and the presence of centrilobular micronodules as well as patchy multifocal GGOs in RB-ILD.

LEARNING POINTS

- RB-ILD can be suspected in patients with progressive respiratory symptoms, long history of cigarette smoking, and a chest HRCT showing GGOs and poorly defined centrilobular nodules.
- HRCT is pivotal in the diagnosis of RB-ILD, differentiating it from other smoking-related ILDs (including IPF), as well as in follow-up.
- Although RB-ILD and HP may have similar clinical and imaging characteristics, heavy exposure to cigarette smoke suggests RB-ILD.
- Bronchoscopy with BAL can be useful in the differential diagnoses of RB-ILD, which usually reveals macrophageal alveolitis with brownish-pigmented macrophages.
- Smoking cessation is the main therapeutic option for RB-ILD patients.

Further Readings

Caminati A, Cavazza A, Sverzellati N, Harari S. An integrated approach in the diagnosis of smoking-related interstitial lung diseases. *Eur Respir Rev.* 2012;21(125):207-217.

Katzenstein AL. Smoking-related interstitial fibrosis (SRIF): pathologic findings and distinction from other chronic fibrosing lung diseases. *J Clin Pathol.* 2013;66:882-887.

Kumar A, Cherian SV, Vassallo R, Yi ES, Ryu JH. Current concepts in pathogenesis, diagnosis, and management of smoking-related interstitial lung diseases. *Chest.* 2018;154(2):394-408.

Nair A, Hansell DM. High-resolution computed tomography features of smoking-related interstitial lung disease. *Semin Ultrasound CT MR.* 2014;35(1):59-71.

Portnoy J, Veraldi KL, Schwarz MI, et al. Respiratory bronchiolitis-interstitial lung disease: long-term outcome. *Chest.* 2007;131(3):664-671.

Reddy TL, John Mayo J, Churg A. Respiratory bronchiolitis with fibrosis. High-resolution computed tomography findings and correlation with pathology. *Ann Am Thorac Soc.* 2013;10(6):590-601.

Sieminska A, Kuziemski K. Respiratory bronchiolitis-interstitial lung disease. *Orphanet J Rare Dis.* 2014; 9:106.

Travis WD, Costabel U, Hansell DM, et al; ATS/ERS Committee on Idiopathic Interstitial Pneumonias. An official American Thoracic Society/European Respiratory Society statement: Update of the international multidisciplinary classification of the idiopathic interstitial pneumonias. *Am J Respir Crit Care Med.* 2013;188(6):733-748.

Walsh SLF, Nair A, Desai SR. Interstitial lung disease related to smoking: imaging considerations. *Curr Opin Pulm Med.* 2015;21(4):407-416.

Watanabe Y, Kawabata Y, Kanauchi T, et al. Multiple, thin-walled cysts are one of the HRCT features of airspace enlargement with fibrosis. *Eur J Radiol.* 2015;84(5):986-992.

CHAPTER 6

Desquamative Interstitial Pneumonia Complicated by Glucocorticoid-Induced Osteonecrosis of the Femoral Head in a Former Smoker

Tomohiro Handa ■ Ryo Sakamoto ■ Akihiko Yoshizawa ■
Claudio Sorino ■ Arata Azuma

History of Present Illness

A 61-year-old man was referred to the department of pulmonary medicine because he had worsening shortness of breath. Chest radiograph showed ground-glass and reticular shadows in both lower lung fields with decreased lung volumes (Fig. 6.1), suggesting a diagnosis of interstitial pneumonia.

Past Medical History

The patient was an office worker and had no exposure to dust or inhaled toxins. He smoked about 20 cigarettes/day for 41 years, until he was age 59. However, he continued to be exposed to

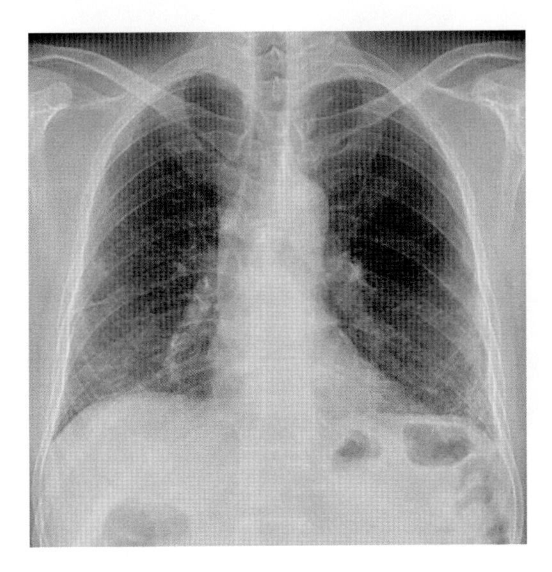

Fig. 6.1 Posteroanterior chest radiograph showing ground-glass and reticular shadows in bilateral lower lung fields.

passive smoke. His family history was negative for interstitial lung diseases. His residence was a 25-year-old wooden house with good sunlight and no mold. He usually wore a down jacket in winter. He has a history of pneumonia and pleurisy at the age of 45. Five years before the current evaluation, he was found to have a chest radiographic abnormality; he was diagnosed with chronic obstructive pulmonary disease and emphysema, and his family doctor prescribed bronchodilators.

Physical Examination and Early Clinical Findings

At his first presentation, the patient had dyspnea with a Modified Medical Research Council (mMRC) score of 2. Oxygen saturation measured by the pulse oximetry (SpO_2) was 95% at rest in room air. Physical examination revealed mild fine crackles on both sides of the back. There were no physical findings suggestive of collagen vascular diseases such as Raynaud phenomenon, arthralgia, skin rash, myalgia, or muscle weakness. Chest computed tomography scan showed bilateral, lower lobe, basal predominant ground-glass shadows around cysts (Fig. 6.2). There was also swelling of the mediastinal lymph nodes, especially below the tracheal bifurcation (Fig. 6.3).

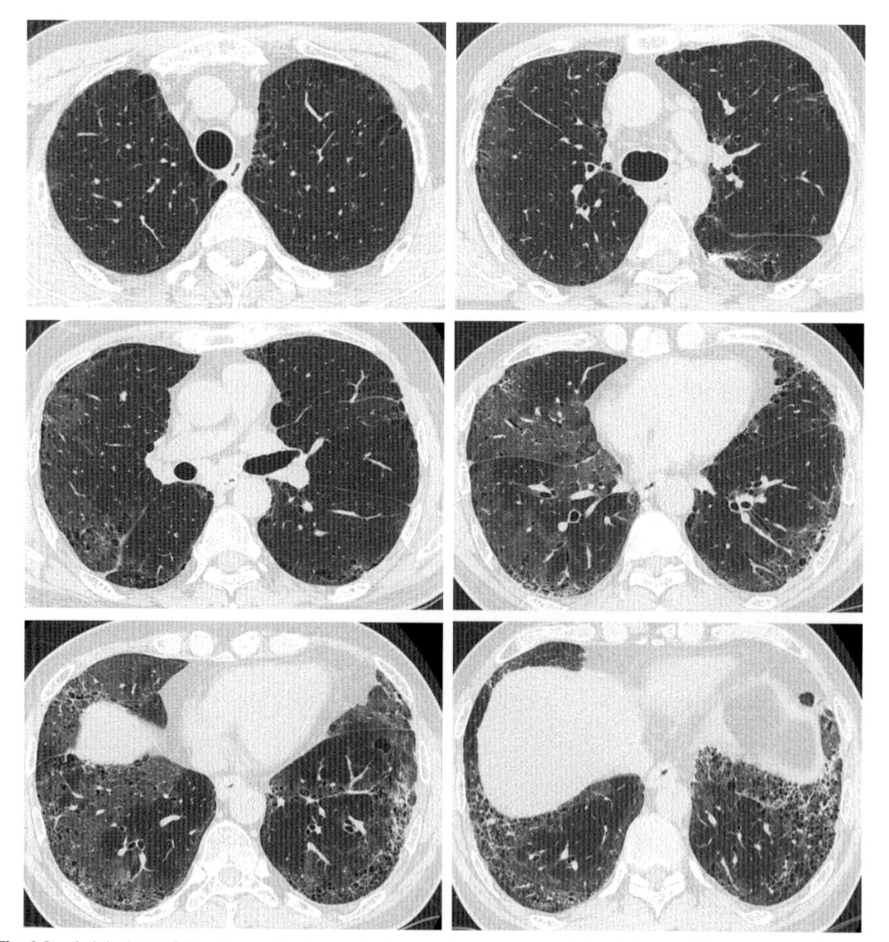

Fig. 6.2 Axial chest CT scan on the lung window setting showing bilateral, lower lobe, basal predominant ground-glass shadows around cysts.

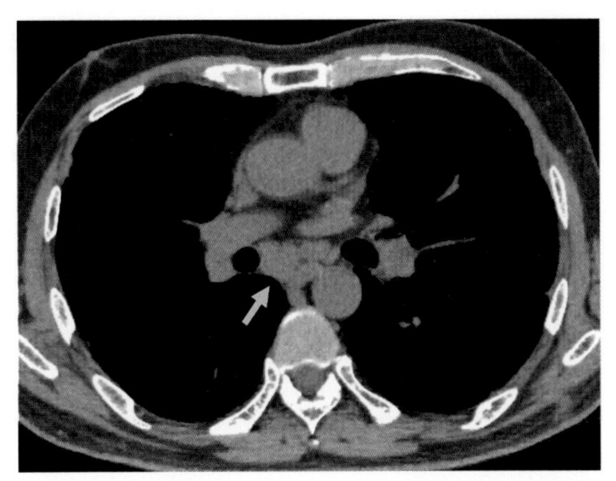

Fig. 6.3 Axial chest CT scan on the mediastinal window setting showing enlarged subcarinal lymph nodes (arrow).

Blood tests showed a mild increase of KL-6 (696 U/mL, reference value < 500 mL), angiotensin-converting enzyme (ACE: 30.5 IU/L, reference value 7.7–29.4 IU/L), IgG4 (134 mg/dL, reference value 4.5–117 mg/dL), and IgE (500 mg/dL, reference value < 170 mg/dL), but soluble interleukin (IL)-2 receptor was within normal range, and all autoantibodies for collagen vascular disease were negative. Pulmonary function tests showed restrictive ventilatory impairment and decreased diffusion capacity as follows: forced expiratory volume in 1 second (FEV_1)/forced vital capacity (FVC) 75.7%, vital capacity (VC) 2.63 L (64.3% predicted), FVC 2.71 L (68.1% predicted), and diffusing capacity of the lungs for carbon monoxide (DLCO) 45.2% predicted. Arterial blood gas analysis showed pH 7.40, PaO_2 83.9 mmHg, $PaCO_2$ 40.4 mmHg, and HCO_3^- 24.5 mEq/L (room air, supine). In the 6-minute walk test, he covered a distance of 420 m, but the SpO_2 decreased to a minimum of 91%.

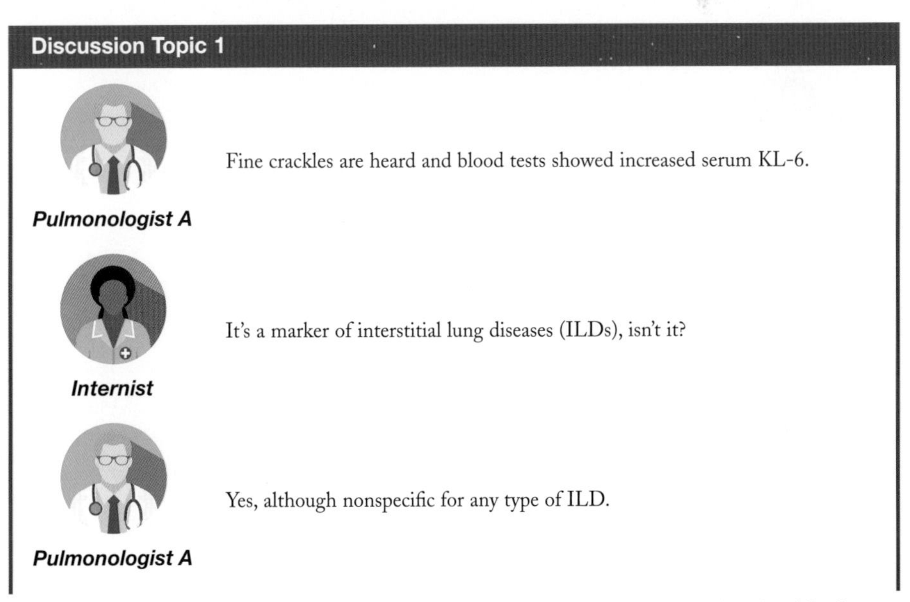

Discussion Topic 1

Pulmonologist A: Fine crackles are heard and blood tests showed increased serum KL-6.

Internist: It's a marker of interstitial lung diseases (ILDs), isn't it?

Pulmonologist A: Yes, although nonspecific for any type of ILD.

Continued on following page

Discussion Topic 1 (Continued)

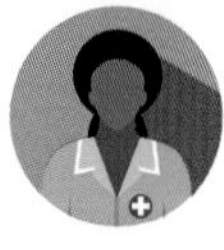

Internist

Is there any finding suggesting lung fibrosis on chest CT? If yes, does it have the usual interstitial pneumonia (UIP) pattern?

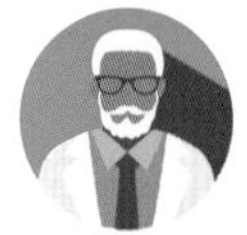

Radiologist

There is mild traction bronchiectasis and a shift of the major fissure to the dorsal side with a volume loss of the right lower lobe. All these findings suggest fibrosis, but there is no typical honeycombing. Moreover, ground glass is the prominent pattern, which is atypical for idiopathic pulmonary fibrosis. Lung emphysema is also found.

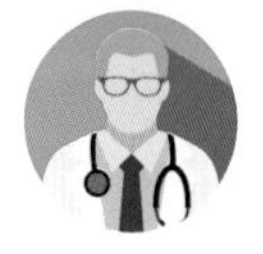

Pulmonologist A

Therefore, the patient would have interstitial pneumonias other than idiopathic pulmonary fibrosis (IPF). What do you think about the enlarged mediastinal lymph nodes?

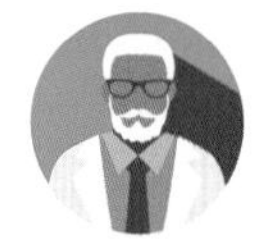

Radiologist

Swollen lymph nodes can also be found in interstitial pneumonia. I think it is necessary to differentiate sarcoidosis, IgG4-related diseases, and metastases from lung cancer or malignant lymphoma.

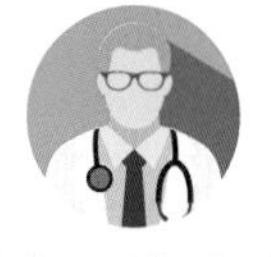

Pulmonologist A

Sarcoidosis and IgG4-related diseases are systemic diseases, so we also need to evaluate organ involvement other than the lungs.

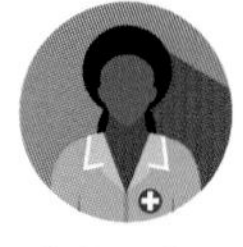

Internist

Physical examination is not suggestive of any collagen vascular disease, nor has the patient had exposure to noxious inhalants or received treatments that may cause drug-induced pneumonia. How about doing a bronchoscopy?

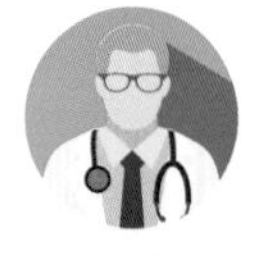

Pulmonologist A

Yes, I agree. Bronchoscopy should be the first diagnostic step. Bronchoalveolar lavage is useful in evaluating sarcoidosis and hypersensitivity pneumonitis (HP).

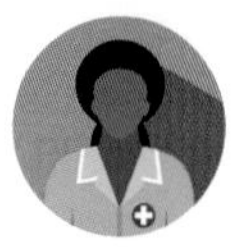

Internist

Do you think lung or lymph node biopsies through bronchoscopy can be helpful?

Discussion Topic 1 (Continued)

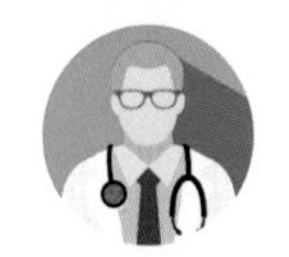

Pulmonologist A

Transbronchial lung biopsy is useful in diagnosing sarcoidosis, although the tissue may be too small for diagnosing interstitial pneumonia. Transbronchial needle aspiration can help evaluate sarcoidosis and rule out malignant diseases. Transbronchial lung cryobiopsy has a higher diagnostic yield than transbronchial biopsy. However, our center is not equipped to do it.

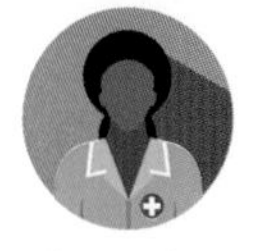

Internist

What if no diagnosis is made?

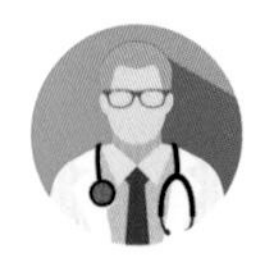

Pulmonologist A

A surgical lung biopsy may be required. It has a risk of acute exacerbation of interstitial pneumonia, but since this patient is relatively young and there is no severe respiratory functional impairment, it can be considered.

Clinical Course

Based on clinical and imaging findings, idiopathic interstitial pneumonia, collagen vascular disease–related interstitial pneumonia, and sarcoidosis and IgG4-related diseases were listed as differential diagnoses. Bronchoalveolar lavage (BAL; right B4) showed a recovery rate of 94/150 mL, and cell fractions were macrophages 86%, lymphocytes 10%, eosinophils 2%, and neutrophils 2%. Transbronchial lung biopsy (TBLB) in the S8 segment of the right lower lung lobe and transbronchial needle aspiration (TBNA) from the subcarinal lymph nodes showed no specific findings.

Discussion Topic 2

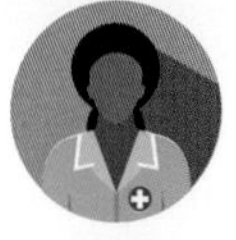

Internist

What is the significance of the predominance of macrophages in BAL?

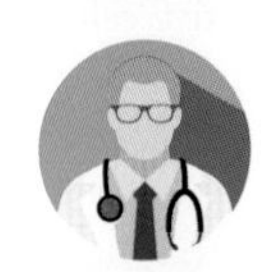

Pulmonologist A

It is not an extraordinary finding. The BAL fluid from a healthy person contains > 85% macrophages. However, a predominance of macrophages containing smoking-related inclusions is compatible with smoking-related ILDs, especially if there is no significant increase in other cell types.

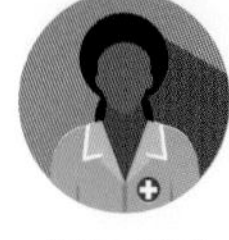

Internist

What are the main smoking-related ILDs?

Continued on following page

Discussion Topic 2 (Continued)

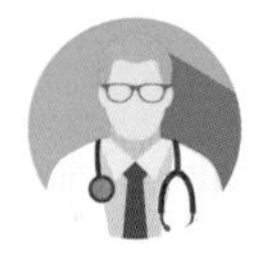

Pulmonologist A

Desquamative interstitial pneumonia (DIP), respiratory bronchiolitis–associated interstitial lung disease (RB-ILD), and Langerhans cell histiocytosis.

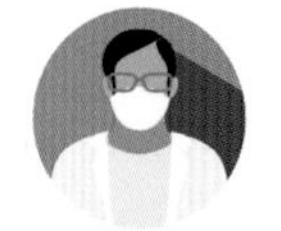

Pulmonologist B

I have already asked the pathologist if there were heavily pigmented alveolar macrophages. Unfortunately, he was unable to give me this information. I think we'll need a biopsy for histology.

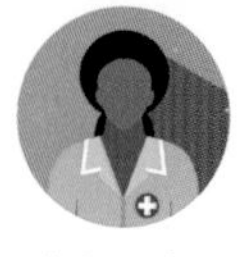

Internist

Could a mediastinoscopy be indicated?

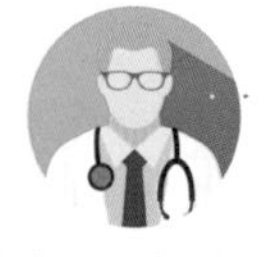

Pulmonologist A

It would allow only mediastinal lymph nodes to be sampled. I think we need a lung parenchyma biopsy.

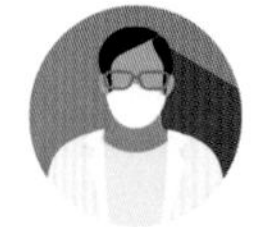

Pulmonologist B

I agree. Surgical lung biopsy remains the gold standard for histopathologic diagnosis of idiopathic interstitial pneumonia.

Surgical lung biopsy and mediastinal lymph node biopsy were performed for further investigation, which revealed aggregates of pigmented macrophages in the alveolar space with thickening of the alveolar wall (Fig. 6.4). There were scattered lymphoid follicles; IgG4 staining showed no significant increase in IgG4-positive cells. Histological examination of the lymph nodes showed nonspecific findings with no granulomas and no significant increase in IgG4-positive cells.

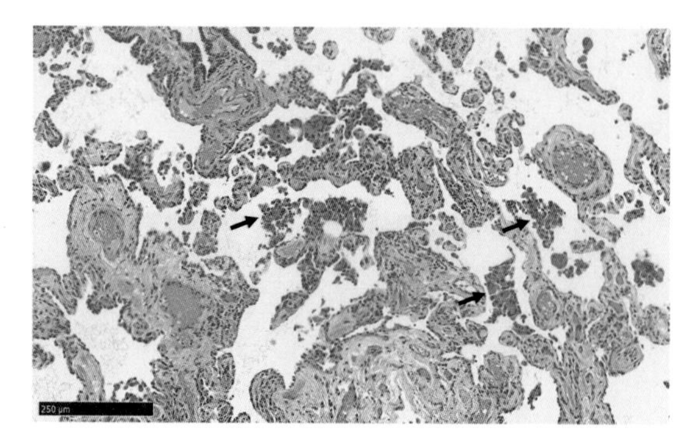

Fig. 6.4 Hematoxylin-eosin stain, ×100 magnification, showing pigmented macrophages in the alveolar space (arrows).

The patient was diagnosed with desquamative interstitial pneumonia (DIP), and treatment was started with prednisolone 1 mg/kg/day (50 mg/day). Chest CT scan performed 2 weeks after the initiation of treatment showed improvement. Thereafter, corticosteroids were tapered at a rate of 10%/week.

Discussion Topic 3

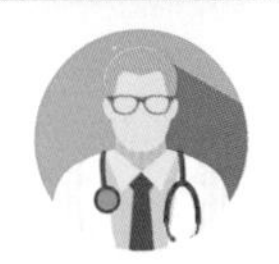

Pulmonologist A

Histological examination confirmed the diagnosis of DIP, with accumulation of numerous pigmented macrophages within the distal airspace of the lung.

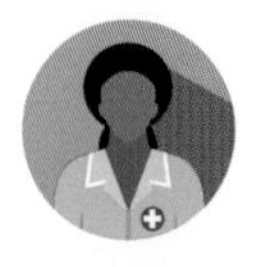

Internist

So the patient will start glucocorticoid therapy, right?

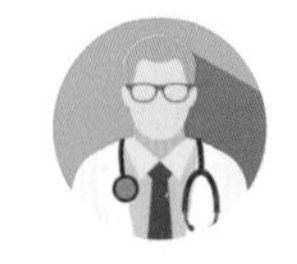

Pulmonologist A

Yes, DIP usually responds well to corticosteroids, with a good prognosis, in contrast to patients with UIP. With treatment, most patients with DIP remain stable or improve, and complete recovery is possible.

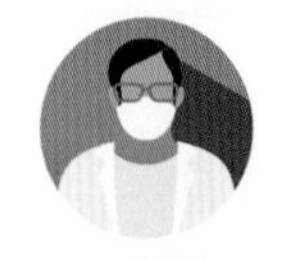

Pulmonologist B

This is particularly true if smoking is discontinued early in the course of the disease.

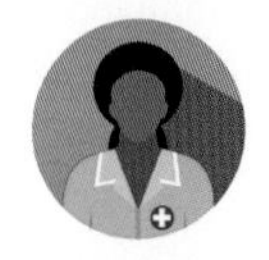

Internist

Which steroid will you use? At what dosage?

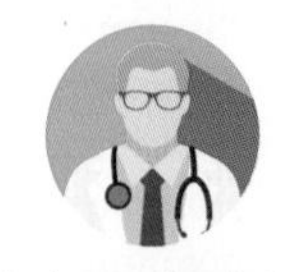

Pulmonologist A

Prednisolone at 1 mg/kg/day. If there is no relapse, it will be tapered off, and, if necessary, maintenance treatment will be planned.

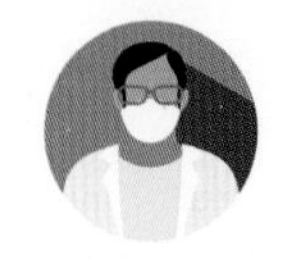

Pulmonologist B

Side effects on bone loss should be prevented.

Continued on following page

Discussion Topic 3 (Continued)

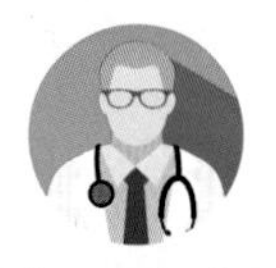

Pulmonologist A

Yes, I'll prescribe bisphosphonates, as well as a calcium and vitamin D supplement. In addition, the patient will perform densitometry annually.

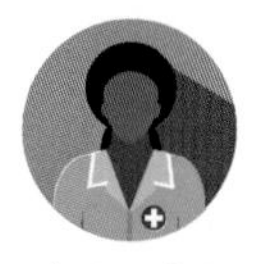

Internist

He doesn't have a history of ulcer disease. Are you going to prescribe a proton pump inhibitor anyway?

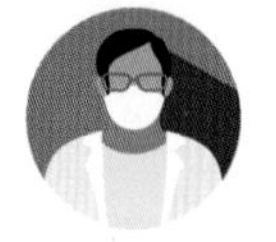

Pulmonologist B

I usually prescribe them if he has other risk factors for gastrointestinal bleeding, such as advanced age or concomitant use of medications such as anticoagulants, antiplatelets, selective serotonin reuptake inhibitors, and nonsteroidal anti-inflammatory drugs.

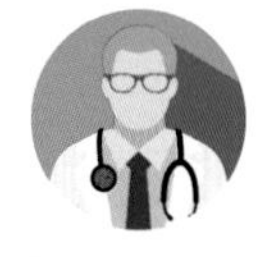

Pulmonologist A

I also suggest testing for *Helicobacter pylori* and relative treatment if positive.

Recommended Therapy and Further Indications at Discharge

The patient was instructed to keep abstaining from cigarette smoking, avoid secondhand smoke, and implement measures for infection control, including influenza and pneumococcal vaccinations. He was scheduled to continue systemic steroid therapy.

Follow-up and Outcome

Glucocorticoids were carefully tapered with attention to relapse, and at 1 year 9 months after the start of treatment, the patient was on prednisolone 3.5 mg/day without worsening. During steroid therapy, the patient developed femoral head necrosis and underwent bilateral cementless total hip arthroplasty surgery. Because follow-up high-resolution computed tomography (HRCT) and pulmonary function tests did not suggest progression of lung fibrosis, an antifibrotic drug was not introduced.

Focus on

Desquamative Interstitial Pneumonia

Desquamative interstitial pneumonia (DIP) is one of the idiopathic interstitial pneumonia (IPP), mostly occurring in male smokers. There are six major IIP types, which are further subclassified into fibrotic interstitial pneumonia, acute/subacute interstitial pneumonia, and smoking-related interstitial pneumonia. The latter include DIP, RB-ILD, and Langerhans cell histiocytosis. These findings may be mixed in the same patient.

Focus on (Continued)

Desquamative Interstitial Pneumonia

According to a systematic review of 362 DIP cases, the most common age for DIP was in the 40s, and the most common symptoms were exertional dyspnea (86%) and cough (65%). Twenty-two percent of the patients had a history of exposure other than smoking, and occupational exposure such as farmer and metal worker was common. In addition, there are cases of drug exposure and collagen vascular diseases.

Histopathology shows diffuse filling of alveolar spaces and septa with pigmented macrophages, which were misidentified as alveolar epithelial cell desquamation in the original report of this disease (hence the misleading DIP's name). Diffuse widening of alveolar septa, showing a fibrotic nonspecific interstitial pneumonia (NSIP) pattern, can also be found.

Chest radiographs are nonspecific. They may show ground-glass shadows in the lower lung zones but are normal in 10% of patients with DIP. HRCT is characterized by bilateral subpleural ground-glass opacities in the lung bases, often associated with fine reticulation. Cysts may also be present, often in the area of the ground-glass shadows. Findings suggesting fibrosis such as irregular linear or reticular shadows, traction bronchiectasis, and honeycombing can be present. DIP usually shows a homogeneous pattern of pneumonia in all lung fields, unlike the primarily bronchiolocentric involvement of respiratory bronchiolitis associated with interstitial lung disease (RB-ILD). Surgical lung biopsy (thoracoscopic or open-lung surgery) is required for definitive diagnosis, whereas the usefulness of cryobiopsy is not clear, especially to differentiate DIP from RB-ILD.

Smoking cessation and avoidance of causative exposures are thought to lead to clinical improvement, but the extent and frequency of this are unclear. For patients who do not improve, corticosteroids are the mainstay of treatment, and immunosuppression may also be used. If HRCT or pulmonary function tests suggest progression of lung fibrosis, the use of antifibrotic drugs may be considered. Although some reports indicate a good long-term prognosis with 10-year survival of approximatly 70%, a systematic review reported a mortality rate of 25%. Patients without smoking history and women have the poorest prognosis.

Focus on

Mediastinal Lymph Node Swelling

The differential diagnosis of mediastinal lymph node swelling includes infections (such as tuberculosis and histoplasmosis), malignancies, autoimmune diseases, sarcoidosis, and IgG4-related diseases, but it can also be seen in idiopathic interstitial pneumonia, and a previous study showed that it is a poor prognostic factor in ILD. Mediastinal lymphadenopathy often is asymptomatic until it compresses or erodes an intrathoracic structure. Chest CT scan is the method of choice to evaluate lymphadenopathy, differentiate it from enlarged pulmonary arteries or pulmonary masses, identify any associated parenchymal lesion, guide the potential biopsy approach. The latter is essential in case of symptoms suggestive of lymphoma (e.g., night sweats, weight loss, low-grade fever) or metastatic malignancy. Both sarcoidosis and IgG4-related disease are systemic disorders. The former may show ocular lesions such as uveitis, skin lesions, kidney stones, joint or muscle pain, and enlarged tender lymph nodes in the neck, axillary, and inguinal regions. The latter may present with enlarged lacrimal and submandibular glands and autoimmune pancreatitis. Histologically, sarcoidosis is characterized by noncaseating epithelioid cell granulomas, whereas IgG4-related disease is characterized by infiltration of IgG4-positive plasma cells and characteristic fibrosis. In the evaluation of sarcoidosis of the mediastinum, it is recommended to perform endobronchial ultrasound–guided lymph node sampling, rather than mediastinoscopy, as the initial sampling procedure.

Focus on

Glucocorticoid-Induced Side Effects

Glucocorticoids are widely used in medicine due to their immunosuppressive and anti-inflammatory effects. Prolonged high-dose glucocorticoid therapy has many potential side effects on different systems; they include the following.

Continued on following page

Focus on (Continued)

Glucocorticoid-Induced Side Effects

Musculoskeletal

Glucocorticoids reduce bone formation and increase bone resorption; thus, bone loss (*osteoporosis*) is one of the most common and debilitating side effects associated with prolonged high-dose therapy. This is most pronounced in the first few months after initiating treatment.

The prevention and treatment of glucocorticoid-induced bone loss include decreasing the doses of glucocorticoid, calcium, and vitamin D supplementation (suggested calcium intake of 1000–1500 mg/day and vitamin D intake of 800 IU/day through either diet or supplements). Pharmacological therapy to prevent further bone loss or increase bone density, such as bisphosphonates, is favorably used (usually if bone mineral density studies reveal a T-score of < -1). Patients who are expected to receive a prednisone equivalent of ≥ 5 mg/day for > 3 months are candidates for therapy if they have any of the following: osteopenia (bone mineral density T-score between -1 and -2.5), osteoporosis (T-score < -2.5), prior fragility fracture, age over 50 years, or postmenopausal. They also should modify lifestyle risk factors (avoiding smoking and ingesting excess alcohol, weight-bearing exercises) and undergo bone densitometry every year as long as glucocorticoid therapy continues.

Glucocorticoids use can cause myopathy by direct catabolic effect on skeletal muscle. Subjects with glucocorticoid-induced myopathy typically present with proximal muscle weakness and atrophy in both the upper and lower extremities. The onset of symptoms is usually subacute and over several weeks or months.

Glucocorticoids are a known cause of avascular necrosis, particularly in the femoral head. It is a type of osteonecrosis due to disruption of blood supply to the proximal femur. The overall incidence is low; the mechanism is not fully understood. Chronic use of steroids or alcohol, coagulopathy, and collagen vascular diseases are recognized as risk factors. Surgery or conservative treatment (e.g., load reduction) depends on the patient's age, complications, unilateral or bilateral involvement, and the size and location of the necrotic area.

Gastrointestinal

The use of systemic glucocorticoids is associated with gastritis, peptic ulcer disease, and gastrointestinal bleeding. There is a synergistic effect with combined use of nonsteroidal anti-inflammatory drugs (NSAIDs).

Endocrine and Metabolic

They include hyperlipidemia, hyperglycemia, adrenal suppression, and Cushing syndrome.

Cardiovascular

Hypertension, together with other side effects of glucocorticoids such as hyperglycemia and obesity, may increase the risk of *ischemic heart disease* and *heart failure*.

Central Nervous System

Behavioral and cognitive changes as well as psychiatric side effects have been noted with glucocorticoid administration such as alterations of mood, memory deficit, or even psychosis.

LEARNING POINTS

- The diagnosis of idiopathic interstitial pneumonia (DIP) is based on clinical, imaging, and histopathological findings.
- The most common chest HRCT pattern of DIP is ground glass with a lower-lung predilection.
- Smoking-related interstitial lung diseases include DIP, RB-ILD, and pulmonary Langerhans cell histiocytosis (PLCH).
- The main histological feature of DIP is the accumulation of numerous pigmented macrophages within most of the distal airspace of the lung.
- The basic DIP treatment is smoking cessation and systemic administration of corticosteroids.
- Femoral head necrosis is an important complication of steroids that worsens quality of life.

Further Reading

Adegunsoye A, Oldham JM, Bonham C, et al. Prognosticating outcomes in interstitial lung disease by mediastinal lymph node assessment. an observational cohort study with independent validation. *Am J Respir Crit Care Med.* 2019;199(6):747-759.

Crouser ED, Maier LA, Wilson KC, et al. Diagnosis and detection of sarcoidosis. An official American Thoracic Society clinical practice guideline. *Am J Respir Crit Care Med.* 2020;201(8):e26-e51.

Cui L, Zhuang Q, Lin J, et al. Multicentric epidemiologic study on six thousand three hundred and ninety-five cases of femoral head osteonecrosis in China. *Int Orthop.* 2016;40(2):267-276.

Grond SE, Little RE, Campbell DA, et al. Oral corticosteroid use and the risk of developing avascular necrosis: a large retrospective review. *Int Forum Allergy Rhinol.* 2022;12(7):903-909.

Hellemons ME, Moor CC, von der Thüsen J, et al. Desquamative interstitial pneumonia: a systematic review of its features and outcomes. *Eur Respir Rev.* 2020;29(156):190181.

Muller R, Habert P, Ebbo M, et al. Thoracic involvement and imaging patterns in IgG4-related disease. *Eur Respir Rev.* 2021;30(162):210078.

Travis WD, Costabel U, Hansell DM, et al. An official American Thoracic Society/European Respiratory Society statement: update of the international multidisciplinary classification of the idiopathic interstitial pneumonias. *Am J Respir Crit Care Med.* 2013;188(6):733-748.

Vassallo R, Ryu JH. Tobacco smoke-related diffuse lung diseases. *Semin Respir Crit Care Med.* 2008;29(6): 643-650.

Wells AU, Nicholson AG, Hansell DM. Challenges in pulmonary fibrosis. 4: smoking-induced diffuse interstitial lung diseases. *Thorax.* 2007;62(10):904-910.

CHAPTER 7

Pulmonary Langerhans Cell Histiocytosis in a Young Man Complaining of a Dry Cough and Exertional Dyspnea

Silvia Pizzolato ■ Sergio Agati ■ Robert Vassallo ■ Claudio Sorino

History of Present Illness

A 38-year-old man went to a pulmonary outpatient clinic complaining of a dry cough and exertional dyspnea without wheezing that began about 1 year earlier. He also reported a recent onset of left-sided chest pain exacerbated by coughing. He had no fever or other notable symptoms in the month leading up to the visit. On the recommendation of the general practitioner, he underwent blood tests and a chest radiograph.

Past Medical History

The patient was a current smoker (> 20 cigarettes/day since he was 18 years of age; 20 pack-years) and worked as a tiler. He had no family history of lung diseases or malignancies. He had hypertension and usually took β-blocker therapy (nebivolol 5 mg once daily).

Physical Examination and Early Clinical Findings

At the time of the visit, the patient was eupneic at rest, with normal oxygen saturation level (SpO_2 97% on room air). On physical evaluation, no significant clinical signs were found in the chest or elsewhere. Blood tests ruled out anemia (hemoglobin level was 15.1 g/dL) and did not suggest an ongoing infection: white blood cell count was normal (8,860 cells/μL) as was the differential count; C-reactive protein was 5 mg/L (normal levels < 10 mg/L).

The electrocardiogram showed sinus tachycardia with a heart rate of 105 beats/min. Chest radiograph revealed a slight reticulonodular pattern in both lungs (Fig. 7.1). Pulmonary function tests (Fig. 7.2) indicated normal lung volumes and diffusion capacity for carbon monoxide.

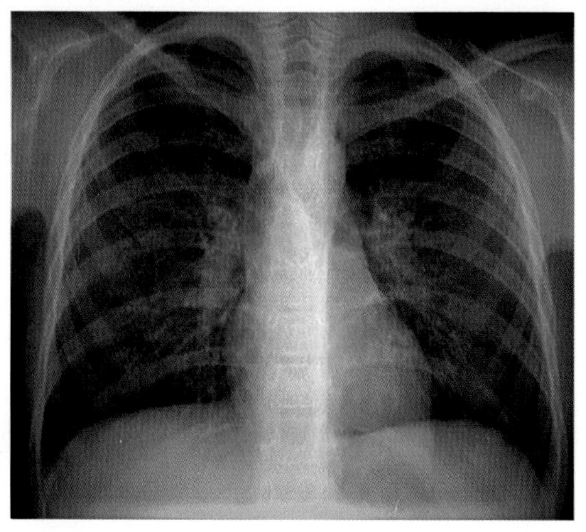

Fig. 7.1 Posteroanterior chest radiograph showing a slight bilateral reticulonodular pattern.

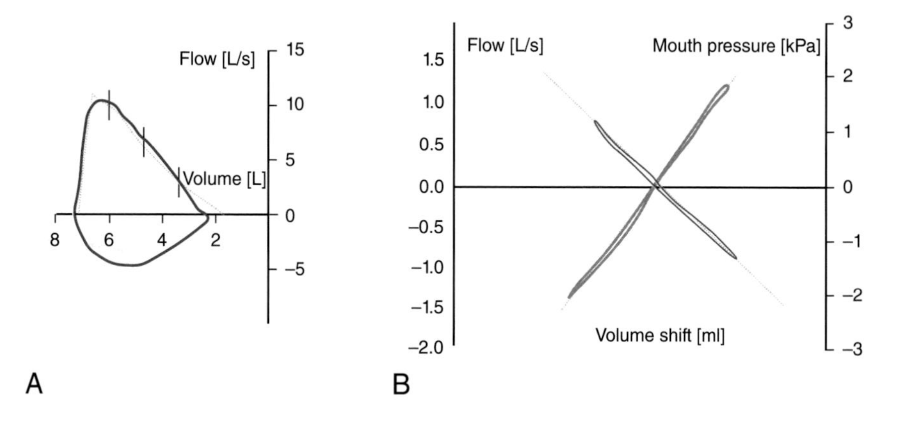

C

ID: ****** ******		Gender: Male		Height: 173 cm
Age: 38 years		**Race: Caucasian**		**Weight: 76 Kg**
	Observed	**Predicted**	**LLN**	**% Observed/Predicted**
FEV_1 (Lit)	3.95	4.03	3.19	98.0
FVC (Lit)	4.81	4.96	3.96	97.0
FEV_1/FVC	0.82	0.81	0.71	101.0
Raw (TkPa*s/L)	0.32	0.30	0.30	106.6
RV (Lit)	1.54	1.48	0.79	104.0
TLC (Lit)	6.55	6.72	5.43	108.8
DLCO (mL/min/mmHg)	26.1	29.8	23.3	87.6

Fig. 7.2 Pulmonary function tests showing no airway obstruction, restriction, or impairment of lung diffusion. (A) Flow-volume curve. (B) Plethysmography. (C) Measured parameters.

Discussion Topic 1

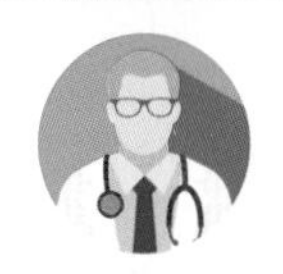

Pulmonologist A

I just visited a 38-year-old patient, current smoker, who has been complaining of exertional dyspnea for about 1 year. He has no anemia and no obvious signs of heart disease. I performed pulmonary function tests and measured diffusion capacity. The results are all normal.

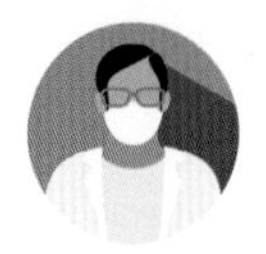

Pulmonologist B

Do you think he may suffer from asthma?

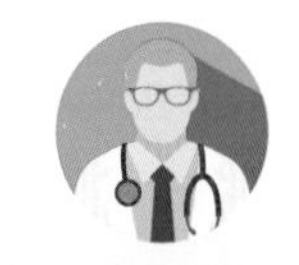

Pulmonologist A

He has never experienced wheezing. However, we could schedule a bronchoprovocation test to see if he has airway hyperreactivity.

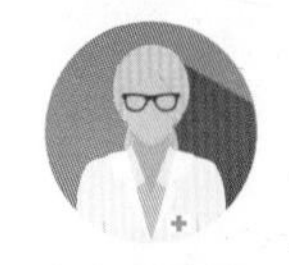

Pulmonologist C

The presence of allergies would increase the clinical suspicion of asthma. Ask for skin tests for inhalants, too. Did he have a chest radiograph?

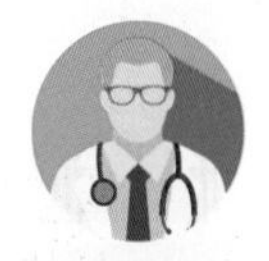

Pulmonologist A

Yes, it shows a reticulonodular pattern. Other possible diagnostic hypotheses should also be considered. I believe a chest high-resolution computed tomography (HRCT) scan is needed.

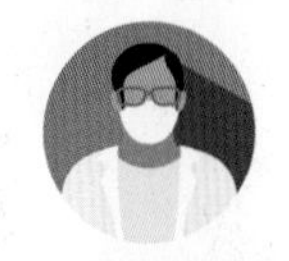

Pulmonologist B

The patient is tachycardic and had chest pain. Don't you think we should rule out pulmonary embolism?

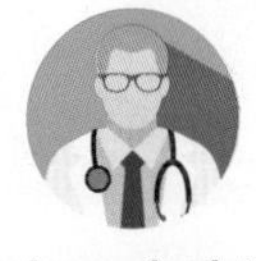

Pulmonologist A

The onset of symptoms is gradual and he has no risk factors for venous thromboembolism. However, let's ask for a plasma D-dimer. If this is negative, we will do an HRCT scan of the chest. Otherwise, I would ask for an urgent CT pulmonary angiography.

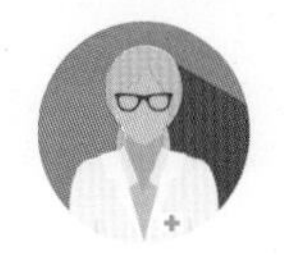

Pulmonologist C

I would also recommend a cardiological evaluation and echocardiography. And for sure, the patient should quit smoking.

Clinical Course

The plasma D-dimer level was normal, and further diagnostic workup was scheduled on an outpatient basis. The patient returned to the pulmonology clinic 1 month later and provided results of the tests requested by the doctors. Symptoms and clinical evaluation were unchanged.

Mantoux tuberculin skin test was negative. An HRCT scan of the chest (Fig. 7.3) revealed the presence of bilateral cavitary nodules and cysts predominantly in a centrilobular and peribronchovascular distribution, with complete sparing of the bases. Some small subpleural bullae were also evident. There was no mediastinal or hilar lymphadenopathy and no pleural effusion.

Echocardiography showed no significant changes in atrial and ventricular size, morphology, and function. Left ventricular ejection fraction and estimated pulmonary arterial pressure were normal.

Skin prick tests showed no allergy to inhalants. The methacholine challenge test was negative (no airway hyperreactivity).

During a 6-minute walk test in ambient air, the patient covered a distance of 560 m, corresponding to 80% of predicted, in the absence of oxygen desaturation (nadir SpO_2 96%). However, he perceived somewhat severe shortness of breath (score 4 on the modified 10-point Borg scale).

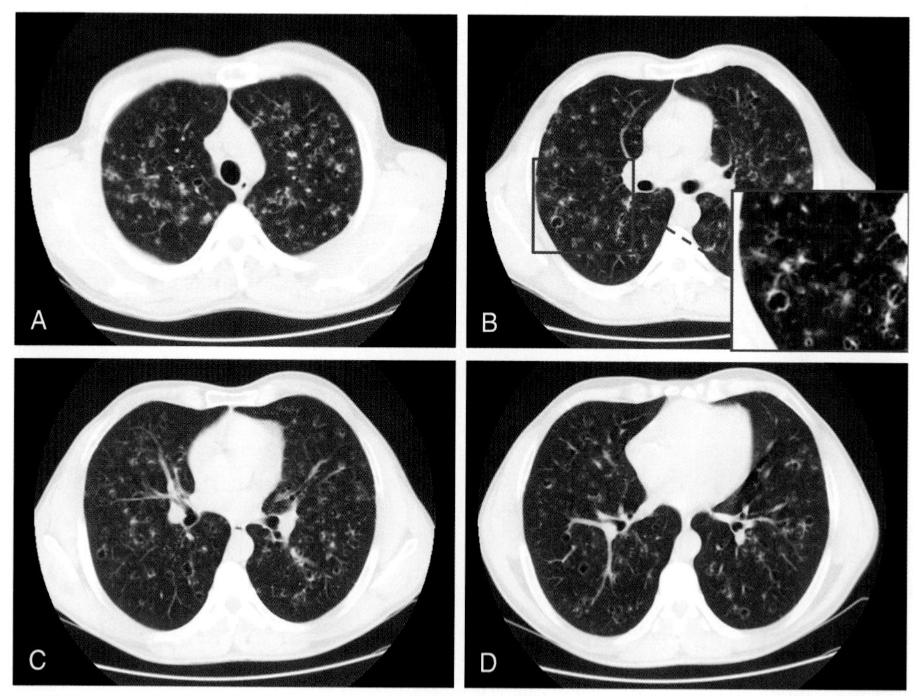

Fig. 7.3 Transverse high-resolution computed tomography of the chest showing bilateral blurred centrilobular nodules, many with central cavitations, with a predominance of the upper and middle fields.

Discussion Topic 2

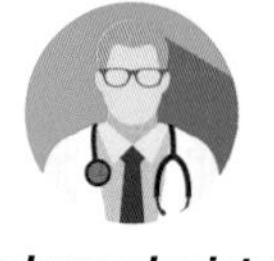

Pulmonologist A

What do you think of the radiological findings? Together with the medical history, they seem compatible with pulmonary Langerhans cell histiocytosis (PLCH).

Discussion Topic 2 (Continued)

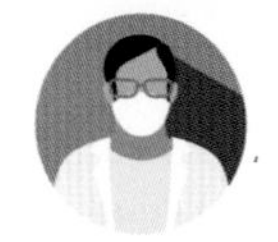

Pulmonologist B

It's a relatively uncommon disease but generally occurs in young smokers like our patient. Imaging can vary depending on the stage of the disease: initially, patients develop small peribronchiolar nodular opacities. Later, these can progress to thick-walled cavitary nodules and finally to multiple irregularly shaped cysts, with normal surrounding lung parenchyma.

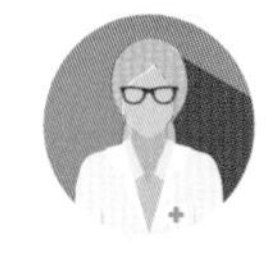

Pulmonologist C

What other differential diagnoses might we consider?

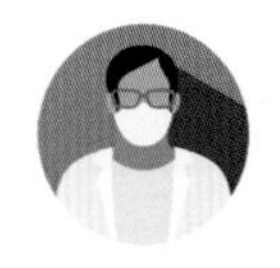

Pulmonologist B

There is complete sparing of the lung bases, as is often the case with pulmonary sarcoidosis.

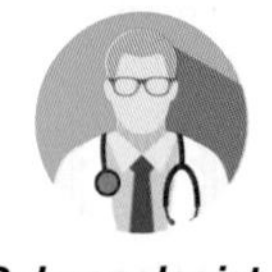

Pulmonologist A

I believe sarcoidosis is much less likely due to the absence of hilar and/or mediastinal lymphadenopathy. In addition, the combination of cystic and nodular lesions as seen in this patient's CT scan would be very unusual in sarcoidosis.

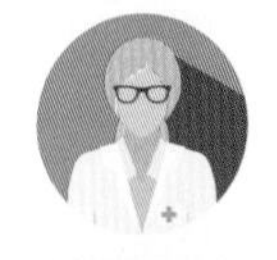

Pulmonologist C

The patient is a tiler; could he have an occupational lung disease such as silicosis?

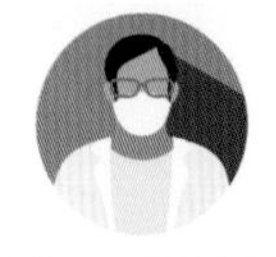

Pulmonologist B

Not impossible, but in my opinion the length of professional exposure is rather short. Moreover, pulmonary silicosis usually causes lung nodules and lymphadenopathy, similarly to sarcoidosis. Here, instead, what I see is mainly cavitary nodules.

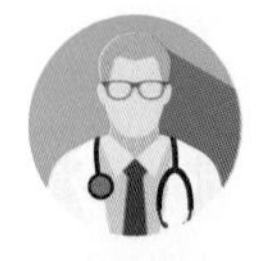

Pulmonologist A

Tuberculosis or nontuberculous mycobacterial infections should be also considered, although even in these cases I would expect mediastinal lymphadenopathy.

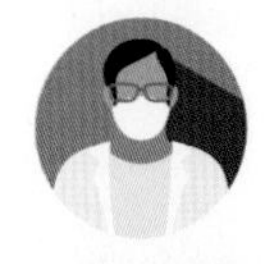

Pulmonologist B

We should perform further investigations. I believe that a bronchoscopy with bronchoalveolar lavage (BAL) analysis can be useful, at least in ruling out infections.

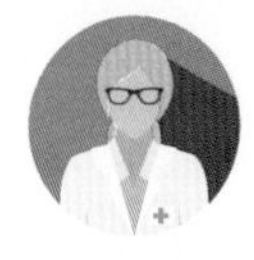

Pulmonologist C

I agree with you. Then we can discuss it in a multidisciplinary meeting.

Bronchoscopy with BAL of the middle lobe was performed. Five aliquots of normal saline (30 mL each) were sequentially instilled, and about 60 mL of BAL fluid were recovered and analyzed. High cellularity (698,000 cells/mL) and a low ratio (1.8%) between squamous epithelial and ciliated columnar epithelial cells were indicative of an optimal sample.

Leukocyte differential count revealed a mild increase in neutrophils (8%) and eosinophils (6%); lymphocytes were 10%, and macrophages were 76%. Lymphocyte subsets analyses showed a $CD4^+$:$CD8^+$ ratio of 1.8 (normal range 0.9–2.5). The amount of CD1a-positive cells was 5% of the total.

The cultures were negative for common pathogens, as well as microscopy for acid-fast bacilli and polymerase chain reaction for Mycobacterium tuberculosis. The cytological analysis of BAL fluid did not reveal malignant cells.

After bronchoscopy, a multidisciplinary team discussed the case. The team included a pulmonologist, a thoracic radiologist, and a pathologist with great experience in interstitial lung diseases (ILDs).

Discussion Topic 3

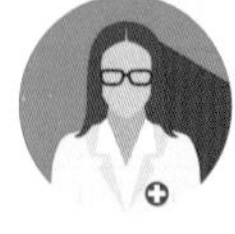

Pathologist

I saw the BAL fluid exams. We could have avoided lymphocyte subset analysis since differential cellular count didn't identify a lymphocytosis, defined as > 15% of lymphocytes. In these cases, lymphocyte subset analysis is rarely helpful and potentially misleading.

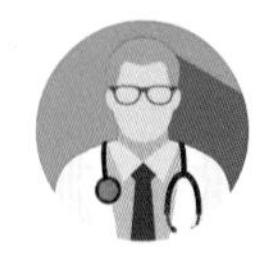

Pulmonologist A

Microbiological testing of BAL fluid did not detect bacterial, mycobacterial, or fungal infections. Cytology was negative for cancer cells.

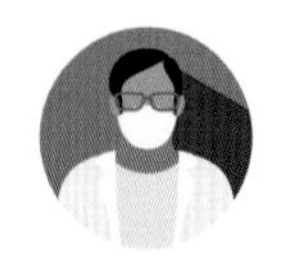

Pulmonologist B

The diagnosis of PLCH remains the most likely. I believe we need no further investigation. Histological confirmation is invasive and can cause complications.

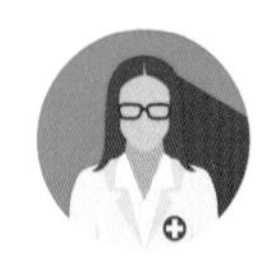

Pathologist

I agree. We also measured CD1a-positive cells, which were beyond the 5% threshold. CD1a is a lipid-presenting molecule that is abundantly expressed on Langerhans cells, although recent evidence suggests that CD1a-positive cells in PLCH might actually reflect an abnormal CD1a expression on activated macrophages, rather than an increase in Langerhans cells in BAL fluid.

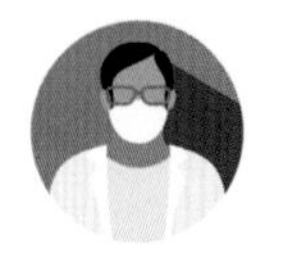

Pulmonologist B

The increase in CD1a-positive cells of ≥ 5% has poor sensitivity but relatively good specificity for PLCH. Although definitive diagnosis requires biopsy, the presence of 5% $CD1a^+$ cells combined with the imaging findings supports this diagnostic hypothesis.

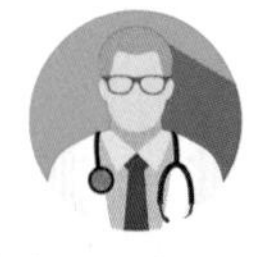

Pulmonologist A

The laboratory, radiology, and anamnestic data are all in agreement and no alternative diagnosis emerged. We can conclude that it is most likely PLCH. The follow-up may provide us with further confirmation.

Recommended Therapy and Further Indications

Since all clinical, radiological, and laboratory data were highly suggestive of PLCH and the main alternative diagnoses were excluded, the multidisciplinary team decided not to continue with invasive investigations. The patient had no signs or symptoms suggesting the coexistence of diabetes insipidus and had no musculoskeletal pain; therefore, he did not undergo further tests.

The doctors advised him of the absolute need to quit smoking and offered him an individualized program with counseling and pharmacological support. Due to his occupational exposure to harmful dust, he was also recommended to use personal protective equipment at work.

Discussion Topic 4

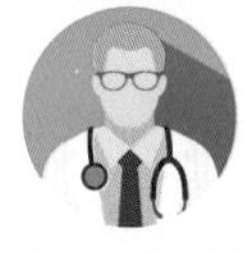

Pulmonologist A

In addition to smoking cessation, will our patient need medication to treat PLCH?

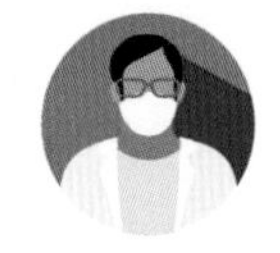

Pulmonologist B

No. Sometime systemic treatments such as oral corticosteroids are given to symptomatic patients or those with impaired lung function or progressive disease. Even in such patients, we have no controlled proof of the efficacy of corticosteroids in inducing or stabilizing disease remission.

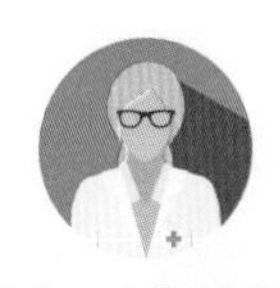

Pulmonologist C

Annual vaccination against influenza and an antipneumococcal vaccine are recommended because the patient is a smoker (which is itself associated with worse outcomes in influenza and pneumococcal pneumonia) and has an underlying diffuse lung disease.

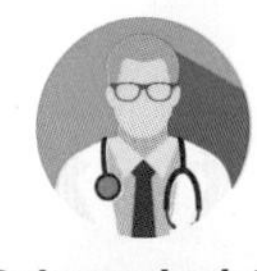

Pulmonologist A

Can we expect the patient to have extrapulmonary involvement?

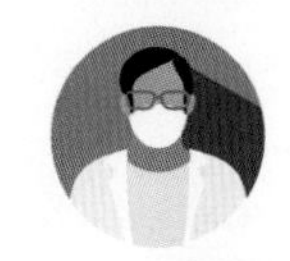

Pulmonologist B

In adult patients, pulmonary lesions are often isolated or the predominant feature. Less frequently, PLCH is part of a systemic disorder that can affect mainly bones, skin, and the pituitary gland. The involved tissues are infiltrated by myeloid cells sharing phenotypic similarities with Langerhans cells, which are often organized into loosely formed granulomas.

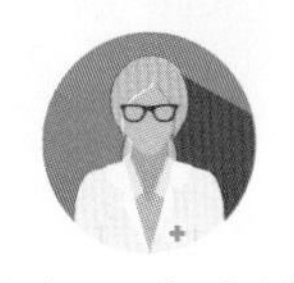

Pulmonologist C

We usually investigate whether the patient has extrapulmonary symptoms (i.e., polyuria-polydipsia for localizations in the pituitary gland, pain for bone localizations, skin or oral mucosa changes). We ascertained that the patient had none of these. If the patient has symptoms that suggest bone involvement or systemic or extrapulmonary disease, consideration may be given to performing a positron-emission tomography (PET) scan.

Continued on following page

Discussion Topic 4 (Continued)

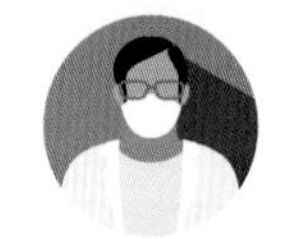

Pulmonologist B

Also, don't forget that > 10% of patients develop pulmonary hypertension, secondary to pulmonary vessel involvement during the course of the disease.

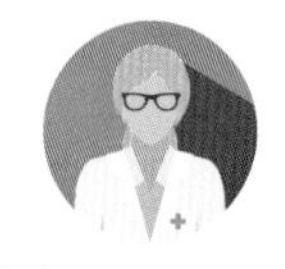

Pulmonologist C

Right! We already performed echocardiography with an estimate of lung pressures. Further tests would be useful only if symptoms get worse, especially dyspnea.

Follow-Up and Outcomes

The patient was monitored from a clinical point of view at 3, 6, and 12 months. He quit cigarette smoking without using medications. Cough and dyspnea subsided and finally disappeared in 3 months. A control HRCT scan of the chest, performed about 6 months later, showed a significant improvement with disappearance of most nodules and cysts (Fig. 7.4). Lung volumes were stable at 6 and 12 months. Further pulmonary function tests were scheduled every 6 months in the following year.

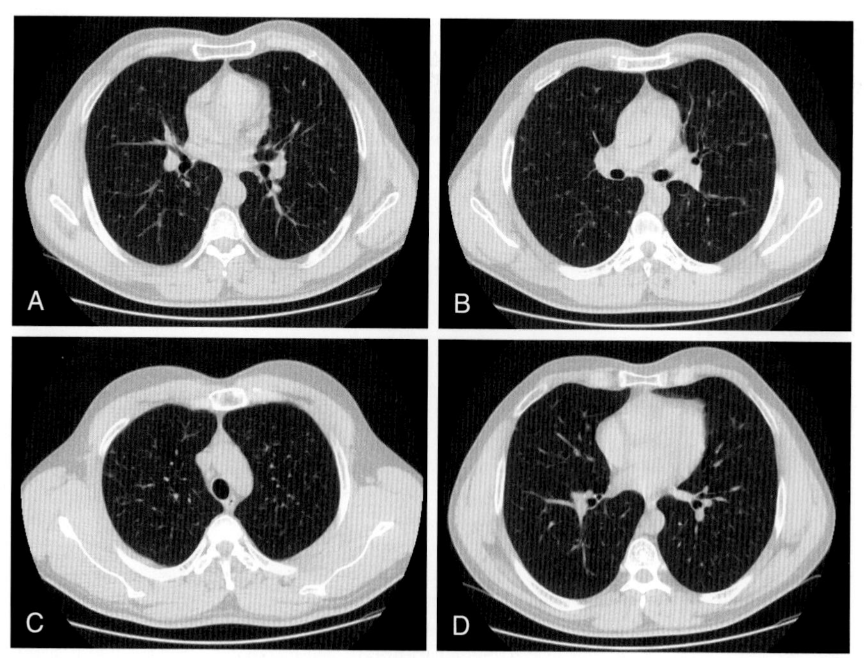

Fig 7.4 Transverse high-resolution computed tomography of the chest (lung parenchyma window) 6 months after smoking cessation. The nodulocystic pattern has almost disappeared. Some residual small cysts are evident.

Focus on

Overview of Pathogenesis and Diagnosis of PLCH

PLCH is a rare disease that generally affects smokers or former smokers with an incidence peak between the ages of 20 and 50 years. The pathogenesis of PLCH appears to be due to recruitment, activation, and persistence of myeloid lineage cells that share morphological features with Langerhans cells (LCs). These cells frequently carry somatic mutations in genes regulating the mitogen-activated protein kinase (MAPK)/extracellular signal-regulated kinase (ERK) signaling pathway, resulting in its activation. The most commonly described activating mutation is the *BRAF-V600E*. These neoplastic myeloid cells accumulate around the small airways, with an accompanying strong inflammatory response that creates small, not well-defined granulomas. This process appears to be triggered by exposure to cigarette smoke. The resulting inflammatory cellular nodular lesions can be of varying sizes, and they infiltrate neighboring tissues and damage their structure.

Typically, chest radiograph shows a reticulonodular pattern. In a coherent clinical setting, HRCT scan may confirm the diagnosis when bilateral symmetric nodular opacities, and cysts are found in the middle and upper lung fields.

LCs can be identified in BAL fluid by immunocytochemical techniques using anti-CD1a antibodies. A small amount of reactive CD1a-positive cells ($< 3\%$ of total cells recovered) can be found in patients with diffuse lung parenchymal diseases other than PLCH. In the proper clinical and radiological context, a count of CD1a-positive cells $> 5\%$ is considered diagnostic of PLCH.

Other BAL findings of patients with PLCH are nonspecific, usually showing a modest increase in neutrophils and eosinophils. The percentage of lymphocytes is normal or reduced and the $CD4^+$:$CD8^+$ ratio can be decreased, as in cigarette smokers. In patients with atypical clinical and/or radiological presentation, BAL can be useful to exclude ILD with more typical lavage findings (e.g., sarcoidosis) as well as lung infections (e.g., *Pneumocystis jirovecii* pneumonia and mycobacterial infections).

The overall sensitivity of the BAL is $< 30\%$, and surgical lung biopsy can be required to confirm the diagnosis. Forceps transbronchial biopsy (TBB) has poor sensitivity (10–40%) because the disease has an irregular distribution and samples collected by TBB are often too small.

Bronchoscopic lung cryobiopsy is a promising technique for the diagnosis of diffuse parenchymal lung diseases, allowing for a sampling of larger amounts of tissue. However, endoscopic biopsies in PLCH patients involve a greater risk of pneumothorax than in other ILDs.

Focus on

Imaging of PLCH

The radiological findings of PLCH can vary according to the stage of the disease. Initially, the disease typically begins with centrilobular micronodules (corresponding to small granulomas). They are commonly bilateral and symmetrical, with preserved lung volume and without distortion of the surrounding parenchyma.

As the granulomas evolve, cellularity may be replaced by cicatricial fibrosis and traction on the central bronchiole so that nodules become cavitated and cyst-like (Table 7.1 shows some of the key features of pulmonary lesions with decreased density).

In the most advanced stages of the disease, the prevailing picture is cystic. The confluence of two or more cysts can give them an irregular or bizarre shape.

Their diameter usually ranges between 1 and 2 cm. They can have thick or thin walls depending on the stage of the disease. In the intermediate stages, small centrilobular nodules can coexist with cysts. Characteristic progression from nodules to cavity nodules, to thick-walled cysts, and eventually to irregular thin-walled cysts may occur when serial chest CT scans are performed. Overall, PLCH lesions (cysts and nodules) have a well-defined distribution with a preference for the upper lobes and common sparing of the costophrenic angles.

^{18}F-Fluorodeoxyglucose positron emission tomography (PET) is of modest value in evaluating patients with PLCH. Only 20% to 25% of patients show significant uptake in the lungs, especially at the level of thick-walled cysts and nodular lesions. PET shows greater sensitivity than CT scan to identify bone lesions, in particular subclinical lymph node, hepatic, thyroid, or spleen lesions. PET can be used to assess early response to treatment and to monitor for disease recurrence.

TABLE 7.1 ■ **Main Characteristics of Pulmonary Lesions With Decreased Density**

Lesions	Features	Comments
Blebs	Rounded, subpleural bulla usually no more than 1 or 2 cm in diameter. More frequent in the upper lobes.	More common in thin patients, often young, and cigarette smokers. Usually found incidentally or after spontaneous pneumothorax (due to a ruptured bleb).
Bullae	Rounded lucencies (air spaces), often several centimeters in diameter, with an imperceptible wall (< 1 mm).	Frequently seen in emphysema. Can occupy a whole hemithorax. Possible causes: cigarette smoking, indoor cooking fires, alpha-1 antitrypsin deficiency.
Cysts	Thin-walled (<2 mm thick) round or irregular lucencies. Can have variable sizes. May be associated with nodules.	Possible causes: Birt-Hogg-Dubé syndrome, lymphangioleiomyomatosis, lymphocytic interstitial pneumonia, pulmonary Langerhans cell histiocytosis.
Cavities	Thick-walled (>4 mm) abnormal gas-filled spaces, seen as a lucency or low-attenuation area, within the lung. Usually associated with a nodule, mass, or area of consolidation. May be partially filled with fluid, debris, mycetoma.	Possible causes: necrotizing bacterial pneumonia, mycobacterial or fungal infection, primary or metastatic cancer, vasculitides (e.g. granulomatosis with polyangiitis).
Bronchiectasis	Dilated, thick-walled bronchi. Can look cystic, but are in communication with airway. Can be clustered.	Possible causes: cystic fibrosis, primary ciliary dysfunction, common variable immunodeficiency, postinfectious.
Honeycombing	Clustered lucencies (cystic air spaces), 3–10 mm in diameter, with well-defined walls (1–3 mm thick). Usually subpleural. Can be associated with traction bronchiectasis and septal thickening.	Possible causes: idiopathic pulmonary fibrosis (IPF), asbestosis, ILD associated with rheumatic disease, fibrosing hypersensitivity pneumonitis.
Pneumatocele	Intrapulmonary gas-filled cystic space. May contain gas-fluid levels. May be solitary or multiple, typically transient.	Possible causes: Can be post-traumatic, due to ventilator-induced lung injury, post-infectious (e.g., *Staphylococcus aureus, Pneumocystis jirovecii*, coccidioidomycosis), or due to hydrocarbon inhalation.

Focus on

Prognosis of PLCH

The long-term prognosis and overall survival of patients with PLCH vary, and evolution is difficult to predict. Some patients have minimially symptomatic disease that can resolve spontaneously; others are stable; and others progress toward parenchymal destruction with coalescence of the cysts, fibrosis, and honeycombing. The most severe forms can cause respiratory failure and death and may require lung transplantation. The development of pulmonary hypertension in patients with PLCH has been associated with worse outcomes. Continued smoking has a deleterious impact on the course of the disease, and successful smoking cessation has been shown to reduce the rate of disease progression. Retrospective case series have reported median survival times of 12.5 to 13 years from the time of diagnosis; however, more recent data suggest better survival, especially for patients who quit smoking and have preservation of lung function on serial pulmonary function testing. Several factors are predictive of an adverse outcome: extremes of age, multiorgan involvement, extensive cysts, honeycombing, and impaired respiratory function tests (reduced DLCO, air trapping, airway obstruction). It is

Focus on (Continued)

Prognosis of PLCH

recommended that patients undergo follow-up with pulmonary function testing every 6 months for the first 2 years following diagnosis to determine whether the disease has a stable trajectory or if there is progression and decline in lung function. These can help identify patients who will benefit from aggressive early treatment. Although no specific pharmacological interventions have been shown to prolong survival in prospective trials, vigorous effort to help patients stop smoking is mandatory. There is evidence that, for selected patients with more severe or symptomatic disease, therapy with cladribine may be associated with disease stabilization or improvement. Comanagement with an oncologist or hematologist is important for patients with more severe or symptomatic disease, as targeted therapy with novel agents like BRAF or MEK inhibitors may provide opportunities for therapy in selected cases.

LEARNING POINTS

- HRCT chest findings of middle and upper lobe cysts and/or nodules in a smoker highly suggest PLCH.
- A count of CD1a-positive cells ≥ 5% in BAL fluid usually confirms the diagnosis of PLCH, especially if imaging is suggestive with nodular and cystic change.
- Lung biopsy is indicated when imaging is inconclusive for the diagnosis of PLCH.
- Smoking cessation is the main first-line intervention to improve disease course, imaging, and respiratory function in PLCH patients.
- PLCH patients should be followed with 6 monthly pulmonary function testing for at least 2 years after diagnosis.
- Prognosis of PLCH may vary from spontaneous resolution to progression with advanced respiratory failure and need for lung transplantation.

Further Reading

Baqir M, Vassallo R, Maldonado F, et al. Utility of bronchoscopy in pulmonary Langerhans cell histiocytosis. *Bronchology Interv Pulmonol.* 2013;20(4):309-312.

Bellia M, Sorino C, Spatafora M. Chest computed tomography for the evaluation of respiratory diseases. In: Sorino C, ed. *Diagnostic Evaluation of the Respiratory System.* New Delhi: Jaypee Brothers Medical Publishers; 2017:234-253.

Lorillon G, Tazi A. How I manage pulmonary Langerhans cell histiocytosis. *Eur Respir Rev.* 2017;26(145): 170070.

Radzikowska E. Pulmonary Langerhans' cell histiocytosis in adults. *Adv Respir Med.* 2017;85(5):277-289.

Radzikowska E. Update on pulmonary Langerhans cell histiocytosis. *Front Med (Lausanne).* 2021;7:582581.

Shaw B, Borchers M, Zander D, Gupta N. Pulmonary Langerhans cell histiocytosis. *Semin Respir Crit Care Med.* 2020;41(2):269-279.

Tazi A, Marc K, Dominique S, et al. Serial computed tomography and lung function testing in pulmonary Langerhans' cell histiocytosis. *Eur Respir J.* 2012;40(4):905-912.

Tazi A. Adult pulmonary Langerhans' cell histiocytosis. *Eur Respir J.* 2006;27(6):1272-1285.

Torre O, Harari S. The diagnosis of cystic lung diseases: a role for bronchoalveolar lavage and transbronchial biopsy? *Respir Med.* 2010;104(suppl 1):S81-S85.

Vassallo R, Ryu JH. Smoking-related interstitial lung diseases. *Clin Chest Med.* 2012;33(1):165-178.

Vassallo R, Ryu JH, Schroeder DR, et al. Clinical outcomes of pulmonary Langerhans'-cell histiocytosis in adults. *N Engl J Med.* 2002;346(7):484-490.

CHAPTER 8

Combined Pulmonary Fibrosis and Emphysema in a Smoker With Apparently Normal Lung Volumes

Claudio Sorino ■ Sergio Agati ■ Stefano Elia ■ Giulio Melone ■ Vincent Cottin

History of Present Illness

A 63-year-old man went to the outpatient pulmonology clinic complaining of shortness of breath on exertion, which progressively worsened during the past year.

A previous chest radiograph revealed hyperexpanded lungs with a slightly increased transparency in the upper fields and a coarse reticular interstitial pattern in the lung bases and subpleural areas (Fig 8.1).

Past Medical History

The patient was a heavy smoker (about 30 cigarettes a day for 40 years equals to 60 pack-years; in the past 3 months he had reduced to 4 or 5 cigarettes a day). He had worked as a construction worker for many years with professional exposure to cement dust and asbestos.

Moreover, the patient was overweight with a body mass index of 29 and had high blood pressure and type 2 diabetes. He routinely took metformin and ramipril.

For some years, he had been experiencing acute bronchitis episodes in the winter months, for which he usually took antibiotics.

About 1 year earlier, his general practitioner (GP) prescribed spirometry, which showed preserved lung volumes. In particular, the values of forced expiratory volume in 1 second (FEV_1), forced vital capacity (FVC), and their ratio (FEV_1/FVC) were within the normal limits. Thus, no long-term inhalation therapy was prescribed. The GP and pulmonologist advised the patient to quit smoking.

Due to the persistence of breathlessness and productive cough, the GP ordered a chest radiograph and an outpatient pulmonology visit.

Physical Examination and Early Clinical Findings

At the time of the visit to the pulmonology clinic, the patient was eupneic at rest but complained of shortness of breath under moderate efforts such as walking at a fast pace or climbing stairs. He often coughed with some sputum, especially in the morning, but he considered this normal as he used to smoke a lot. His wife referred that he usually snored a lot at night. When the doctors asked if he was sleepy during the day, he replied that he fell asleep easily in many circumstances such as when watching TV, sitting in an armchair, or even while in the hospital waiting room.

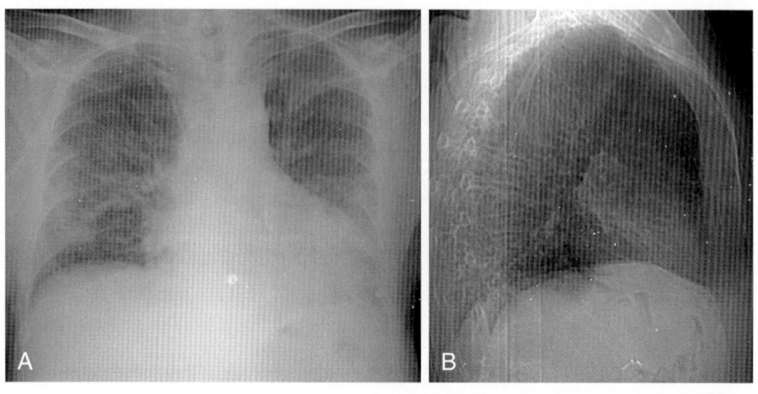

Fig 8.1 Posteroanterior (A) and lateral (B) chest radiograph showing a coarse reticular interstitial pattern in the lung bases and subpleural areas as well as an increased and irregular radiolucency of the lungs in the upper zones. A pulmonary hyperexpansion is also evident with an increase in chest anteroposterior diameter and retrosternal airspace. The contours of the diaphragm are almost normal.

Oxygen saturation measured by pulse oximetry (SpO_2) was 92% in room air. Chest examination revealed a diffuse reduction in vesicular breath sounds and crackles in both lung bases. He had no pallor or finger clubbing. Recent blood tests showed quite high values of hemoglobin (Hb 18.2 g/dL; normal range for adult males 13.8–17.2 g/dL) and hematocrit (Hct 54.8%; normal range for adult males 42–52%). Leukocytes, platelets, liver and kidney function, electrolytes, and inflammatory indices were all normal.

Discussion Topic 1

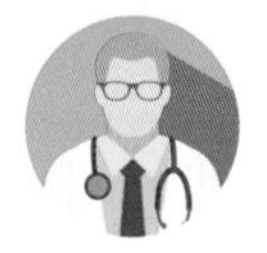

Pulmonologist A

The patient has an important smoking history, I wouldn't be surprised if he really does have a chronic obstructive pulmonary disease (COPD).

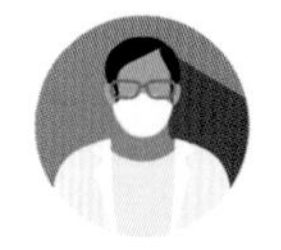

Pulmonologist B

Yet previous lung function tests don't support the diagnosis: the FEV_1:FVC ratio is normal, as well as isolated FEV_1 and FVC.

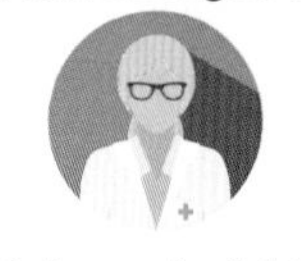

Pulmonologist C

Those results baffle me. I'd repeat the spirometry and add the measurement of lung volumes and diffusing capacity to better understand the situation.

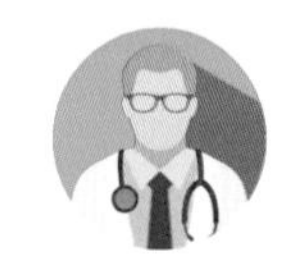

Pulmonologist A

And what about the lung bases? There is a reticular pattern on the chest x-ray and we heard crackles. Do you think he could have just fibrotic outcomes of previous lung infections?

Discussion Topic 1 (Continued)

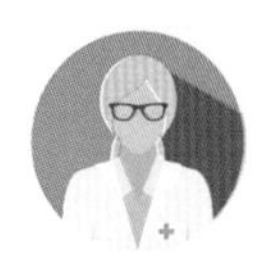

Pulmonologist C

We can't do without a chest high-resolution computed tomography (HRCT) scan, especially because of crackles at auscultation.

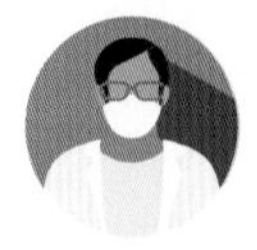

Pulmonologist B

Blood tests showed polycythemia, and SpO_2 is barely sufficient at rest. I'd also suggest asking for an arterial blood gas analysis and evaluating desaturation during sleep and exercise.

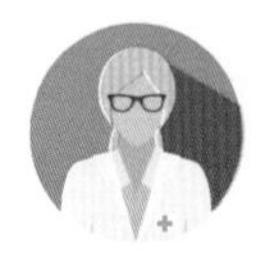

Pulmonologist C

I agree. He has symptoms and risk factors for obstructive sleep apnea. It could be a secondary polycythemia, as hypoxemia triggers the production of erythropoietin and consequently the production of red blood cells.

Clinical Course

The patient repeated pulmonary function tests (PFTs, Fig 8.2), which showed again preserved lung volumes and airflow rates, although they were near the lower limits of normal. Moreover, there was a severe increase in airway resistances and an impairment of the diffusing capacity for carbon monoxide (DLCO 48% predicted).

An arterial blood gas analysis confirmed just sufficient arterial oxygen levels at rest (pO_2 63.5 mmHg), with normal acid-base balance and partial pressure of carbon dioxide (pH 7.39, pCO_2 41 mmHg).

At the 6-minute walk test (6MWT, Fig 8.3), the patient covered a distance of 510 m, corresponding to 85% of predicted, experienced somewhat severe dyspnea (score 4 on the 10-point Borg dyspnea scale), and had oxygen desaturation (lowest SpO_2 85%, mean SpO_2 89%).

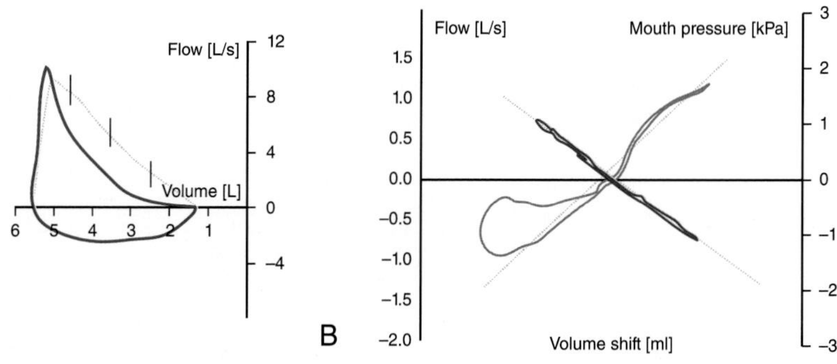

Fig 8.2 Pulmonary function tests (post-bronchodilator values). (A) Flow-volume curve; (B) body plethysmography;

Continued on following page

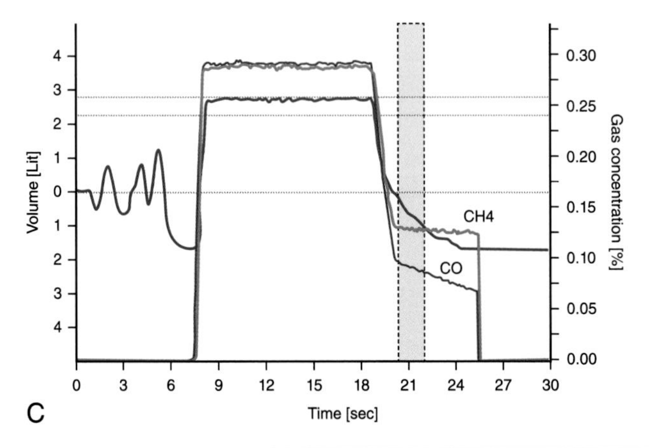

D

ID: ****** ******		Gender: Male		Height: 185 cm
Age: 63 years		**Race: Caucasian**		**Weight: 101 Kg**
	Observed	**Predicted**	**LLN**	**% Observed/Predicted**
FEV_1 (Lit)	3.12	3.80	2.82	82.2
FVC (Lit)	4.38	4.98	3.77	87.9
FEV_1/FVC	71.2	76.5	64.2	93.1
Raw (TkPa*s/L)	0.95	0.30	0.30	316
RV (Lit)	2.44	2.54	1.55	96.1
TLC (Lit)	7.63	7.89	6.31	96.6
DLCO (mL/min/mmHg)	14.2	29.3	21.8	48.4

Fig 8.2, cont'd (C) lung diffusion test; (D) measured parameters. Main lung volumes are within the normal limits, whereas airway resistances are very high, and diffusing capacity is severely impaired. FEV_1, forced expiratory volume in 1 second; LLN, lower limit of normal; FVC, forced vital capacity; RV, residual volume; TLC, total lung capacity; DLCO, diffusing capacity of the lungs for carbon monoxide.

6-Minute Walk Test						
Distance covered (meters)	510			**Shortness of breath**	**Initial**	**Final**
				0 Nothing at all	☐	☐
	85% predicted			1 Very slight (just noticeable)	☒	☐
SpO_2 (%)	Initial 92	Final 87		2 Slight	☐	☐
				3 Moderate	☐	☐
	Lowest 85; mean 89			4 Somewhat severe	☐	☒
Heart rate (beats/min)	Initial 78	Final 110		5 Severe	☐	☐
				6	☐	☐
	Highest 114; mean 95			7 Very severe	☐	☐
Blood pressure (mm Hg)	Initial 115/80	Final 150/90		8	☐	☐
				9 Very, very severe (almost maximal)	☐	☐
				10 Maximal	☐	☐

Fig 8.3 Parameters before and after the 6-minute walk test. Dyspnea was measured by a 10-point Borg dyspnea scale.

Discussion Topic 2

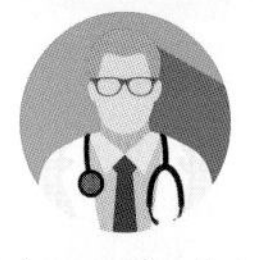

Pulmonologist A

Oxygen levels at rest are quite low, the DLCO is severely impaired, and exercise causes desaturation. The patient has a respiratory problem and we need to understand what it is.

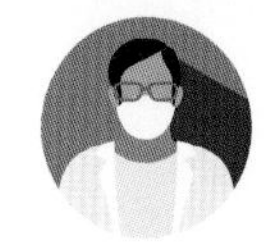

Pulmonologist B

I continue to be perplexed about imaging and chest examination. The patient could be affected by lung fibrosis.

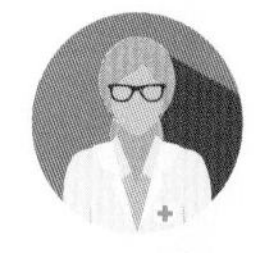

Pulmonologist C

Wouldn't we have noticed a reduction in lung volumes?

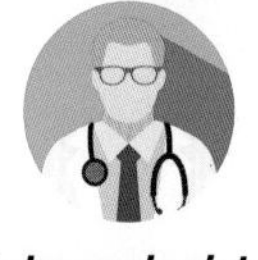

Pulmonologist A

It's usually present in the more advanced stages.

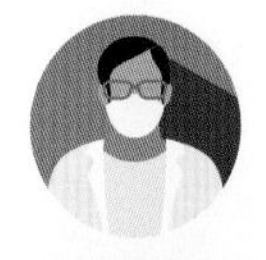

Pulmonologist B

Maybe we'll have some answers to our doubts when he performs the HRCT of the chest.

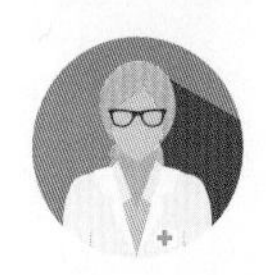

Pulmonologist C

Also, an echocardiogram would be useful to look for other possible causes behind the patient's symptoms and rule out pulmonary hypertension.

The patient underwent HRCT of the chest, which revealed bilateral emphysema, mainly in the upper lobes, and fibrosis with a usual interstitial pneumonia (UIP) pattern including honeycombing in the dorsal and peripheral areas of the lower lobes (Fig 8.4).

The echocardiography showed a left ventricular ejection fraction (LVEF) of 55% and a mild elevation in mean pulmonary artery pressure (mPAP 30 mmHg; normal values 14 + 3.3 mmHg; values ≥25 mmHg usually define pulmonary hypertension).

After the examinations indicated by the doctors were completed, the case was discussed by a multidisciplinary team.

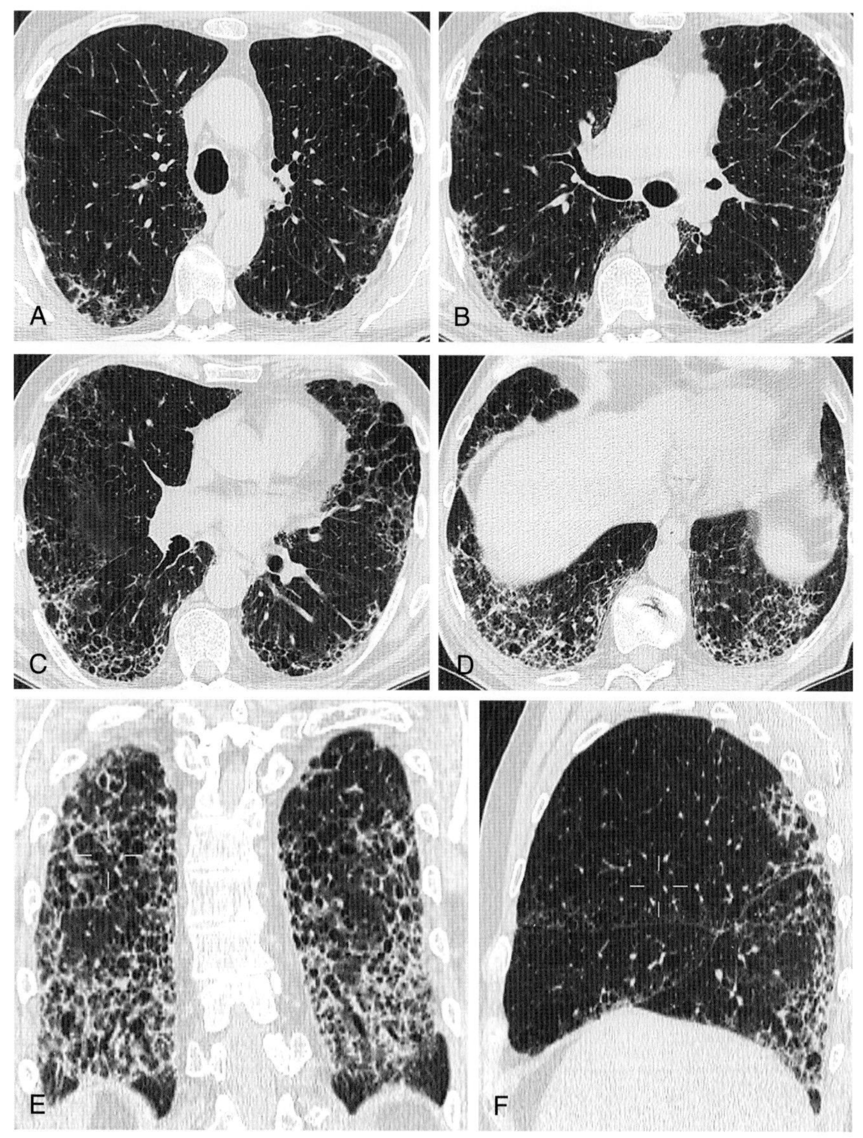

Fig 8.4 Chest CT images (lung window setting), showing the coexistence of emphysema (prevalent in the middle-upper fields) and pulmonary fibrosis with honeycombing (prevalent in the dorsal and lower areas). (A–D) Axial scan; (E) dorsal coronal scan; (F) right sagittal scan.

Discussion Topic 3

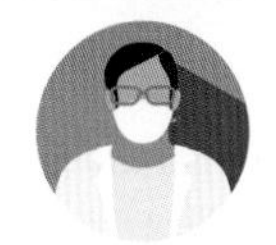

Pulmonologist B

What do you think about the chest CT scan? There is a UIP pattern with peripheral honeycombing as in idiopathic pulmonary fibrosis (IPF).

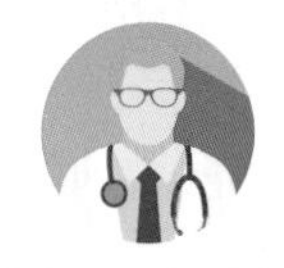

Pulmonologist A

Yes, but there's also a diffuse emphysema.

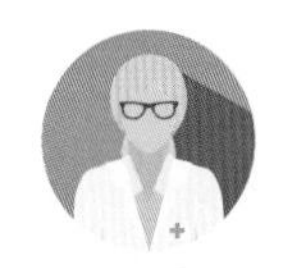

Pulmonologist C

A consolidation due to lung infection could create radiological images resembling honeycombing in patients with emphysema.

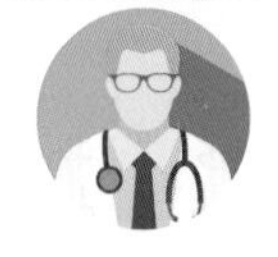

Pulmonologist A

In our patient, the symptoms slowly worsened. He had no fever or other signs of acute infection. Furthermore, the inflammatory indices are normal.

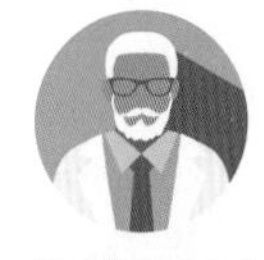

Radiologist

It's most likely a combined pulmonary fibrosis and emphysema (CPFE) syndrome.

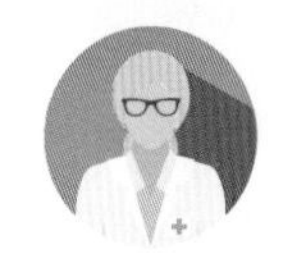

Pulmonologist C

The concomitant presence of emphysema and lung fibrosis would explain the findings of the PFTs. The two diseases act in the opposite direction on lung volumes, which are therefore counterbalanced. However, both concur to affect the diffusion capacity, which is severely reduced.

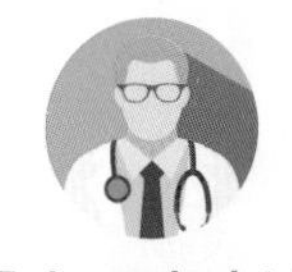

Pulmonologist A

Fibrosis in CPFE is often unclassifiable. Other times it is an IPF or another classifiable interstitial lung disease (ILD). Do we need histological confirmation?

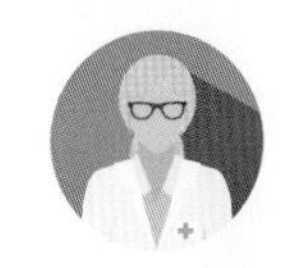

Pulmonologist C

In such a patient, the risks of a surgical lung biopsy may be excessive. A cryobiopsy could be considered as an alternative.

Continued on following page

Discussion Topic 3 (Continued)

Radiologist

I believe histology is not needed here. The interstitial component of the disease has UIP features on the chest HRCT, with subpleural and basal honeycombing and reticular abnormalities.

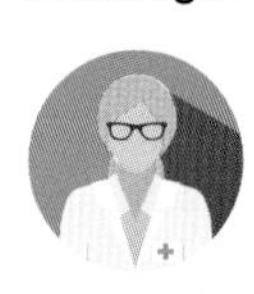

Pulmonologist C

However, I suggest excluding the presence of ILD secondary to connective tissue diseases (CTDs).

The search for antinuclear antibodies (ANAs) and autoantibodies against extractable nuclear antigens (ENAs) was negative. The rheumatological evaluation did not find signs of CTDs. The multidisciplinary team, with a pulmonologist, radiologist, and pathologist, confirmed the diagnosis of CPFE.

Overnight pulse oximetry (Fig 8.5) showed a mean SpO_2 of 88.9% with the lowest value of 69%. The patient spent 50.2% of the night with SpO_2 <90%. The number of desaturations per hour of sleep (oxygen desaturation index [ODI]) was 34.6.

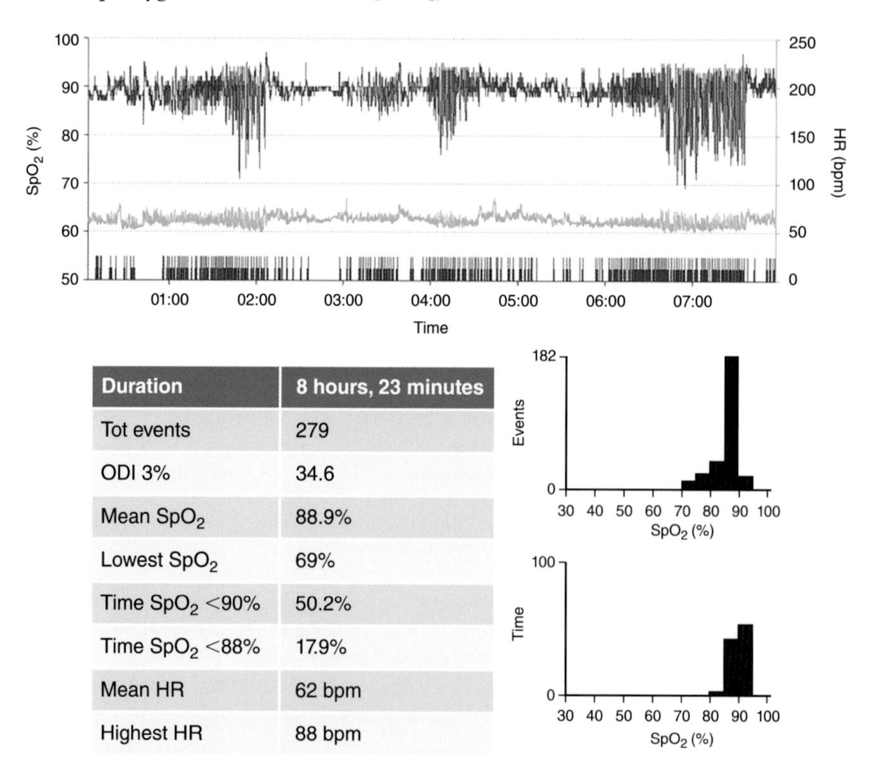

Duration	8 hours, 23 minutes
Tot events	279
ODI 3%	34.6
Mean SpO_2	88.9%
Lowest SpO_2	69%
Time SpO_2 <90%	50.2%
Time SpO_2 <88%	17.9%
Mean HR	62 bpm
Highest HR	88 bpm

Fig 8.5 Overnight pulse oximetry showing oxygen desaturation index (ODI: Oxygen Desaturation Index = number of desaturations per hour of sleep). ODI 3% considers a reduction in SpO_2 ≥3% for at least 10 seconds as a desaturation event.

A subsequent polysomnography study confirmed the presence of severe obstructive sleep apnea (OSA) syndrome with apnea-hypopnea index (AHI: apneas + hypopneas / total sleep time in hours) of 39.

Discussion Topic 4

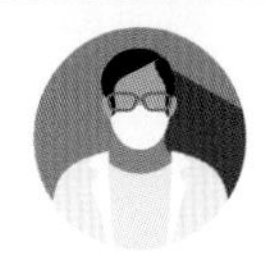

Pulmonologist B

Could antifibrotic drugs such as pirfenidone or nintedanib be effective in CPFE?

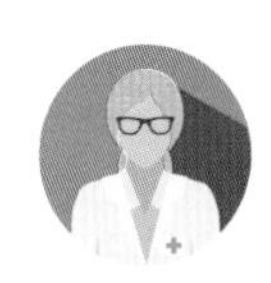

Pulmonologist C

Antifibrotics are indicated when CPFE is composed of emphysema and IPF (nintedanib or pirfenidone), or emphysema and progressive pulmonary fibrosis (nintedanib). More precisely, in IPF trials, antifibrotics slowed the decline in FVC, although this was not accompanied by meaningful changes in measures of health-related quality of life (HRQoL). Conversely, the INBUILD trial showed that in patients with progressive fibrosing ILD, nintedanib can reduce symptoms and worsening of HRQoL. Overall, available data are insufficient to indicate a role of antifibrotic treatments in CPFE in general and should be discussed on a case-by-case basis.

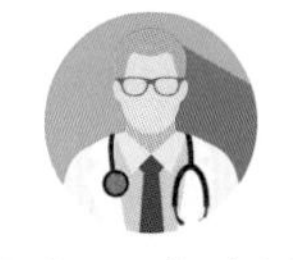

Pulmonologist A

Pulmonary hypertension (PH) can be a serious problem in CPFE. Should we perform a right heart catheterization to accurately measure the mPAP and cardiac index?

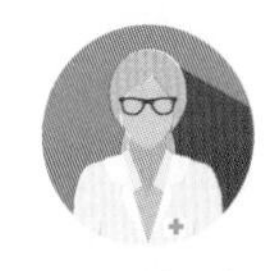

Pulmonologist C

At this moment I would say no. The systolic PAP estimated by transthoracic echocardiography is not very high, and there is no suspicion of left heart disease.

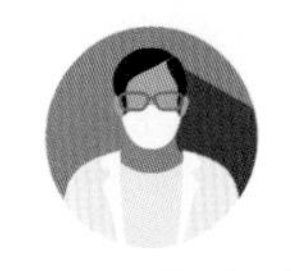

Pulmonologist B

The value obtained by the right catheterization would be more precise.

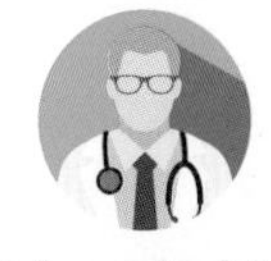

Pulmonologist A

Yes, but it is an invasive procedure. In this case, what would we do with the precise data?

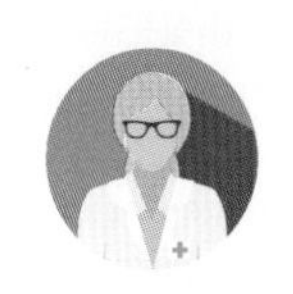

Pulmonologist C

I believe that right catheterization is of little use now, except if there is clinical data suggesting a post-capillary PH, that is, due to left heart disease. If PH is precapillary, the patient would be classified as group III, that is PH due to chronic lung disease or hypoxia. The efficacy of pulmonary arterial hypertension (PAH)-directed drugs in this group is limited and in some cases may be harmful. This seems to be partially due to the vasodilatory effects of such agents, which may worsen ventilation–perfusion abnormalities and gas exchange in individuals with lung disease.

Continued on following page

Discussion Topic 4 (Continued)

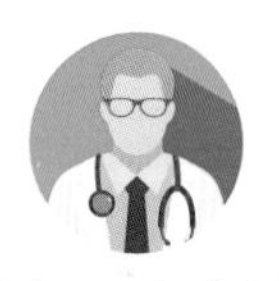

Pulmonologist A

I agree. Only in rare circumstances is PAH-directed therapy considered for such patients, usually only when general measures have failed or when there is a severe PH despite mild lung disease.

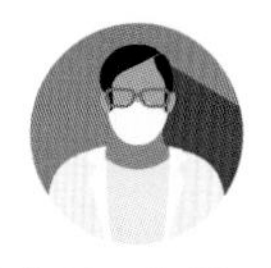

Pulmonologist B

We could give him inhaled therapy. Even if lung volumes are preserved, we may expect that inhaled corticosteroids and bronchodilators relieve dyspnea and reduce the risk of acute exacerbations.

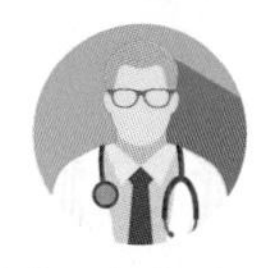

Pulmonologist A

How will we assess the progression of the disease? FVC is not the best longitudinal lung function parameter.

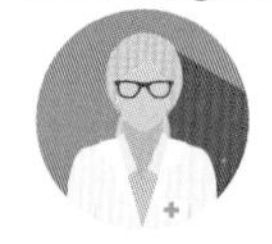

Pulmonologist C

We may monitor a combination of indicators including symptoms, 6MWT, and lung function and periodically measure the diffusion capacity. To repeat CT scan of the chest will be necessary, too. This will also be useful because, unfortunately, a large proportion of the patients with CPFE develop lung cancer.

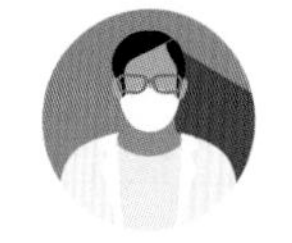

Pulmonologist B

Do you think he could benefit from a period of pulmonary rehabilitation?

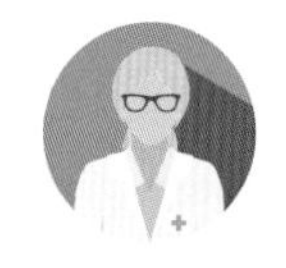

Pulmonologist C

Data on the effects of pulmonary rehabilitation in CPFE are scarce, but it appears to improve quality of life and exercise capacity, albeit somewhat less than in patients with emphysema alone.

Recommended Therapy and Further Indications

Doctors strongly encouraged the patient to quit smoking and prescribed a combined inhaled corticosteroid (ICS)/long-acting β_2-agonist (LABA)/long-acting antimuscarinic agent (LAMA).

A good correction of the apneas (reduction of AHI to 5) was obtained with a continuous positive airway pressure (CPAP) 12 cm H_2O. However, overnight oxygen saturation remained fairly low (mean SpO_2 89.8%; SpO_2 <90% for about one-third of sleep time).

The patient was prescribed an oxygen supplement of oxygen 1 L/min both under exertion and when using CPAP. A short-term comprehensive inpatient pulmonary rehabilitation was planned.

Vaccinations against influenza virus and *Streptococcus pneumoniae* were also recommended.

Follow-up and Outcomes

In the following 6 months, the patient did not smoke. He completed a 3-week inpatient pulmonary rehabilitation program. Subsequent regular light exercise was recommended. PFTs and echocardiography were unchanged, but he felt a slight reduction in dyspnea and improvement in exercise tolerance. An annual low-dose chest CT scan was scheduled to monitor for disease and to screen for lung cancer. In consideration of the nocturnal and exercise respiratory failure, the impaired DLCO (48% predicted), and the age (<65 years old), he was referred to evaluation for lung transplantation.

Focus on

Overview of Combined Pulmonary Fibrosis and Emphysema

Combined pulmonary fibrosis and emphysema (CPFE) is a syndrome characterized by the coexistence of emphysema and interstitial fibrosis. It almost always occurs in current or former heavy smokers and is strongly predominant in males. The disease presents with worsening dyspnea on exertion, cough, hypoxemia, and recurrent exacerbations and can evolve rapidly.

Pulmonary hypertension (World Health Organization Group 3) and lung cancer are frequent comorbidities contributing to a poor prognosis. Their incidence is 47% to 90% and 46.8%, respectively (higher than in idiopathic pulmonary fibrosis or emphysema alone).

Typically, chest CT scan shows emphysema predominantly in the upper zones and fibrosis in the lower ones.

Emphysema can be centrilobular, paraseptal, or (most frequently) mixed. Fibrosis can have different patterns, such as usual interstitial pneumonia, nonspecific interstitial pneumonia, chronic hypersensitivity pneumonitis like smoking-related interstitial fibrosis, or unclassifiable. The clinical interstitial lung disease (ILD) causing CPFE may be idiopathic pulmonary fibrosis, unclassifiable, or classifiable (e.g., connective tissue disease–related ILD).

A relatively preserved lung function can be observed in patients with CPFE due to the counterbalancing effects of fibrosis and emphysema (respectively causing a restrictive and obstructive disorder). However, both components concur to impair the diffusing capacity of the lung.

Smoking cessation is the most important intervention. For the obstructive pulmonary disease or emphysema component, inhaled long-acting bronchodilators may be effective. Inhaled corticosteroids seem able to reduce exacerbation frequency and severity. Data on antifibrotics in CPFE are currently not available. Lung transplantation is sometimes considered when no medical options have been successful.

Focus on

Honeycombing

Honeycombing, or "honeycomb lung," is a term used to describe the radiological appearance of a destroyed and fibrotic pulmonary tissue. It represents the end-stage of chronic interstitial lung diseases (ILDs), regardless of etiology.

On chest HRCT, honeycombing is defined as the presence of multiple air-filled cystic spaces, usually 3 to 10 mm in diameter, grouped in clusters or staked in rows. These are often subpleural, peripheral, and basal in distribution and have thick (1–3 mm), well-defined walls.

Honeycombing can be subdivided into microcystic (<4-mm cysts), macrocystic (>4-mm cysts), or mixed.

Notably, airspace consolidation in the presence of pulmonary emphysema can mimic this appearance. Multiplanar reconstruction of CT images can help differentiate honeycombing from traction bronchiectasis and paraseptal emphysema.

Honeycombing is the most specific sign associated with usual interstitial pneumonia (UIP) pattern and occurs in up to 90% of the patients with a diagnosis of idiopathic pulmonary fibrosis (IPF).

A diagnosis of UIP can be established when the HRCT imaging shows predominantly peripheral and lower lobe bilateral reticulation, traction bronchiectasis, and honeycombing.

Continued on following page

Focus on (Continued)

Honeycombing

Honeycombing can be present in other conditions such as fibrosing hypersensitivity pneumonitis (HP) and, although less common, nonspecific interstitial pneumonia (NSIP). The extent of honeycombing is one of the most useful HRCT features for distinguishing IPF from NSIP. Indeed, ground-glass opacities dominate in NSIP while honeycombing, if present, is usually minimal.

Similarly, even if HP can also occur with honeycombing, other features such as centrilobular nodules, mosaic attenuation, and upper lobe predominant fibrosis are often present, discriminating it from UIP.

Sometimes honeycombing represents >70% of the fibrotic portions of the lungs, and this can be referred to as "exuberant honeycomb sign." This feature is more commonly associated with connective tissue disease–related ILD rather than IPF-UIP.

Focus on

Pulmonary Hypertension (PH) Due to Chronic Lung Disease

The World Health Organization (WHO) differentiates five groups of PH based on different causes. Patients in Group 1 are considered to have pulmonary arterial hypertension (PAH). Group 2 (the most common) includes patients with PH due to left heart disease; Group 3 includes PH due to lung disorders and/or hypoxemia; Group 4 includes PH due to pulmonary artery obstructions (pulmonary embolism); and Group 5 includes patients who have PH associated with different or mixed mechanisms.

Group 3 PH is classified as a precapillary form of PH, defined on right heart catheterization (RHC) by a mean pulmonary artery pressure (mPAP) >20 mmHg, pulmonary vascular resistance (PVR) of ≥2 Wood units (WU), and pulmonary capillary wedge pressure ≤15 mmHg in the setting of underlying lung disease.

Group 3 PH can be caused by several lung disorders including:

- Obstructive lung diseases (e.g., chronic obstructive pulmonary disease)
- Restrictive lung diseases (e.g., interstitial lung disease, kyphoscoliosis)
- Lung diseases with mixed obstruction and restriction (e.g., combined pulmonary fibrosis and emphysema)
- Hypoxia without parenchymal lung disease (e.g., sleep-disordered breathing, obesity hypoventilation, living in an area of high altitude for a long time)
- Developmental lung disorders (e.g., bronchopulmonary dysplasia, congenital lobar emphysema)

Currently, there are no specific therapies approved for Group 3 PH. Treatment of the underlying condition and/or supplemental oxygen are recommended in all these patients, as they are assumed to improve alveolar hypoxia, which is thought to contribute to the pathogenesis and progression of PH.

LEARNING POINTS

- CPFE is a smoking-related lung disease characterized by the coexistence of emphysema and interstitial fibrosis.
- Fibrosis in CPFE can be IPF, a classifiable ILD (e.g., CTD related, fibrosing HP, asbestosis, etc.), smoking-related interstitial fibrosis, or unclassifiable.
- DLCO is often severely impaired in CPFE, while lung volumes can be preserved due to a counter-balancing effect of emphysema and fibrosis on lung elastance and compliance.
- Chronic respiratory failure, acute exacerbations, PH, and lung cancer are the major causes of mortality in patients with CPFE.
- Treatment of the underlying condition and/or supplemental oxygen are the basic therapy of PH due to lung disorders and/or hypoxemia (WHO Group 3).

Further Reading

Amariei DE, Dodia N, Deepak J, et al. Combined pulmonary fibrosis and emphysema: pulmonary function testing and a pathophysiology perspective. *Medicina (Kaunas)*. 2019;55(9):580.

Benfante A, Brown RH, Sorino C, Scichilone N. High-resolution computed tomography for the evaluation of airways distensibility. In: Sorino C, ed. *Diagnostic Evaluation of the Respiratory System*. New Delhi: Jaypee Brothers Medical Publishers; 2017:254-259.

Champtiaux N, Cottin V, Chassagnon G, et al; Groupe d'Etudes et de Recherche sur les Maladies "Orphelines" Pulmonaires (GERM"O"P). Combined pulmonary fibrosis and emphysema in systemic sclerosis: a syndrome associated with heavy morbidity and mortality. *Semin Arthritis Rheum*. 2019;49(1):98-104.

Cottin V, Selman M, Inoue Y, et al. Syndrome of combined pulmonary fibrosis and emphysema: an official ATS/ERS/JRS/ALAT research statement. *Am J Respir Crit Care Med*. 2022;206(4):e7-e41.

Hage R, Gautschi F, Steinack C, Schuurmans MM. Combined pulmonary fibrosis and emphysema (CPFE) clinical features and management. *Int J Chron Obstruct Pulmon Dis*. 2021;16:167-177.

Nasrullah A, Fadl S, Ahuja J, Xu H, Kicska G. Radiographic signs and patterns in interstitial lung disease. *Semin Roentgenol*. 2019;54(1):66-72.

Shioleno AM, Ruopp NF. Group 3 pulmonary hypertension: a review of diagnostics and clinical trials. *Clin Chest Med*. 2021;42(1):59-70.

Swigris JJ. Towards a refined definition of combined pulmonary fibrosis and emphysema. *Respirology*. 2019;24(1):9-10.

PART III

Granulomatous Lung Diseases

CHAPTER 9

Swollen Cervical Lymph Nodes and Centrilobular Pulmonary Nodules Due to Sarcoidosis

Silvia Pizzolato ■ Sergio Agati ■ Stefano Negri ■ Claudio Sorino

History of Present Illness

A 44-year-old Caucasian man went to his general practitioner because of persistent swelling in the left submandibular area (Fig. 9.1). The symptom disturbed him a lot, both aesthetically and because it affected chewing and swallowing. He was prescribed an ultrasound and then a magnetic resonance imaging (MRI) of the neck, which showed the presence of large confluent lymph nodes suspected of malignancies such as lymphoproliferative disease or metastases. The parotid gland had no morphological and/or structural changes. An enlargement of the inferior nasal turbinate was also found.

A couple of weeks later, the patient underwent biopsies of a lateral cervical lymph node and the nasal mucosa. In both sites, chronic granulomatous inflammation with lymphocyte prevalence and some necrotizing areas were found. The acid-fast bacilli (AFB) smears were negative, and cultures showed no mycobacterial growth. Then, the patient underwent a chest-abdomen computed tomography (CT) scan with intravenous contrast medium (Fig. 9.2). This showed bilateral pulmonary nodules with centrilobular distribution and "tree-in-bud" pattern, most evident in the middle lobe. Enlarged partially necrotic lymph nodes were found in the mediastinum. There was no pleural or pericardial effusion. In the right kidney, there was a small (5 mm) nonobstructing kidney stone.

Active tuberculous was suspected; thus, the patient was admitted to the pulmonology ward.

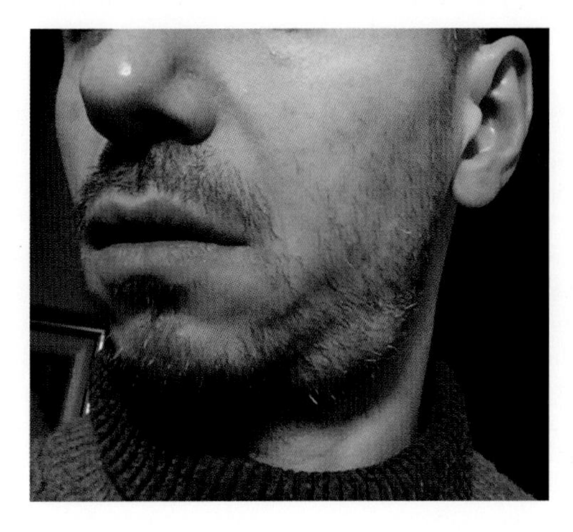

Fig. 9.1 Clinical presentation with swelling in the left submandibular area.

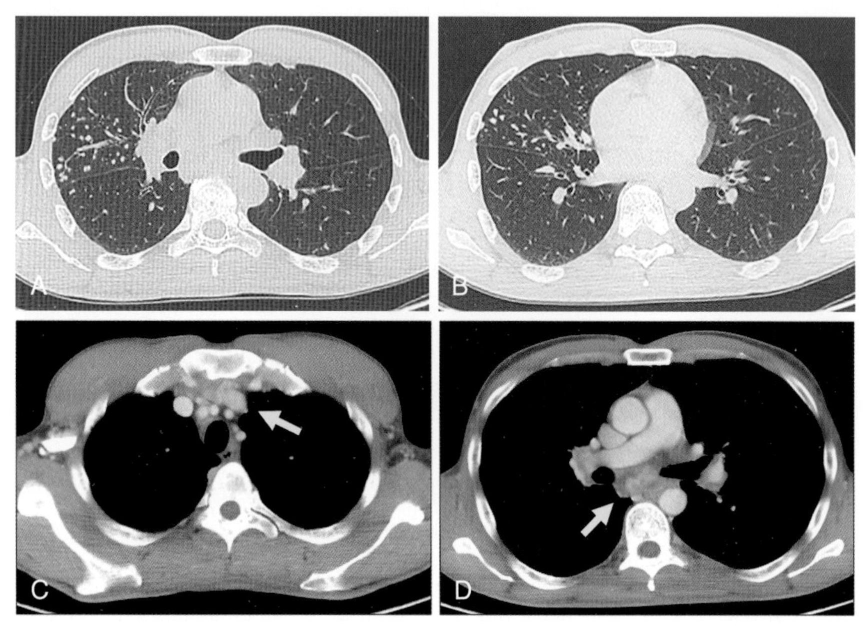

Fig. 9.2 Axial chest CT scan showing centrilobular pulmonary nodules with tree-in-bud pattern mainly in the middle lobe (A and B, lung window setting) and partially necrotic mediastinal lymph nodes (B and C, mediastinal window).

Past Medical History

The patient was a lifelong nonsmoker, without previous significant exposure to noxious particles or gases. His body mass index (BMI) was normal (height 178 cm, weight 71 kg, BMI 22.4), and he had no recent weight loss or reduced appetite. No drug or inhalant allergies were known. He had no contact with people who had pulmonary tuberculosis or other respiratory infections.

He suffered from nephrolithiasis and underwent extracorporeal shock wave lithotripsy due to a calcific kidney stone in his right kidney. He also had a deviation of the nasal septum and turbinate hypertrophy. He was not on any medication at the time of evaluation.

Physical Examination and Early Clinical Findings

At admission, the patient had no fever (body temperature was 36.5°C [97.7°F]). In addition to the symptoms related to neck swelling, he complained of exertional dyspnea, sporadic dry cough, and a somewhat stuffy nose. Oxygen saturation (SpO_2) was 97% while at rest in room air, with a respiratory rate of 17 breaths/min. Blood pressure was 130/85 mmHg, and heart rate was 75 beats/min.

Chest examination revealed no pathological sounds. No clubbing or peripheral edema was observed.

Blood tests showed a mild increase in inflammation indices (C-reactive protein [CRP] 35 mg/L; normal values < 5 mg/L), normal white blood cell (WBC) count (6,450 cells/μL), and normal differential count. Basic autoimmunity blood pattern (antinuclear antibodies, extractable nuclear antigen, anti-neutrophil cytoplasmic antibody) was negative.

Arterial blood gas analysis confirmed normal respiratory exchanges at rest (pH 7.41, pO_2 89 mmHg, pCO_2 36 mmHg).

Discussion Topic 1

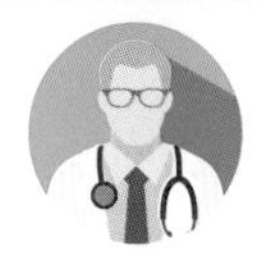

Pulmonologist A

Our patient has cervical lymphadenopathy with evidence of granulomas and signs of necrosis. Chest CT shows centrilobular nodules and tree-in-bud pattern. We should quickly perform a bronchoscopy to rule out active tuberculosis!

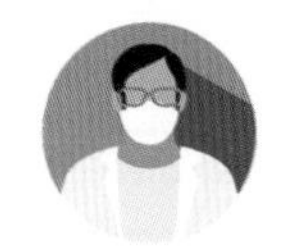

Pulmonologist B

I agree. We should also explore other possible causes of that radiological pattern.

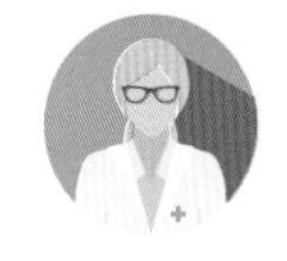

Pulmonologist C

What other diseases are you thinking about?

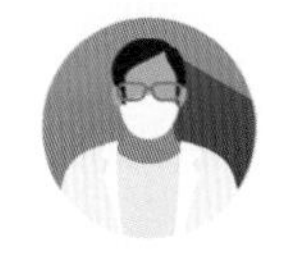

Pulmonologist B

Centrilobular nodules and "tree-in-bud" are usually expressions of an endobronchial spread of infection, but not necessarily Mycobacterium tuberculosis. We'll search for atypical mycobacteria, fungi, and bacteria.

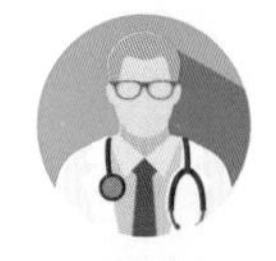

Pulmonologist A

Even noninfectious conditions can cause centrilobular nodules, for instance, connective tissue diseases such as rheumatoid arthritis (RA), or obliterative bronchiolitis.

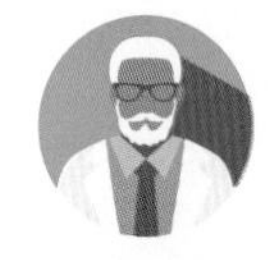

Radiologist

Given the proximity of small pulmonary arteries and small airways, a rarer cause of tree-in-bud sign is the infiltration of arterioles or axial interstitium by neoplasms. I would not neglect this hypothesis. Let's not forget that the patient has mediastinal lymph nodes with a necrotic appearance. Cytological examination of bronchial lavage is necessary.

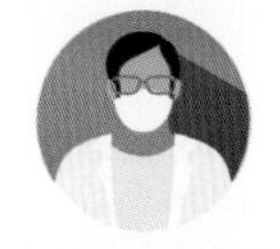

Pulmonologist B

Necrotic lymph nodes can also be found in infectious diseases such as mycobacterial and fungal infections. And even sarcoidosis can occasionally cause epithelioid cell granuloma with necrosis.

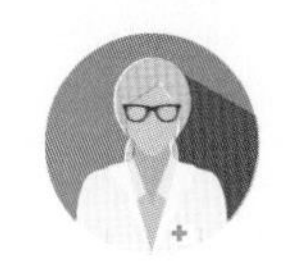

Pulmonologist C

I suggest doing a bronchoalveolar lavage (BAL) with cell count to investigate the underlying pulmonary alveolitis and other possible causes. I'd also consider an ultrasound-guided transbronchial needle aspiration (EBUS-TBNA).

Continued on following page

Discussion Topic 1 (Continued)

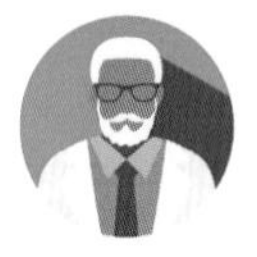

Radiologist

How does BAL differ from bronchial lavage?

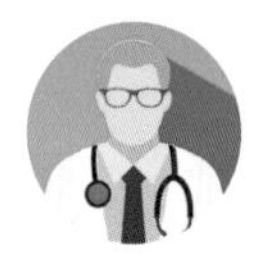

Pulmonologist A

In bronchial lavage, saline is instilled into the large airways and then aspirated for fluid analysis. This sampling is used primarily to detect cytological abnormalities such as cancer or to identify infectious pathogens. In contrast, during BAL, the bronchoscope is directed into a smaller airway and the distal alveolar surfaces are washed. Thus, BAL provides information on the different components of lung biology.

Clinical Course

During hospitalization, tuberculin skin test and QuantiFERON-TB test were performed and turned out negative. The search for HIV antibodies was negative, too. Serum angiotensin-converting enzyme (ACE) levels were normal (40 μg/L, suggested cutoff 68 μg/L), whereas the soluble interleukin 2 receptor (sIL-2R) was slightly increased (3760 pg/mL, suggested cutoff 3550 pg/mL).

A bronchoscopy with BAL was performed. A total volume of 200 mL of saline was instilled in the middle lobe (4×50 aliquots), with a satisfactory fluid retrieval (110 mL).

No ultrasound-guided transbronchial needle aspiration (EBUS-TBNA) attempt was made as the patient had a worsening cough during the procedure, despite sedation (intravenous midazolam 7 mg) and instillation of local anesthetic into the upper airways (lidocaine 2%).

Since inflammatory indices slightly raised (CRP 62 mg/L), empiric antibiotic therapy was started just after the bronchoscopy (ceftriaxone 2 g/day intravenously).

BAL fluid analyses revealed lymphocytic alveolitis (lymphocytes 85%), with an increase in the $CD4^+$:$CD8^+$ ratio (7.8; normal value < 2). A nucleic acid amplification test (NAAT) for Mycobacterium tuberculosis complex was negative, as well as the acid-fast bacilli smear. No malignant cells were found on cytology. The general culture examination did not show the growth of microorganisms, and the search for the galactomannan antigen was negative.

Discussion Topic 2

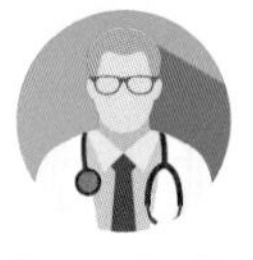

Pulmonologist A

BAL fluid analysis showed lymphocytic alveolitis and an increase in the $CD4^+$:$CD8^+$ ratio. Other tests were all negative. In particular, no infection or malignancy was found.

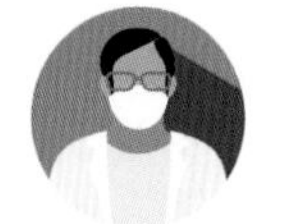

Pulmonologist B

The results point to sarcoidosis, right?

Discussion Topic 2 (Continued)

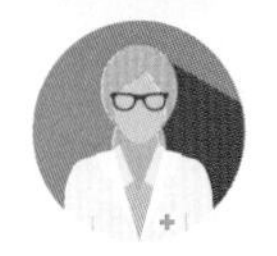

Pulmonologist C

Yes, they do. Most patients with sarcoidosis have a $CD4^+$:$CD8^+$ ratio > 3.5.

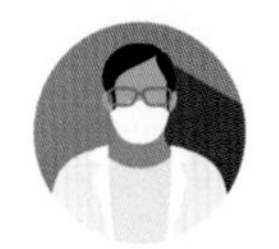

Pulmonologist B

Does this finding differentiate sarcoidosis from other diffuse parenchyma lung diseases?

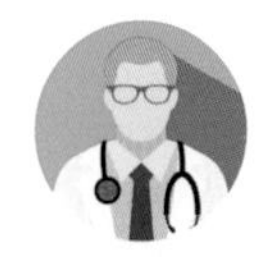

Pulmonologist A

Often, but not always. Specificity is between 60% and 80%.

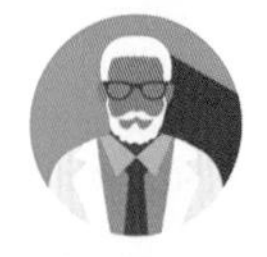

Radiologist

The combination of noncaseating granulomas in one organ and clinical evidence of another organ involvement significantly increases the likelihood of sarcoidosis.

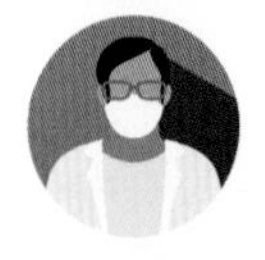

Pulmonologist B

So, in this case, the tree-in-bud pattern would be due to small noncaseating parenchymal granulomas?

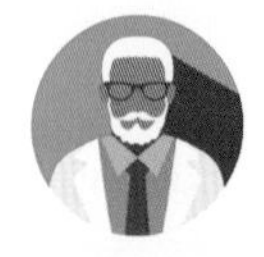

Radiologist

It could be. "Sarcoid clusters" have been described. They are rounded, oval, or tree-in-bud clusters of multiple lung nodules. Occasionally these nodules are so small and confluent that they produce a ground-glass appearance.

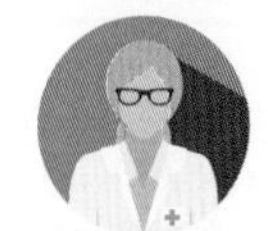

Pulmonologist C

Are the findings so far obtained sufficient to exclude other pathologies, in particular, infections and tumors?

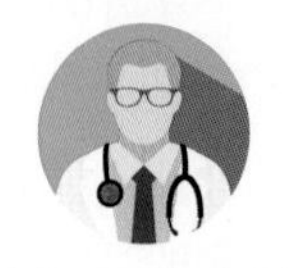

Pulmonologist A

Biopsies from a laterocervical lymph node had already been done and didn't show cancer.

Continued on following page

Discussion Topic 2 (Continued)

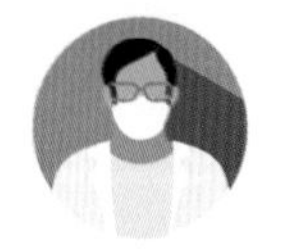

Pulmonologist B

I continue to be worried about necrosis within granulomas and mediastinal lymph nodes. The needle biopsy samples were very small, just a few millimeters! A sarcoidosis-like granulomatous inflammatory reaction could also be found at the edge of a tumor.

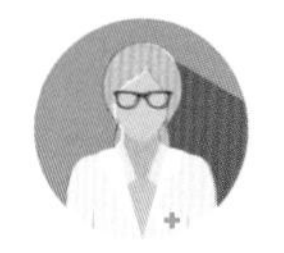

Pulmonologist C

For a better histological definition, I propose to entirely remove a laterocervical lymph node. This is the best way to rule out malignancies as well as the gold standard to diagnose active sarcoidosis.

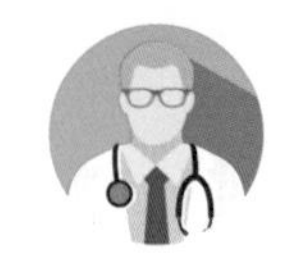

Pulmonologist A

Should we first do an ^{18}F-fluorodeoxyglucose (FDG)–positron emission tomography (PET)/CT to evaluate the uptake of the lymph nodes and choose the best site for a biopsy?

Radiologist

PET/CT exposes the patient to radiation. A laterocervical lymph node is palpable. It is already an easy biopsy site with a high probability of providing a diagnosis.

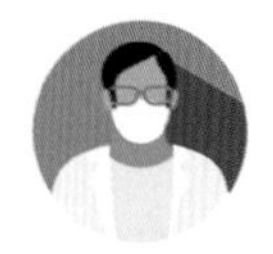

Pulmonologist B

It's true, but PET is also the best method to assess disease activity and distribution, as well as to monitor therapeutic response, whether it is lymphoma or sarcoidosis.

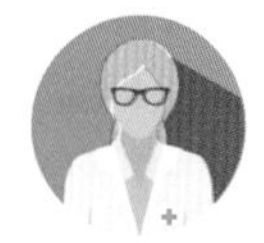

Pulmonologist C

I usually reserve it for patients in whom cardiac sarcoidosis is suspected, and this is not the case. However, we can do a PET since conventional imaging has not provided diagnostic certainty.

In the following days, a total body PET/CT scan (Fig. 9.3) showed a moderate FDG uptake of mediastinal lymph nodes, particularly in the left paratracheal, pretracheal, and subcarinal areas (maximum standardized uptake value [SUV_{max}] 4–6.2) and in bilateral pulmonary hila (SUV_{max} 3.9 on the right). A minimal accentuation of radiopharmaceutical uptake (SUV_{max} 1.8) was also present at the nodules with tree-in-bud appearance in the right upper lobe, the middle lobe, and the lateral basal segment of the left lobe.

An entire laterocervical lymph node was removed (excisional biopsy). Histology was negative for malignancy and confirmed the presence of a focal necrotizing granulomatous inflammation (Fig. 9.4). A polymerase chain reaction (PCR) for the detection of Mycobacterium tuberculosis was negative.

Thus, the patient was diagnosed with pulmonary and extrapulmonary sarcoidosis, with involvement of the lung parenchyma, mediastinal and laterocervical lymph nodes, and nasal mucosa.

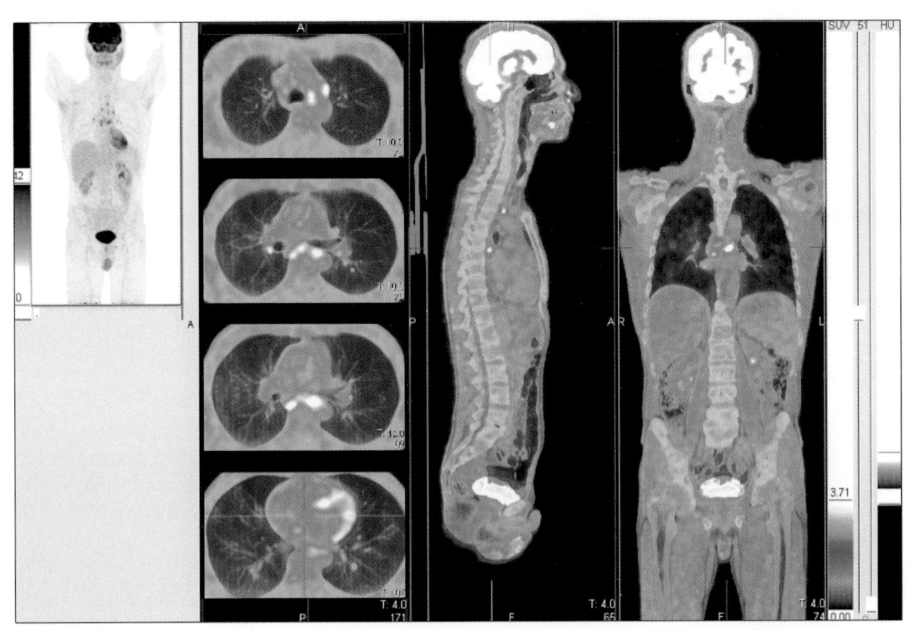

Fig. 9.3 FDG-PET showing uptake of cervical and mediastinal lymph nodes. A very low FDG uptake of lung parenchyma is observed.

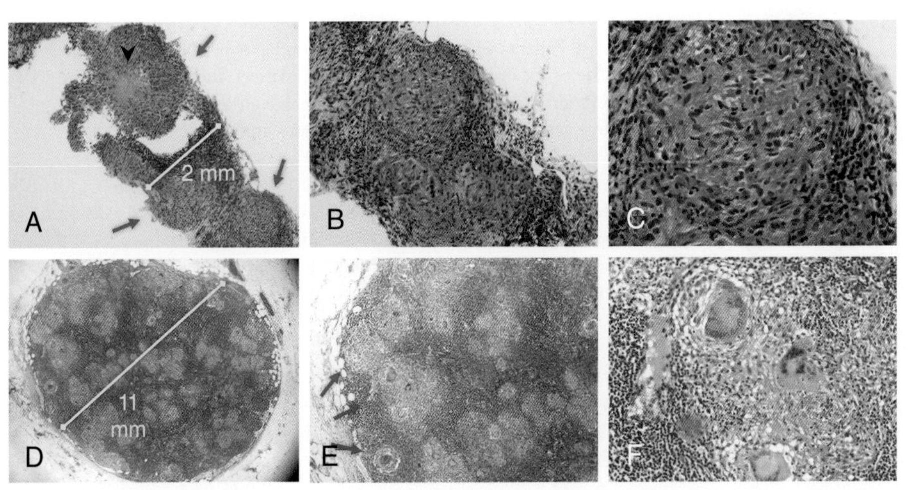

Fig. 9.4 Histological examinations (H&E stain) of the needle biopsy of a laterocervical lymph node (A, B, C with progressive enlargement) and excisional biopsy of the same lymph node (D, E, F with progressive enlargement). There are evident epithelioid granulomas with multinucleated giant cells and focal necrotic areas. Note the different sizes of the needle biopsy sample, which is a few millimeters thick (A) compared to the excisional biopsy of the entire lymph node, which is over a centimeter thick (D).

Discussion Topic 3

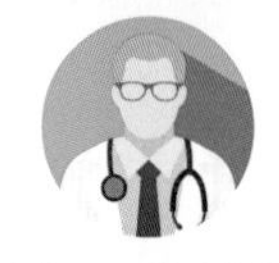

Pulmonologist A

Now we have no doubts: the patient has sarcoidosis.

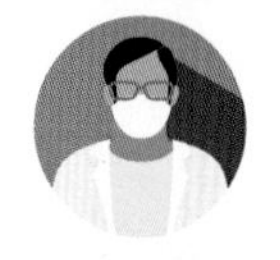

Pulmonologist B

He'll need to perform pulmonary function tests. Also, I'll prescribe echocardiography with a pulmonary pressure assessment.

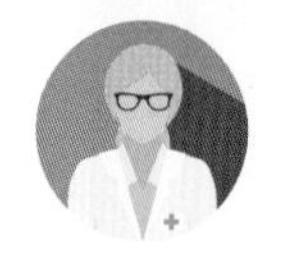

Pulmonologist C

We usually do an abdomen ultrasound to evaluate if there is splenomegaly or renal stones, but we can avoid it as our patient already underwent a chest-abdomen CT scan during the diagnostic process.

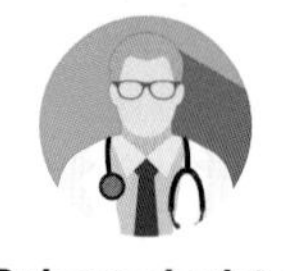

Pulmonologist A

So, his history of nephrolithiasis could be related to this diagnosis!

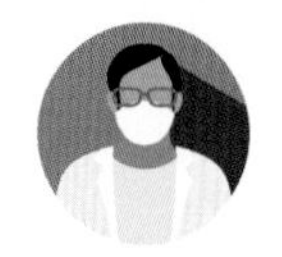

Pulmonologist B

Probably yes. Patients with sarcoidosis may develop hypercalcemia and hypercalciuria due to the overproduction of 1,25-dihydroxy vitamin D_3 by pulmonary alveolar macrophages. This leads to increased absorption of calcium in the intestine and increased resorption of calcium in the bones.

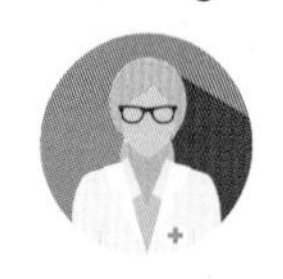

Pulmonologist C

We should test serum and urine electrolytes to screen for abnormal calcium metabolism, then monitor their trend over time.
Also, serum alkaline phosphatase and transaminases will be enough to monitor liver function.

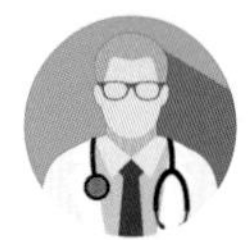

Pulmonologist A

The patient never had symptoms attributable to uveitis, which is one of the most frequent manifestations when sarcoidosis involves the eyes. However, an ophthalmological evaluation could be useful to assess possible retinal vascular changes or conjunctival nodules.

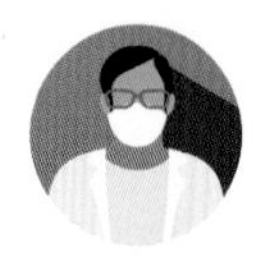

Pulmonologist B

I'd schedule an FDG-PET for follow-up. It is important to know if there is continuous inflammation in the lung parenchyma, because it might lead to progressive destruction of the lung.

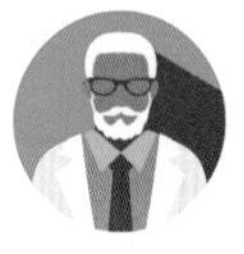

Radiologist

However, integration with CT scan will be necessary, because sarcoidosis in remission as well as end-stage fibrosis may show anatomical abnormalities while FDG-PET shows that the disease itself has become inactive.

Pulmonary function tests performed before discharge showed lung volumes within the limits of normal (forced expiratory volume in 1 second [FEV_1]/forced vital capacity [FVC] 74%, FVC 92% predicted, FEV_1 89% predicted, total lung capacity [TLC] 95% predicted) and a slight reduction in gas exchange (diffusing capacity of the lungs for carbon monoxide [DLCO] 76% predicted).

At the 6-minute walk test (6MWT), the patient covered a normal distance (510 m) without significant oxygen desaturation (mean SpO_2 96%, lowest SpO_2 94%).

Echocardiography also showed no pathological findings. No alterations were found at the eye examination.

Urinary electrolytes were evaluated and hypercalciuria was found, although blood calcium level was still within the upper limits (10.1 mg/dL, normal values 8.6–10.3 mg/dL). There was no significant alteration in serum 25-hydroxyvitamin D_3 (38 ng/mL, normal values 20–40 ng/mL) and parathyroid hormone (14 pg/mL, normal values 11–60 pg/mL). Renal function also was normal (serum creatinine 0.96, glomerular filtration rate 95.7 mL/min/1.73 m^2).

The urologist review indicated only an ultrasound follow-up of the kidneys for nephrolithiasis.

Discussion Topic 4

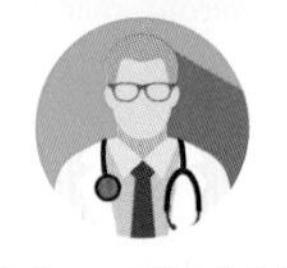

Pulmonologist A

Our patient has pulmonary and extrapulmonary involvement of sarcoidosis. Should we start drug treatment?

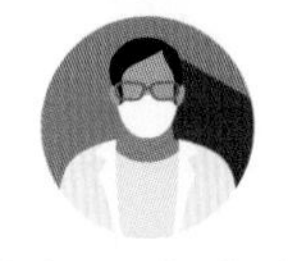

Pulmonologist B

Usually, we treat individuals with lung parenchyma abnormalities and significant respiratory symptoms or progressive lung disease or those with severe extrapulmonary disease. The goal of sarcoidosis management is to prevent or control organ damage, relieve symptoms, and improve the patient's quality of life.

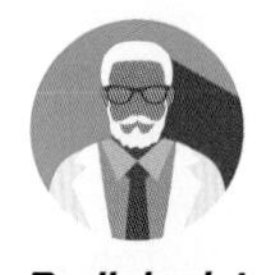

Radiologist

Imaging of our patient suggests stage II sarcoidosis, for evidence of lymphadenopathy and pulmonary infiltrates. If he were asymptomatic, he could only undergo a follow-up because spontaneous resolution is common.

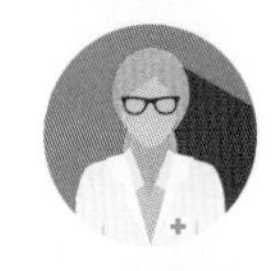

Pulmonologist C

Our patient complains of exertional dyspnea, and the swelling of his neck bothered him a lot. Furthermore, he has hypercalciuria.

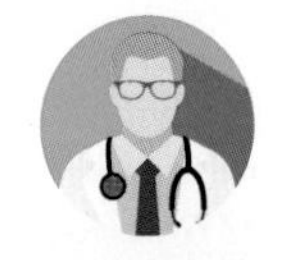

Pulmonologist A

I'd start oral glucocorticoids; they are the mainstay of therapy. I generally start with 0.3 to 0.6 mg/kg/day of prednisone or equivalent, corresponding to about 20 to 40 mg/day in a 70-kg person. After 4 to 6 weeks, if the patient achieves clinical improvement, we should start tapering the initial dose.

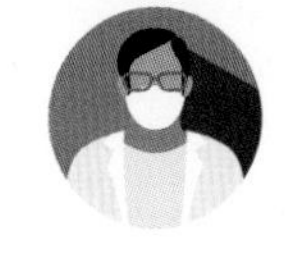

Pulmonologist B

Fortunately, the patient has no involvement of the eye, nervous system, or heart, which are the most troubling complications of sarcoidosis and which require prompt and aggressive management.

Continued on following page

Discussion Topic 4 (Continued)

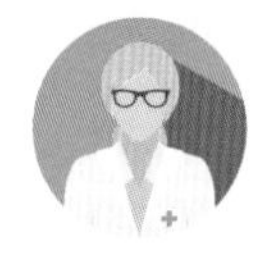

Pulmonologist C

In fact, lung involvement is poor. Since treatment is introduced mainly for quality-of-life reasons, I suggest using low to medium doses with a highly flexible patient-centered approach.

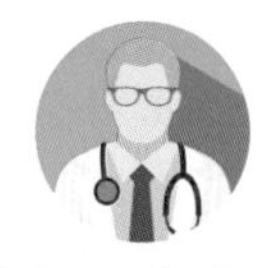

Pulmonologist A

I agree. The higher the cumulative dose of prednisone, the more toxicity that will be encountered.

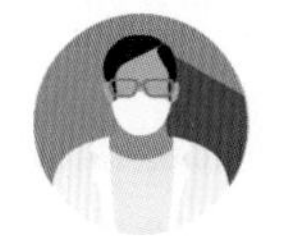

Pulmonologist B

We should verify if he has osteopenia. If so, we should also give bisphosphonates to prevent further corticosteroid-induced bone loss. If we fail to reduce prednisone to < 10 mg/day within 6 months, we should start steroid-sparing agents such as methotrexate or azathioprine.

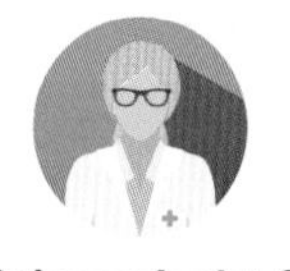

Pulmonologist C

In any case, before starting a long-term treatment, we need to communicate clearly to the patient, involve him in decision-making, and ask him to weigh-up treatment benefits against adverse effects.

Recommended Therapy and Further Indications at Discharge

Although the patient had only mild respiratory symptoms and serum calcium within limits, a pharmacological therapy was proposed because the swelling of cervical lymph nodes had a noticeable effect on his quality of life. After he was given an explanation of the possible benefits and side effects of systemic corticosteroid therapy, the patient agreed to undergo the treatment and was placed on prednisone 37.5 mg/day, corresponding to about 0.5 mg/kg.

Clinicians indicated bone densitometry and scheduled pulmonology outpatient visits after 4 weeks. Subsequent follow-up included pulmonary function tests, blood tests, and FDG-PET/CT scan after 12 weeks, as well as pulmonology visits every 2 months.

Follow-Up and Outcomes

The patient began to observe clinical improvement after about 1 month. Swollen lymph nodes in the neck shrank, and exertional dyspnea progressively disappeared. No further extrapulmonary symptoms appeared. Clinicians maintained the induction dose of prednisone for 6 weeks; then, it was reduced to 35 mg/day, and subsequently a tapering of 5 mg every 4 weeks was scheduled.

Bone densitometry showed femoral and lumbar osteopenia. To prevent further corticosteroid-induced bone loss, bisphosphonates (alendronate 70 mg every 7 days) were prescribed.

FDG-PET/CT scan showed minimal residual uptake in cervical and mediastinal lymph nodes and nasal mucosa (SUV_{max} 1.8–3.5). Pulmonary nodules disappeared. Lung volumes were relatively stable, and diffusion capacity improved slightly (DLCO 82% predicted).

Hypercalciuria disappeared. Follow-up echocardiography showed stable normal findings.

An otolaryngologist review described an improvement of the nasal mucosal endoscopic features.

Tapering of prednisone continued until a daily dose of 10 mg prednisone was reached; then the patient was placed at this maintenance dose for 6 months. Finally, prednisone was lowered again at 5 mg/day (4 weeks) and then discontinued. No relapse occurred after a 6-month follow-up after prednisone suspension. The patient achieved normalization of chewing and swallowing. Body weight remained stable despite corticosteroid therapy.

Focus on

Overview of Sarcoidosis and Clinical Manifestations

Sarcoidosis is a systemic inflammatory disease of unknown etiology that can affect any organ.

It is characterized by the formation of epithelioid granulomas, usually nonnecrotizing. If there is necrosis, this is noncaseating. Incidence is highest for individuals younger than 40 years.

Lungs and lymph nodes are most commonly affected. About 90% of patients have pulmonary involvement, and 5% to 15% have progressive fibrosis of the lung parenchyma.

Less commonly affected are the skin (erythema nodosum, plaques, subcutaneous nodules, and lupus pernio), eyes (mainly uveitis), liver (granulomas cholestasis), heart (patchy granulomatous infiltration of the myocardium surrounded by reactive edema, with possible scarring and remodeling of the heart, dilatation of heart cavities, and thinning of heart muscle), central nervous system (inflammation and abnormal cell deposits in any part of the nervous system, called neurosarcoidosis, with cranial nerves most commonly affected), and spleen.

Sarcoidosis can be asymptomatic. When symptomatic, patients can experience fatigue, shortness of breath, dry cough, joint aches and pains, arthritis, dry eyes, blurry vision, and skin lesions.

Lofgren syndrome is an acute form of sarcoidosis characterized by fever, erythema nodosum, hilar lymphadenopathy, and polyarthralgia. The prognosis is relatively good, as it usually resolves spontaneously without the need for therapy other than symptomatic medications such as nonsteroidal anti-inflammatory drugs.

The combination of anterior uveitis, parotitis, cranial nerve VII paralysis, and fever is called uveoparotid fever or Heerfordt syndrome. It can also resolve spontaneously.

Focus on

Staging of Thoracic Sarcoidosis

Thoracic sarcoidosis can be studied by a chest radiograph, although high-resolution CT and FDG-PET provide more precise information. The most common radiological finding of thoracic sarcoidosis is bilateral hilar adenopathy. Usually, the pulmonary hila are equally enlarged, although sometimes the right one is larger. Unilateral adenopathy is rare and occurs in $< 5\%$ of patients.

When sarcoidosis involves the lung parenchyma, it can cause nodules or interstitial lung disease with ground-glass, reticular, or, seldom, honeycombing pattern.

Thoracic sarcoidosis has been classically divided into five radiological stages, which just indicate the areas affected by it. Unlike many other diseases, the consecutively numbered stages do not reflect the disease's activity or progression.

- Stage 0: no chest abnormalities.
- Stage 1: hilar or mediastinal nodal enlargement only. There is often a right paratracheal node enlargement. It is the most commonly observed, involving nearly half of the patients at initial diagnosis. In 60% to 80% of cases, these adenopathies spontaneously regress in 1 to 3 years, while about 10% of patients develop chronic adenopathy, persisting for > 10 years.
- In stage 2: hilar adenopathies and parenchymal disease. These are often reticular opacities, mainly in the upper lobes. These findings are present at initial diagnosis in 25% of patients.

Continued on following page

Focus on (Continued)

Staging of Thoracic Sarcoidosis

About 50% to 60% of these patients have a spontaneous resolution, while in the others there is often a disease progression. They are usually patients with mild to moderate symptoms (fever, dyspnea, cough, fatigue).

- Stage 3: parenchymal disease only. Spontaneous remission is observed in < 30% of patients.
- In stage 4: fibrotic lung disease. It comprises radiological findings of pulmonary fibrosis, mostly involving upper fields, including irregular interstitial thickening, traction bronchiectasis, lung volume loss, confluent masses, calcifications, cavitations, cysts, and sometimes honeycombing. Spontaneous resolution of sarcoidosis in the fibrosing phase has never been observed.

Focus on

Management of Sarcoidosis

Sarcoidosis management aims to prevent or control organ damage, relieve symptoms, and improve the patient's quality of life. Sarcoidosis may be self-limiting and remit spontaneously, and a significant percentage of patients never need therapy. Pharmacological treatment of sarcoidosis should be reserved for individuals with lung parenchyma abnormalities and significant respiratory symptoms or progressive lung disease or severe extrapulmonary involvement. In particular, eye, nervous system, and heart involvement may require prompt aggressive management due to their potentially serious clinical consequences.

Systemic glucocorticosteroids are the first choice in the treatment of sarcoidosis. The initial dose generally ranges from 0.3 to 0.6 mg/kg/day of prednisone in acute disease. Most responses to therapy are seen within 4 to 6 weeks. In this case, tapering of oral glucocorticoids should begin, usually by 5 mg, targeting a maintenance dose of 5 to 10 mg of prednisone by approximately 6 months after initiation of treatment, often continued for 6 to 12 months.

Prolonged use of prednisone at ≥ 10 mg/day or equivalent is associated with frequent severe side effects.

Antimetabolites (e.g., methotrexate) and biologics (e.g., infliximab) are useful additions to corticosteroids in refractory sarcoidosis or as steroid-sparing options.

In patients with advanced pulmonary fibrosis with respiratory failure and/or pulmonary hypertension, referral for lung transplantation should be considered.

In patients with airway obstruction, which can occur in up to 30% to 40% of patients, inhaled corticosteroids can be used.

LEARNING POINTS

- The diagnosis of sarcoidosis should not routinely be made on clinical grounds alone, particularly if pharmacological treatment is needed or if there is diagnostic uncertainty.
- Diagnostic workout of sarcoidosis requires excluding malignancies (lymphoma) and infections (tuberculosis) where there are enlarged lymph nodes or other forms of ILD where there is pulmonary involvement.
- Tissue should be obtained from the most accessible site such as a peripheral lymph node if abnormal findings are present; otherwise, intrathoracic sampling is indicated via bronchoscopy.
- Granulomas in sarcoidosis are usually nonnecrotizing; when there is necrosis, it is noncaseating.
- Radiological stages of sarcoidosis describe the pulmonary involvement but do not reflect the activity, progression, or functional deficit of the disease.
- Pharmacological treatment of sarcoidosis should be reserved for individuals with significant respiratory symptoms or progressive lung disease or severe extrapulmonary involvement.
- Inhaled corticosteroids may be an alternative to systemic corticosteroids in selected patients.

Further Reading

Baughman RP, Valeyre D, Korsten P, et al. ERS clinical practice guidelines on treatment of sarcoidosis. *Eur Respir J.* 2021;58(6):2004079.

Belperio JA, Shaikh F, Abtin FG, et al. Diagnosis and treatment of pulmonary sarcoidosis: a review. *JAMA.* 2022;327(9):856-867.

Casal A, Suárez-Antelo J, Soto-Feijóo R, et al. Sarcoidosis. Disease progression based on radiological and functional course: predictive factors. *Heart Lung.* 2022;56:62-69.

Crouser ED, Maier LA, Wilson KC, et al. Diagnosis and detection of sarcoidosis. An official American Thoracic Society clinical practice guideline. *Am J Respir Crit Care Med.* 2020;201:e26-e51.

Keijsers RGM, Grutters JC. In which patients with sarcoidosis is FDG PET/CT indicated? *J Clin Med.* 2020;9(3):890.

Lee GM, Pope K, Meek L, et al. Sarcoidosis: a diagnosis of exclusion. *AJR Am J Roentgenol.* 2020;214(1):50-58.

Sellarés J, Francesqui J, Llabres M, et al. Current treatment of sarcoidosis. *Curr Opin Pulm Med.* 2020;26(5):591-597.

Shaikh F, Abtin FG, Lau R, et al. Radiographic and histopathologic features in sarcoidosis: a pictorial display. *Semin Respir Crit Care Med.* 2020;41(5):758-784.

Wessendorf TE, Bonella F, Costabel U. Diagnosis of sarcoidosis. *Clin Rev Allergy Immunol.* 2015;49(1):54-62.

CHAPTER 10

Relapsing Pulmonary Infiltrates, Severe Asthma, and Eosinophilia With Systemic Manifestations

Claudio Sorino ■ Dina Visca ■ Martina Zappa ■ Marco Vanetti ■ Antonio Spanevello

History of Present Illness

A 68-year-old Caucasian woman arrived at the emergency department (ED) due to a severe cough with sputum, breathlessness, and wheezing. The symptoms had started 4 weeks earlier, and the general practitioner had given her an oral antibiotic (amoxicillin/clavulanic acid 750/250 mg every 8 hours) and mucolytic (carbocisteine 2.7 g every 24 hours) for 10 days. She was also suggested to use bronchodilators (salbutamol and ipratropium) and glucocorticoids (beclomethasone) through a nebulizer in addition to the medications she usually took for asthma. Despite such treatment, the patient had poor improvement of the symptoms.

Past Medical History

The patient was a nonsmoker housewife with no history of exposure to noxious substances. She reported no adverse drug reactions. At the age of 55, she was diagnosed with type 2 bronchial asthma (blood eosinophilia and increased fractional exhaled nitric oxide [FeNO]) requiring long-term therapy with medium dose of inhaled corticosteroids (ICS-) associated with long-acting β_2-agonist (LABA): beclomethasone/formoterol 100/6 μg, two inhalations at morning and two in the evening.

No allergen sensitization was found.

At the age of 65, she was hospitalized due to pneumonia and asthma exacerbation. In this circumstance, chest radiograph and computed tomography (CT) scan showed large bilateral opacities (Fig 10.1; Fig 10.2), and the patient received both antibiotic and systemic corticosteroid therapy. Notwithstanding the complete radiological resolution of pneumonia, she experienced poor asthma control and two acute exacerbations requiring oral corticosteroids (OCS-) over the next 6 months.

Thus, the patient was successively placed on progressively major therapy including high-dose ICS/LABA (beclomethasone/formoterol 200/6 μg, two inhalations in the morning and two in the evening), long-acting muscarinic antagonist (LAMA: tiotropium 2.5 μg, two inhalations every 24 hours), and anti–interleukin-5 (IL-5) biological therapy for severe eosinophilic asthma: mepolizumab 100 mg subcutaneous once every 28 days.

The patient also had arterial hypertension, gastroesophageal reflux disease (GERD), and glaucoma. Mild obstructive sleep apnea (apnea-hypopnea index [AHI] 14 without nocturnal

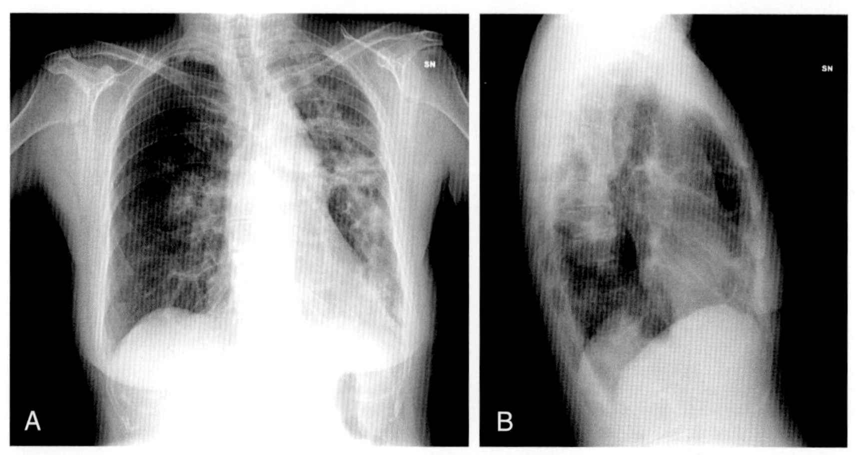

Fig 10.1 Chest radiograph performed when the patient had pneumonia at age 65. Posteroanterior (A) and lateral (B) views show multiple bilateral opacities.

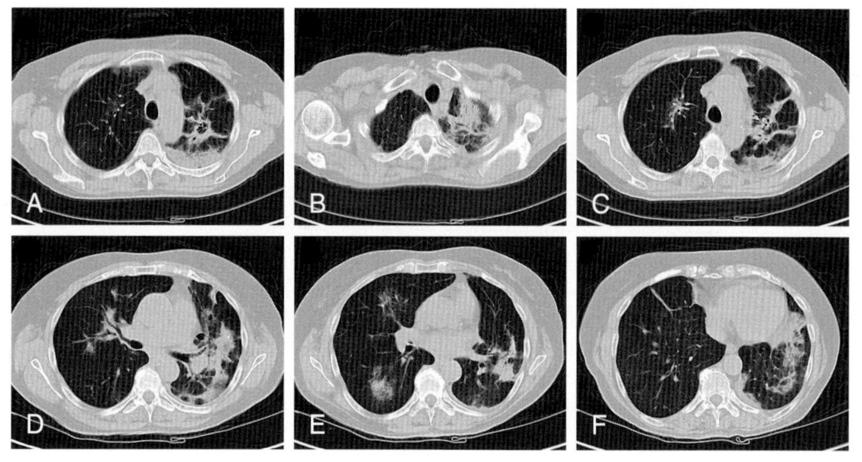

Fig 10.2 Axial CT scan of the chest performed when the patient had pneumonia at age 65. Images on the lung window setting (A–F) show multiple bilateral hyperdensities in all the lung lobes, with greater involvement of the left side.

desaturation) was diagnosed a few years earlier, but only positional therapy was undertaken (lateral recumbency).

Her home medication list also included omeprazole 20 mg and valsartan 80 mg in the morning, Travoprost 40 μg/mL 1 drop in each eye in the evening. She frequently took topical decongestants for nasal obstruction and nonsteroidal anti-inflammatory drugs (NSAIDs) due to both headache and pain in the four limbs with distal paresthesia.

Physical Examination and Early Clinical Findings

Upon arrival at the ED, the patient was dyspneic and tachycardic (heart rate 105 beats/min), had a low-grade fever (body temperature 37.5°C [99.5°F]), and low oxygen saturation (SpO_2 88% at

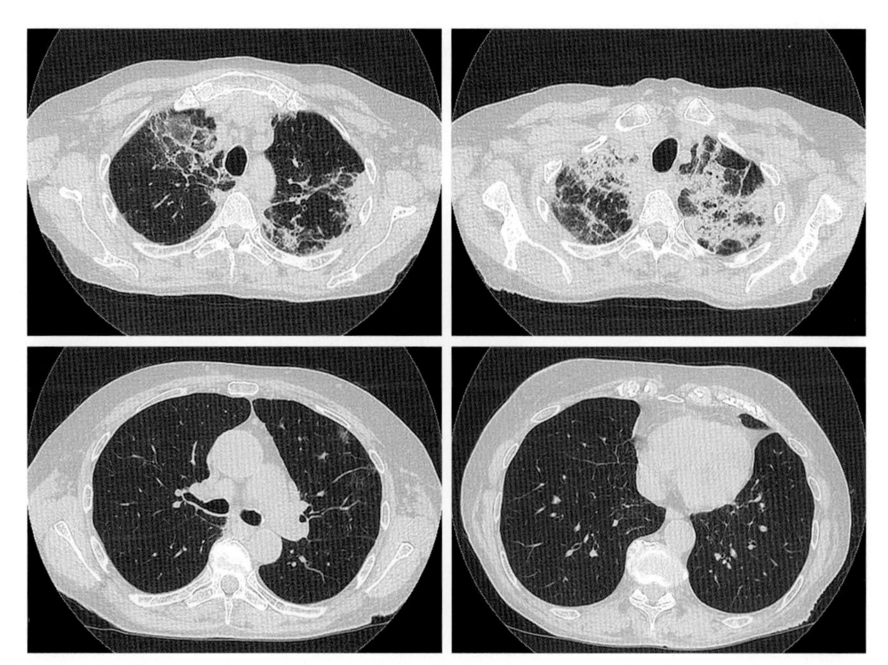

Fig 10.3 Axial CT scan of the chest (lung window setting) performed at the ED. Hyperdensities were present in the upper lobes, while the remaining lobes were spared.

rest while breathing in ambient air). Arterial blood gas analyses revealed acute partial respiratory failure (pH 7.44, pCO_2 36.9 mmHg, pO_2 58.4 mmHg, HCO_3^- 22 mmol/L). The respiratory rate was 24 breaths/min, and arterial pressure was 135/80 mmHg.

On auscultation, the breath sounds were slightly reduced and wheezing was present in the middle and lower fields.

Blood tests showed mild leukocytosis (white blood cell [WBC] count 11,420 cells/mm^3) with relative eosinophilia (eosinophils 983 cells/mm^3, 8.6%), increase in the indices of inflammation (C-reactive protein [CRP] 183 mg/L, normal values <10 mg/L; erythrocyte sedimentation rate [ESR] 56 mm/h, normal values <10 mm/h), no anemia (Hb 13.8 g/dL), normal brain-type natriuretic peptide (proBNP 320 pg/mL; normal values <400 pg/mL), and normal kidney and liver functions.

Due to an increased D-dimer (976 ng/mL), chest CT-angiography was done. This excluded pulmonary embolism and detected bilateral opacities in the upper lobes (Fig 10.3).

Low-flow oxygen supplement (2 L/m by nasal cannula) was able to grant good SpO_2.

ED doctors gave a bolus of methylprednisolone 40 mg and started intravenous antibiotic therapy (ceftazidime 1 g 3 times daily). The patient was admitted to the pulmonology guard.

Discussion Topic 1

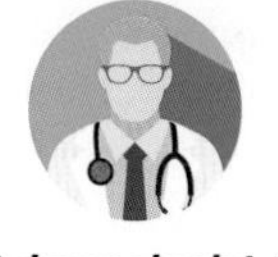

Pulmonologist A

The patient once again has bilateral pneumonia. Her concomitant severe asthma doesn't help: she has an acute respiratory failure.

Continued on following page

Discussion Topic 1 (Continued)

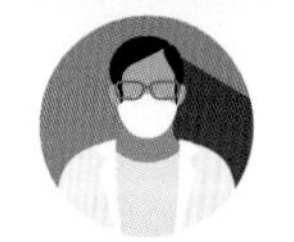

Pulmonologist B

Did you notice that blood eosinophils are very high despite anti–IL-5 treatment?

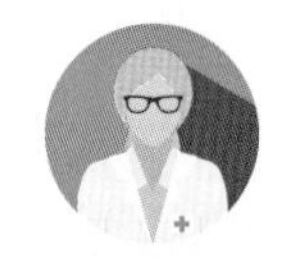

Pulmonologist C

Mepolizumab does not completely clear blood eosinophils, but this patient continues to have particularly high values.

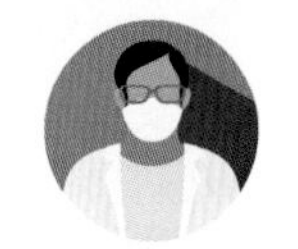

Pulmonologist B

She had a similar event about 3 years ago. What if she has non-infectious pneumonia?

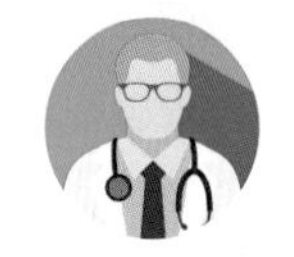

Pulmonologist A

Are you thinking about eosinophilic pneumonia?

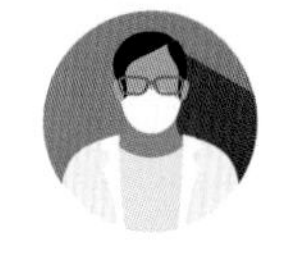

Pulmonologist B

Yeah. I think we should have a bronchoscopy with bronchoalveolar lavage (BAL). It would allow us to understand if she needs corticosteroids more than antibiotics.

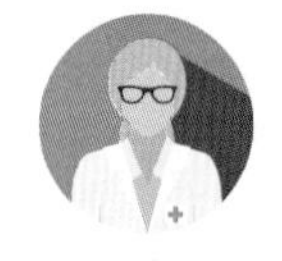

Pulmonologist C

The patient also has severe airway hyperresponsiveness and currently has respiratory failure. We should be careful not to aggravate her condition with bronchoscopy and BAL.

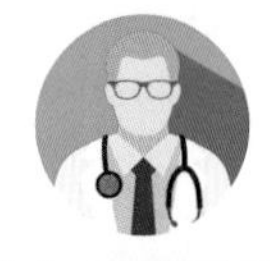

Pulmonologist A

She needs only a 2 L/m oxygen supplement, and wheezing decreased after the intravenous bolus of methylprednisolone.

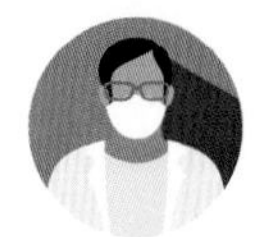

Pulmonologist B

I believe that the information provided by bronchoscopy is important.
If a subject had pulmonary opacities and blood hypereosinophilia, i.e., >1,500 cells/mm^3, the diagnosis of eosinophilic pneumonia would be almost certain even without performing BAL. This is not the case, and we need confirmation as well as ruling out a bacterial or parasitic infection.

Discussion Topic 1 (Continued)

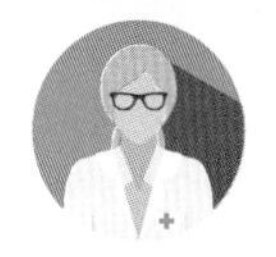

Pulmonologist C

Just before the procedure, we can give bronchodilators, and soon after we will begin empirical treatment with daily systemic glucocorticoids.

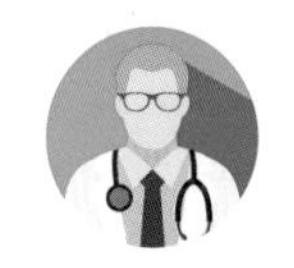

Pulmonologist A

Ok. Bronchoscopy should be performed as soon as possible and before further administration of systemic corticosteroids. I will speak to the patient, and if she accepts the procedure, I will schedule it for tomorrow morning.

Clinical Course

The patient underwent bronchoscopy with BAL in the left upper lobe, then she was placed on methylprednisolone 20 mg intravenously every 12 hours and oral acetylcysteine 600 mg daily. Ceftazidime intravenous was continued, as well as her usual home therapy that included bronchodilators and a proton pump inhibitor. The total amount of BAL fluid recovered was 47 mL (39.2% of saline instilled): 9 mL in the first aliquot and 38 mL in the remaining aliquots. Total cellularity of BAL fluid was 1,483,000 cells/mL, and cell differential count revealed a marked eosinophilia (eosinophils 74%, alveolar macrophages 18%, neutrophils 1%, lymphocytes 7%; CD4:CD8 ratio 0.9). No eggs, larvae, or adult parasites were found on microscopy of the BAL fluid, and no organisms grew on the culture. The polymerase chain reaction for the detection of Mycobacterium tuberculosis was negative.

Discussion Topic 2

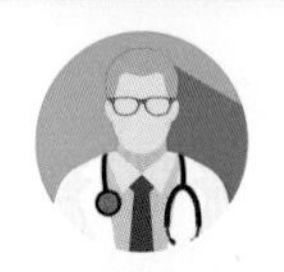

Pulmonologist A

The characteristics of BAL fluid analysis leave no doubt. This is eosinophilic pneumonia.

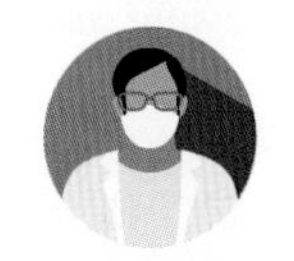

Pulmonologist B

It's probably chronic eosinophilic pneumonia (CEP). In acute forms, the onset is relatively sudden, the clinical picture is usually more severe, and peripheral eosinophilia is often initially absent.

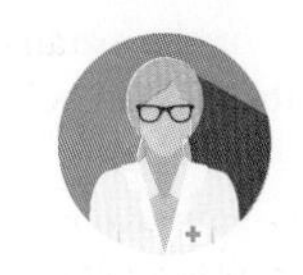

Pulmonologist C

There is no correlation with drugs or evidence of parasitic infections. We can also conclude that it is idiopathic.

Continued on following page

Discussion Topic 2 (Continued)

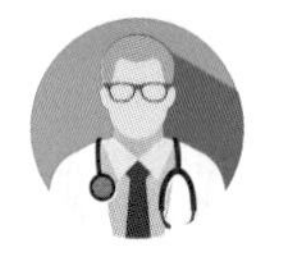

Pulmonologist A

The presence of asthma also makes this diagnosis more likely. Furthermore, this could be a relapse. The patient had previous pneumonia along with asthma exacerbation treated with systemic corticosteroids.

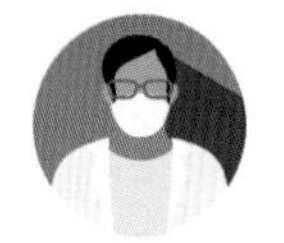

Pulmonologist B

CEP may be a presenting feature of eosinophilic granulomatosis with polyangiitis (EGPA). A careful clinical evaluation should be made to evaluate this hypothesis. In particular, we should explore the possible involvement of the heart, kidneys, nose, nervous system, and gastrointestinal tract.

The patient's clinical condition progressively improved. After 5 days of hospitalization, she no longer needed supplemental oxygen, while blood tests showed a clear reduction in eosinophils and inflammation indices: WBC 10,650/mm^3 with eosinophils 576/mm^3 (5.4%), CRP 16.2 mg/L, and ESR 21 mm/h. The anti-neutrophil cytoplasmic antibody (ANCA) essay was negative. Serum total IgE was 98.2 IU/mL (normal range for adults <200 IU/mL). The corticosteroid was switched to oral administration at a lower dosage (prednisone 35 mg daily).

After 10 days of treatment, parenchymal opacities were no longer recognizable on the chest radiograph, and inflammatory indices were negative. The patient was much better; the antibiotic was stopped, and the oral prednisone was gradually tapered. Given the current and previous extensive use of corticosteroids, she underwent dual-energy x-ray absorptiometry (DXA) to measure bone mineral density (BMD). This revealed osteoporosis in the femoral neck and lumbar spine (T-score −2.7 and −2.5, respectively). A 25-hydroxyvitamin D deficiency was also highlighted (14 ng/mL, normal range 20–40 ng/mL).

Recommended Therapy and Further Indications

The patient was discharged with the diagnosis of idiopathic chronic eosinophilic pneumonia (ICEP). She was prescribed oral prednisone 25 mg daily, to be reduced by 5 mg every 4 weeks. Oral cholecalciferol (5,000 IU weekly for 6 weeks) and oral bisphosphonate (once-weekly alendronate 70 mg) were added to the therapy. A continuation of the diagnostic process for suspected EGPA was scheduled on an outpatient basis.

The patient underwent several further investigations. An esophagogastroduodenoscopy (EGD) with biopsy of the esophageal mucosa showed eosinophilic esophagitis (eosinophilic infiltration of the esophageal epithelium).

The parasitological examination of the stool was negative.

A CT scan of the sinuses (Fig 10.4) revealed diffuse mucous thickenings in the paranasal cavities due to chronic inflammation. There was also turbinate hypertrophy without nasal polyps.

Four-limb electromyography documented a symmetrical axonal peripheral neuropathy.

Pulmonary function tests (Fig 10.5) showed severe airflow obstruction with post-bronchodilator FEV_1 0.91 L (42.6% of predicted; z-score −3,43) and marked increase in airway resistance (Raw; total 206% of predicted). Most values were slightly worse than those obtained about 1 year earlier.

A cardiological evaluation showed a normal left ventricular ejection fraction (LVEF > 55%) with no sign of pericarditis; no rhythm abnormalities were found at the Holter-electrocardiogram evaluation. Urine tests did not reveal proteinuria.

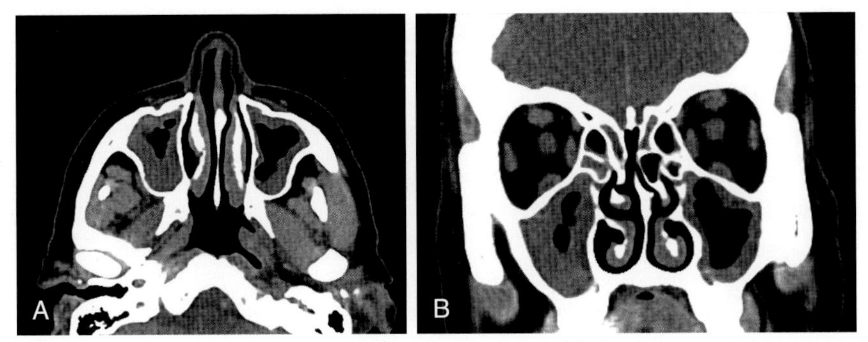

Fig 10.4 CT scan of the sinuses in the axial (A) and coronal plane (B) showing mucosal thickening in the paranasal sinus cavities, and obstruction of the ostiomeatal complexes.

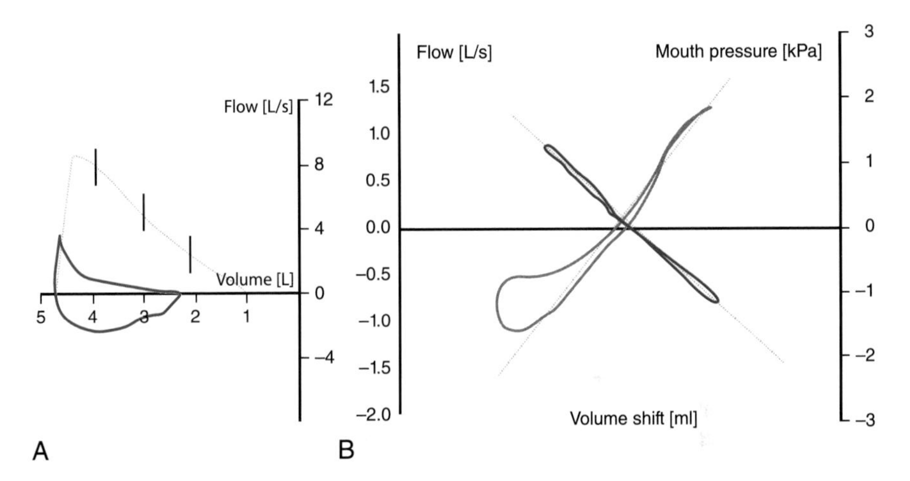

ID: ****** ******		Gender: Female		Height: 158 cm		
Age: 68 years		**Race: Caucasian**		**Weight: 62 Kg**		
Index	**Observed**	**Predicted**	**Z-score**	**LLN**	**ULN**	**% Observed/ Predicted**
FEV_1 (Lit)	0.91	2.14	−3.43	1.57	2.68	42.63
FVC (Lit)	2.34	2.73	−0.88	2.01	3.49	85.65
FEV_1/FVC	0.39	0.79	−4.10	0.66	0.90	49.46
FEF25–75 (Lit)	0.58	1.87	−2.35	0.88	3.25	31.03
DLCO	16.80	18.27	−0.51	13.81	23.76	91.94
VA (Lit)	4.45	4.31	0.26	3.46	5.25	103.26
TLC (Lit)	4.62	4.70	−0.13	3.75	2.78	98.26
RV (Lit)	2.09	1.79	0.59	1.08	2.70	117.07
RV/TLC	45.24	37.74	0.98	25.84	50.45	119.86
Raw (TkPa*s/L)	0.62	0.30	-	-	-	206

FEV_1: Forced expiratory volume in 1 second; LLN: Lower limit of normal; FVC: Forced vital capacity; RV: Residual volume; TLC: Total lung capacity. DLCO: Diffusing capacity of the lungs for carbon monoxide.

C

Fig 10.5 Pulmonary function tests performed 1 month after discharge at the severe asthma center (post-bronchodilator values). (A) Flow-volume curve; (B) plethysmography; (C) measured parameters. There is a severe airflow obstruction with $FEV_1/FVC <$ LLN and $FEV_1 < 50\%$ predicted (z-score between −3 and −4), normal diffusing capacity, and a marked increase in airway resistance.

Discussion Topic 3

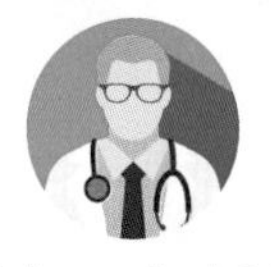

Pulmonologist A

Our patient has asthma, eosinophilia, peripheral neuropathy, non-fixed pulmonary infiltrates, sinusitis, and oesophageal extravascular eosinophils. The criteria for EGPA are largely satisfied.

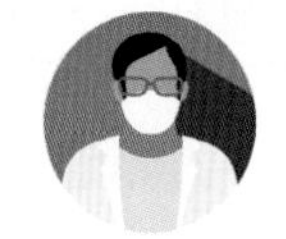

Pulmonologist B

So, her chronic eosinophilic pneumonia was a manifestation of this systemic disease!

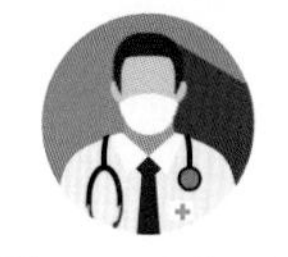

Rheumatologist

Corticosteroids should be very carefully reduced and preferably maintained for many months; otherwise, the risk of relapse of eosinophilic pneumonia would be very high.

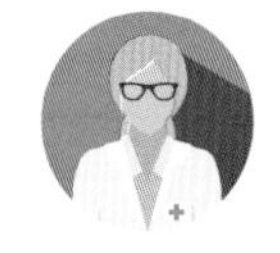

Pulmonologist C

She is already in treatment with an anti–IL-5 biological. However, compared with the dosage of 100 mg every 4 weeks, patients with concomitant EGPA can receive mepolizumab 300 mg every 4 weeks. This appears to ensure an improvement in symptoms and respiratory function.

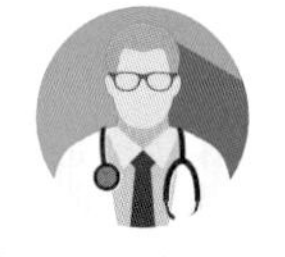

Pulmonologist A

Should this dosage be held forever?

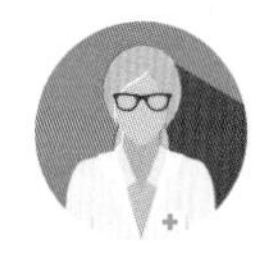

Pulmonologist C

No, mepolizumab can again be reduced to 100 mg every 4 weeks in severe asthmatic patients with EGPA in the remission phase.

Follow-Up and Outcomes

A multidisciplinary discussion with pulmonologists, otorhinolaryngologists, and rheumatologists led to the diagnosis of severe eosinophilic asthma with EGPA. Due to the frequent acute exacerbations and recurrent eosinophilic pneumonia with the use of systemic corticosteroids, the biological therapy was enhanced by increasing the dose of mepolizumab to a subcutaneous injection of 300 mg once every 4 weeks.

In 3 months, prednisone was reduced to 10 mg/day; then the patient continued on this maintenance dose for another 3 months, when doctors further reduced it to 5 mg/day. She experienced an improvement in asthma symptoms control as confirmed by Asthma Control Test (ACT) and Asthma Control Questionnaire (ACQ). Lung function also improved significantly (Fig 10.6). Over the first year of biological treatment, the patient did not report further asthma exacerbations and pulmonary function tests were steadily improved; thus, the OCS maintenance therapy was stopped.

Variables	1 month	6 months	12 months
FEV_1 [Lit (%)]	0.91 (42.6)	1.37 (64.2)	1.45 (67.9)
FVC [Lit (%)]	2.34 (85.6)	2.53 (92.6)	2.64 (96.6)
FEV_1/FVC	0.39	0.54	0.55
Eosinophils [cells (%)]	504 (4.8)	109 (1.2)	58 (0.6)
FeNO	56	48	34
OCS (mg)	10	7.5	5
ACT	11	22	23
ACQ	3	1.67	0.16

Fig 10.6 Trending of respiratory function and asthma control indicators 1, 6, and 12 months after hospitalization for eosinophilic pneumonia. FeNO, fractional exhaled nitric oxide; OCS, oral corticosteroid; ACT, asthma control test (the score ranges from 5 to 25; < 16: very poorly controlled asthma; 16 to 19: not well controlled; 20 to 24: well controlled; 25: completely controlled; minimally important difference: 3 points between 2 groups or for changes over time); ACQ, asthma control questionnaire (the score ranges from 0, i.e., totally controlled, to 6, i.e., severely uncontrolled).

Focus on

Eosinophilic Disorders

Eosinophilic diseases include a broad spectrum of pathological conditions characterized by varying degrees of persistently increased blood and/or tissue eosinophils.

The upper limits of normal in the peripheral blood are considered between 350 and 500/mm³ for the absolute eosinophil count (AEC) or 3% to 5% of the total white blood cell count.

The term "eosinophilia" is preferred for a small increase of AEC (from the upper limit to 1,500/mm³), while "hypereosinophilia" (HE) is defined as an AEC >1,500/mm³ on two consecutive occasions, persistent for a minimum of 1 month. HE is considered moderate when AEC is between 1,500 and 5,000/mm³ and severe if AEC is >5,000/mm³.

A peripheral HE along with organ damage and extensive tissue infiltration by eosinophils allows a diagnosis of hypereosinophilic syndrome (HES). In case of life-threatening conditions (e.g., myocardial ischemia or respiratory failure), the patient deserves immediate care without waiting for a second blood examination.

Pathophysiology, clinical manifestations, and outcomes of eosinophilic disorders are highly heterogeneous as they sometimes occur with mild symptoms, whereas severe forms may cause end-organ dysfunction and are potentially fatal. The most frequent symptoms are cutaneous (e.g., urticaria and angioedema) and respiratory (e.g., asthma and sinusitis). Gastrointestinal, cardiovascular, and neurological involvement is also possible, with cardiac manifestations having the greatest impact on morbidity and mortality.

Therapeutic advances have recently been made, and biological therapies against eosinophilic inflammation are available.

Idiopathic, hematological (primary), and nonhematological (reactive or secondary) eosinophilic syndromes have been described (Table 10.1). The secondary causes of eosinophilia have significant geographical influences, including parasitic infections in tropical settings and allergic diseases in more developed and Western countries.

Focus on

Eosinophilic Lung Diseases

Some lung diseases with a primary pathogenetic role of eosinophils are called eosinophilic lung diseases (ELDs). They include eosinophilic pneumonias, allergic bronchopulmonary mycoses, and hypereosinophilic obliterative bronchiolitis. In normal conditions, very few eosinophils are found in the lungs (<2% on BAL), whereas in ELDs they are usually >5% and reach a very high ratio (>25%) in cases of eosinophilic pneumonia.

Eosinophilic pneumonia is usually referred to as idiopathic when no cause is found. Idiopathic eosinophilic pneumonias include simple eosinophilic pneumonia (Loeffler syndrome), chronic eosinophilic pneumonia (CEP), and acute eosinophilic pneumonia (AEP).

Other forms are associated with systemic conditions such as EGPA or induced by infections (mainly parasitic), smoking, airborne dust, medications, illicit drugs, and radiation therapy.

AEP is a rare but serious lung disease. It occurs with rapid onset of fever, cough, tachypnea, and dyspnea in previously healthy individuals and progresses to acute respiratory failure within a few days. Imaging shows bilateral diffuse lung opacities. Unlike idiopathic CEP, patients have no prior history of

Continued on following page

TABLE 10.1 ■ **Pathological Conditions Associated With Eosinophilia**

Allergic diseases	Eosinophilic asthma, allergic rhinitis, non-allergic rhinitis with eosinophilia syndrome (NARES), food allergies, atopic dermatitis, drug allergies (e.g., DRESS: Drug Reaction with Eosinophilia and Systemic Symptoms), allergic bronchopulmonary aspergillosis (ABPA), eosinophilic chronic rhinosinusitis (ECRS), eosinophilic otitis media, eosinophilic laryngitis
Infections	Parasites (Toxocara, Toxoplasma, Strongyloides, Ascariasis, Trichinella, Echinococcus, Scabiae, Microflaria) Fungi (*Coccidioides mycoses*) Viruses (HIV, HCV)
Autoimmune diseases	Connective tissue disorders, sarcoidosis, inflammatory bowel disease, bullous pemphigoid, systemic vasculitis (e.g., EGPA)
Endocrine diseases	Addison disease
Hematological neoplasms	Myeloid: acute/chronic eosinophilic leukemia, chronic myeloid leukemia Ph+, myelodysplastic syndromes, systemic mastocytosis, aggressive mastocytosis, mast cell leukemia lymphoid: Hodgkin lymphoma, non-Hodgkin lymphoma, T-cell lymphoma
Solid neoplasms	Lung, gastrointestinal tract and pancreas adenocarcinoma, thyroid, genital and skin tumors
Organ-restricted diseases with HE	Esophagitis, gastroenteritis, cystitis, pneumonia, dermatological conditions
Immunodeficiencies	Hyper-IgE syndrome (Job syndrome), Omenn syndrome
Rare diseases	Gleich syndrome (episodic angioedema, eosinophilia, polyclonal IgM), eosinophilia-mialgia syndrome
Other	Graft-versus-host disease, cholesterol embolization, radiation exposure

Adapted from Leru PM. Eosinophilic disorders: evaluation of current classification and diagnostic criteria, proposal of a practical diagnostic algorithm. *Clin Transl Allergy.* 2019;9:36.

Focus on (Continued)

Eosinophilic Lung Diseases

asthma and there is no peripheral eosinophilia, which is typically delayed. Two-thirds of patients with AEP are smokers. The prognosis of AEP is usually good as it responds to corticosteroids. A treatment duration of 2 weeks is usually sufficient. Complete resolution of both symptoms and x-ray abnormalities occurs within 14 days in most patients and by 1 month in almost all. The initial dose of corticosteroids depends on the severity of the disease. Most patients receive prednisone 40 to 60 mg orally once a day. In the most severe cases, methylprednisolone 60 to 125 mg IV every 6 hours can be used.

CEP has a gradual onset (over 2–4 weeks), but it is not a truly chronic disorder. Rather, it is an acute or subacute disease that recurs (a better name might be *recurrent eosinophilic pneumonia*). Women develop CEP about twice as often as men. The clinical presentation is similar to community-acquired pneumonia. Asthma precedes or accompanies the illness in >50% of cases. Blood tests typically show peripheral eosinophilia and very high ESR. Iron deficiency, anemia, and thrombocytosis are frequent. Eosinophilia >40% in BAL fluid is highly suggestive of CEP. Response to oral corticosteroids is very high and rapid. An initial dose of prednisone 20 to 60 mg/day or equivalent led to symptom relief within 48 hours and resolution of pulmonary opacities within 1 week in about 80% of patients. However, most patients need very prolonged treatment due to the high frequency of relapse below a daily dose of prednisone 10 mg/day or equivalent.

Focus on

EGPA- and ANCA-Associated Vasculitides

Eosinophilic granulomatosis with polyangiitis (EGPA) is a rare multisystemic disease characterized by granulomatous and eosinophil-rich inflammation and systemic necrotizing vasculitis affecting small to medium-sized vessels.

The disease combines asthmatic symptoms with eosinophilic manifestations and vasculitis.

Antineutrophil cytoplasm antibodies (ANCAs), mainly specific for myeloperoxidase (MPO), can be detected in 30% to 35% of patients with EGPA.

Two distinct phenotypes have classically been described according to ANCA status. The main eosinophil-driven complications such as lung infiltrates, myocardiopathy, and gastrointestinal manifestations are most frequently found in ANCA-negative individuals. Conversely, MPO-ANCA–positive patients have more vasculitic manifestations, such as palpable purpura, peripheral neuropathy, rapidly progressive glomerulonephritis, and, rarely, alveolar hemorrhage.

MPO-ANCA should be tested in any patient with eosinophilic asthma and clinical features suggesting EGPA. However, in EGPA patients, ANCA status is not recommended to guide treatment decisions, and monitoring ANCA is useful only when they are found positive at disease onset.

Other ANCA-associated vasculitides are granulomatosis with polyangiitis and microscopic polyangiitis.

LEARNING POINTS

- More than 25% eosinophils in BAL are indicative of eosinophilic pneumonia.
- Unlike acute eosinophilic pneumonia, chronic eosinophilic pneumonia (CEP) typically has a gradual onset, and patients have a history of asthma and high blood eosinophils.
- CEP responds dramatically to corticosteroids but recurs frequently when prednisone is reduced to <10 mg/day.
- CEP can be a manifestation of eosinophilic granulomatosis with polyangiitis (EGPA).
- Mepolizumab 300 mg every 4 weeks may improve symptoms and lung function in patients with severe asthma and EGPA.

Further Reading

Bel EH, Wenzel SE, Thompson PJ, et al; SIRIUS Investigators. Oral glucocorticoid-sparing effect of mepolizumab in eosinophilic asthma. *N Engl J Med.* 2014;371(13):1189-1197.

Bettiol A, Urban ML, Dagna L, et al; European EGPA Study Group. Mepolizumab for eosinophilic granulomatosis with polyangiitis: a European multicenter observational study. *Arthritis Rheumatol.* 2022;74(2): 295-306.

Caminati M, Crisafulli E, Lunardi C, et al. Mepolizumab 100 mg in severe asthmatic patients with EGPA in remission phase. *J Allergy Clin Immunol Pract.* 2021;9(3):1386-1388.

Chung SA, Langford CA, Maz M, et al. 2021 American College of Rheumatology/Vasculitis Foundation guideline for the management of antineutrophil cytoplasmic antibody-associated vasculitis. *Arthritis Rheumatol.* 2021;73(8):1366-1383.

Cottin V. Eosinophilic lung diseases. In: Broaddus VC, Ernst JD, King Jr TE., eds. *Murray & Nadel's Textbook of Respiratory Medicine.* 7th ed. Philadelphia: Elsevier – OHCE; 2021.

Pavord ID, Korn S, Howarth P, et al. Mepolizumab for severe eosinophilic asthma (DREAM): a multicentre, double-blind, placebo-controlled trial. *Lancet.* 2012;380(9842):651-659.

Wechsler ME, Akuthota P, Jayne D, et al; EGPA Mepolizumab Study Team. Mepolizumab or placebo for eosinophilic granulomatosis with polyangiitis. *N Engl J Med.* 2017;376(20):1921-1932.

Yancey SW, Ortega HG, Keene ON, et al. Meta-analysis of asthma-related hospitalization in mepolizumab studies of severe eosinophilic asthma. *J Allergy Clin Immunol.* 2017;139(4):1167–1175.e2.

CHAPTER 11

Diffuse Parenchymal Lung Disease With Granulomas in the Colon and Cervical Lymph Nodes Due to Tuberculosis

Claudio Sorino ■ Federico Giussani ■ Michele Mondoni ■ Sergio Agati

History of Present Illness

A 53-year-old Caucasian male was admitted to the surgical ward due to bowel obstruction and suspected colon cancer. He underwent right hemicolectomy in one stage, with end-to-end anastomosis. The histological examination of the resected bowel showed no cancer but did show tissue inflammation with non-necrotizing granulomas and extensive involvement of the ileocecal valve and terminal ileum (Fig. 11.1). Thus, the patient was diagnosed with terminal ileitis due to Crohn disease.

During hospitalization, a preoperative chest radiograph showed bilateral hazy opacities in the mid- and upper fields (Fig. 11.2). He had no respiratory symptoms; thus, he was discharged, and an outpatient pulmonology visit was scheduled.

Past Medical History

The patient was a plumber and a lifetime nonsmoker and had no allergies. He had a hiatal hernia and mild *Helicobacter pylori*–negative gastritis. Several years earlier, he underwent right saphenectomy and right meniscectomy. The patient did not routinely take drugs. No family members had respiratory diseases.

Physical Examination and Early Clinical Findings

At the pulmonology visit, the patient was afebrile, alert, and cooperative. He had no breathlessness at rest or during exertion. Oxygen saturation measured by pulse oximetry (SpO_2) was 97% on room air, heart rate was 76 beats/min, respiratory rate was 15 breaths/min, and blood pressure was 120/80 mmHg. The physical examination revealed normal respiratory sounds. No pallor, clubbing, or peripheral edema was observed. A chest computed tomography (CT) scan revealed several rounded ground-glass hyperdensities with centrilobular distribution. The central part of the lesions was less dense than the peripheral one (the atoll sign or reversed halo sign). They were mainly located in both the upper lobes and the apical segments of the lower lobes (Video 11.1; Fig. 11.3). Calcific paratracheal and subcarinal lymph nodes were also found (Fig. 11.4).

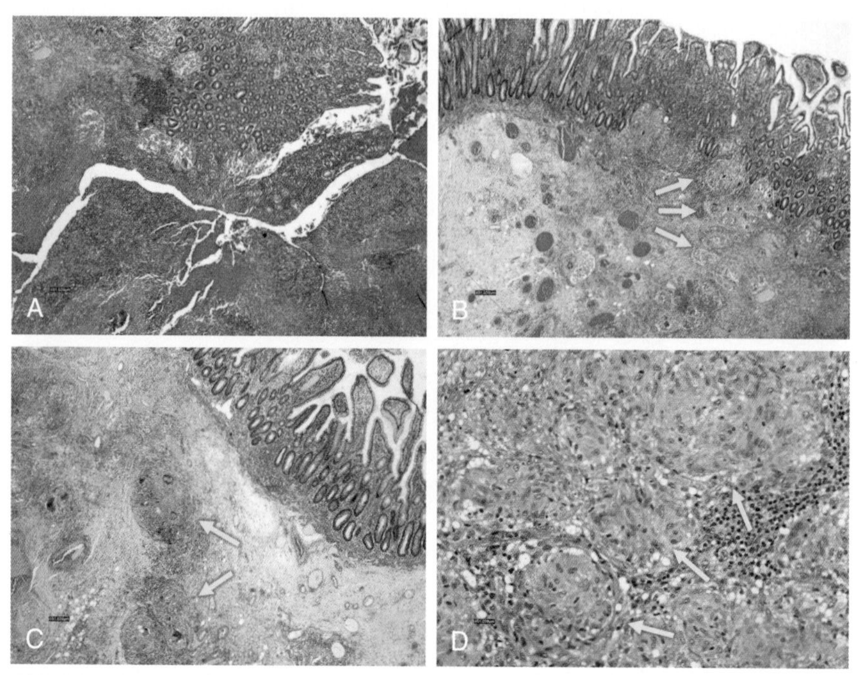

Fig. 11.1 Histological sections from the last ileal tract after right hemicolectomy, showing extensive fissuring of the mucosa (A: hematoxylin and eosin [H&E] stain ×4) and multiple epithelioid non-necrotizing granulomas (arrows) with giant cells (B: H&E stain ×20, C: H&E stain ×40, D: H&E stain ×60).

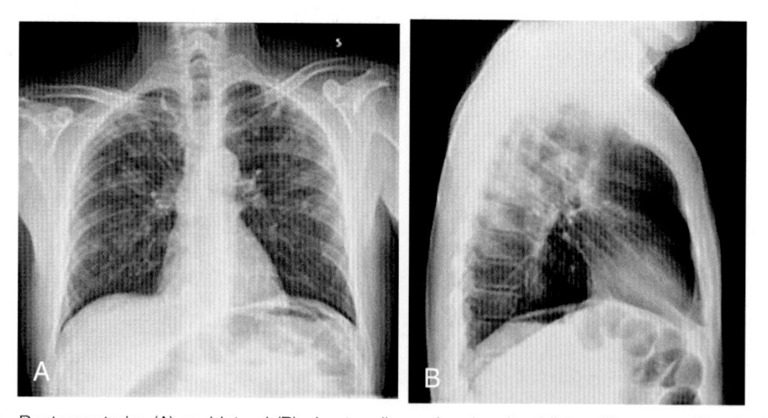

Fig. 11.2 Posteroanterior (A) and lateral (B) chest radiography showing bilateral hazy opacities in the mid- and upper fields.

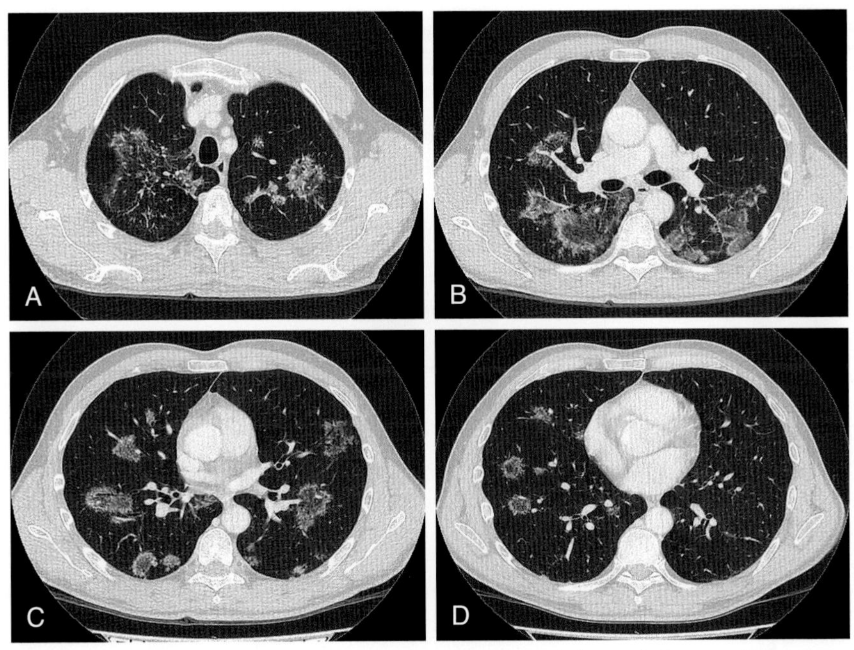

Fig. 11.3 Axial chest CT scan (lung window) showing bilateral rounded ground-glass opacities with centrilobular distribution, surrounded by hyperdense areas (atoll sign or reversed halo sign).

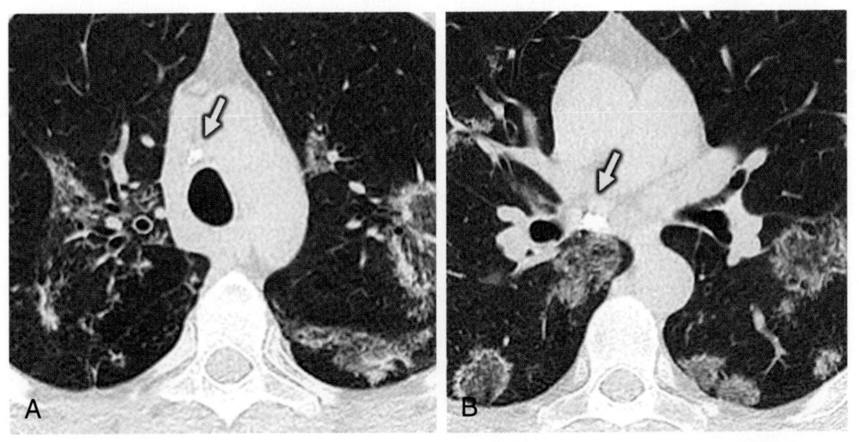

Fig. 11.4 Details of axial chest CT scan showing calcific paratracheal (A) and subcarinal (B) lymph nodes (arrows).

Discussion Topic 1

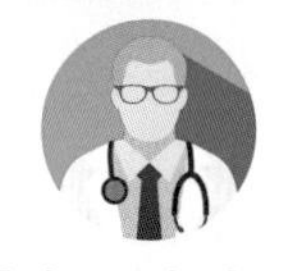

Pulmonologist A

Did you see the chest CT scan? The patient has numerous ground-glass hyperdensities in both lungs.

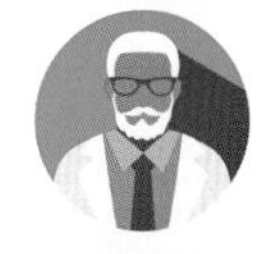

Radiologist

They seem to have a centrilobular distribution. Although there is no clear "tree-in-bud" sign, this pattern suggests something spreading through the airways.

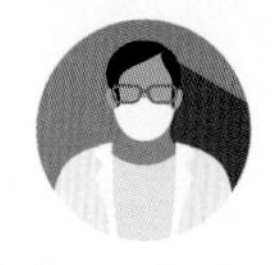

Pulmonologist B

Do you mean an infection? Yet he has no fever.

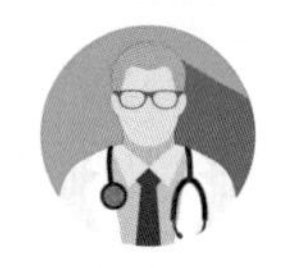

Pulmonologist A

For that matter, he doesn't even have a cough or breathlessness!
We'll need some blood tests, at least blood cell count and inflammatory indexes.

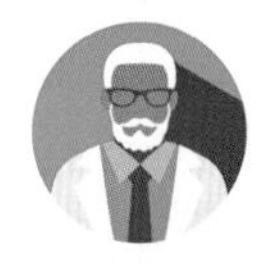

Radiologist

Opacities have a central hypodense area, known as the "atoll sign." This is most commonly seen in organizing pneumonia, which may be cryptogenetic or secondary to specific causes.

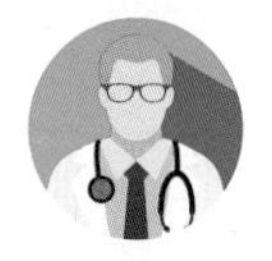

Pulmonologist A

What if they were tumor lesions? That aspect would make me think of a lepidic grow adenocarcinoma. However, it is unlikely that it occurs with multiple bilateral lesions.

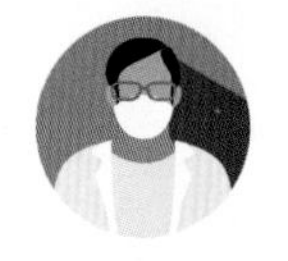

Pulmonologist B

I think it is right not to neglect any hypothesis among the differential diagnoses. Do you know if he has any risk factors for hypersensitivity pneumonitis?

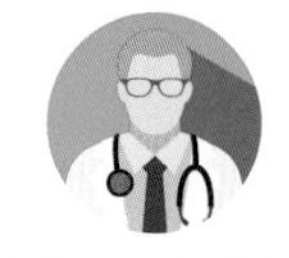

Pulmonologist A

He has no pets or birds, nor is there mold or humidity in the house.
He has never worked as a farmer or bird breeder or poultry farmer.
I don't know if he uses humidifiers, air conditioners, or heating systems.
I'll ask for further anamnestic data.

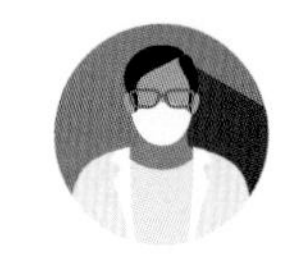

Pulmonologist B

It could also be useful to exclude rheumatic diseases. In any case, bronchoscopy with bronchoalveolar lavage (BAL) should be done.

Discussion Topic 1 (Continued)

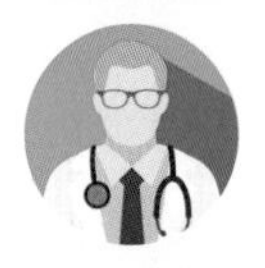

Pulmonologist A

I agree. His clinical condition is good and allows for the procedure to be performed on an outpatient basis.

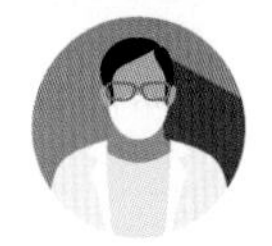

Pulmonologist B

Should we also run pulmonary function tests?

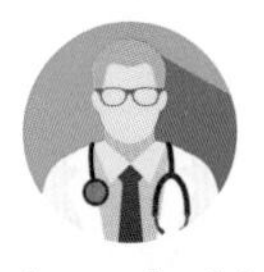

Pulmonologist A

Not before having ruled out a lung infection.

Clinical Course

No clinical signs of rheumatic diseases were found. The search for antibodies against nuclear antigens (ANAs), extractable nuclear antigens (ENAs), and neutrophil cytoplasmic antigens (ANCAs) was negative.

The patient underwent bronchoscopy with BAL. No bronchial abnormalities were found on endoscopic exploration. Lymphocytes in the bronchoalveolar lavage fluid were 9% (normal values 7.5–12.5% for non-smokers, 3.5–7.5% for smokers). The $CD4^+$:$CD8^+$ ratio was fairly increased (4.3; normal value < 2). Cultures for common pathogens and mycobacteria were negative. A nucleic acid amplification test (NAAT) for Mycobacterium tuberculosis was negative. No malignant tumor cells were found.

Discussion Topic 2

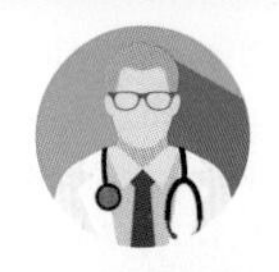

Pulmonologist A

BAL fluid has a normal lymphocyte count but a high $CD4^+$:$CD8^+$ ratio.

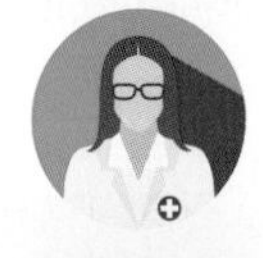

Pathologist

The BAL cell profile can often help, but these values do not clearly point toward a specific diagnosis.

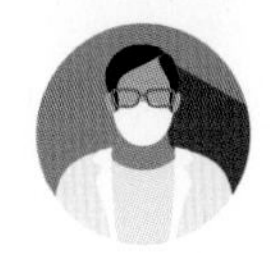

Pulmonologist B

What do you mean?

Continued on following page

Discussion Topic 2 (Continued)

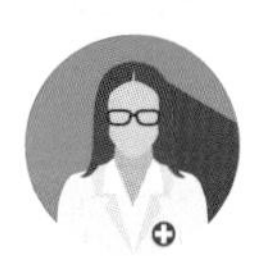

Pathologist

A $CD4^+$:$CD8^+$ ratio > 3.5 is highly specific for sarcoidosis but can also be found in various diseases, including tuberculosis (TB) and malignancies. The percentage of lymphocytes is generally higher in sarcoidosis than in TB. But only a high-grade lymphocytosis (i.e., $> 50\%$) makes the diagnosis of sarcoidosis very likely, as it is rarely seen in patients with TB. Conversely, high-grade neutrophilic alveolitis ($> 20\%$) makes the likelihood of a sarcoidosis diagnosis very low.

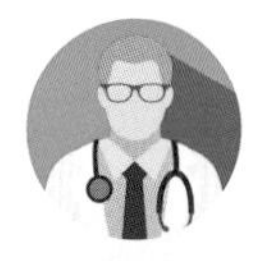

Pulmonologist A

Another finding that usually excludes sarcoidosis is a very low $CD4^+$:$CD8^+$ ratio (< 0.5), particularly when combined with a low percentage of lymphocytes.

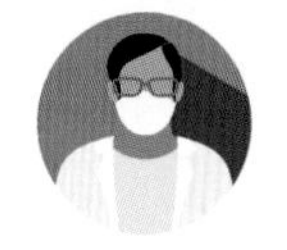

Pulmonologist B

Thus, malignancies and sarcoidosis are unlikely but not ruled out. TB is possible, but there is no evidence of bacilli or genetic material of *M. tuberculosis* in the BAL fluid.

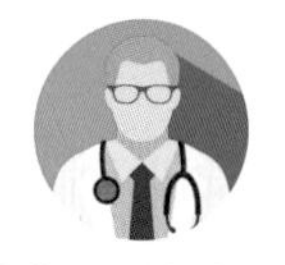

Pulmonologist A

Shall we perform positron emission tomography (PET)/CT? It can be used to better define the extent of the disease and identify possible sites where biological samples can be taken.

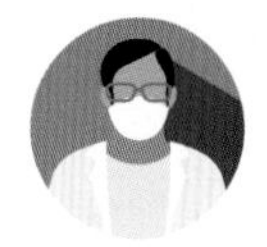

Pulmonologist B

Yes, it is a good idea.

A PET/CT showed significant ^{18}F-fluorodeoxyglucose (FDG) uptake in the multiple lung parenchymal lesions, which was higher in their peripheral area (maximum standardized uptake value [SUV_{max}] 13.79). Several lymphadenopathies with increased FDG uptake were found in the right laterocervical area, in both pulmonary hila and the mediastinum (SUV_{max} up to 19.33). An FDG uptake of abdominal lymph nodes was also found, in particular, in the lumboaortic and mesenteric area (SUV_{max} 10.42) and at the right colonic flexure, near the recent hemicolectomy (SUV_{max} 18.77).

Discussion Topic 3

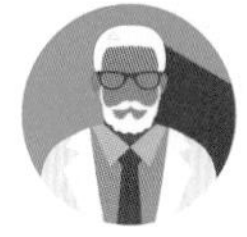

Radiologist

FDG-PET shows intense metabolic activity of lung lesions and lymph nodes in different parts of the body. The findings may be consistent with the clinical suspicion of systemic granulomatous disease.

Discussion Topic 3 (Continued)

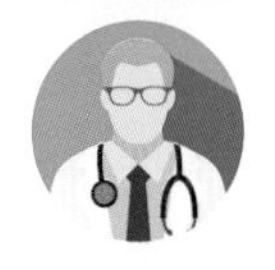

Pulmonologist A

It looks just like sarcoidosis. Do we have to start a corticosteroid treatment?

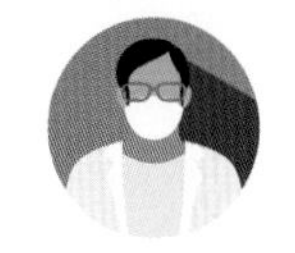

Pulmonologist B

I'm not entirely sure of this. Did the patient have ocular symptoms attributable to uveitis? Skin problems? Or other systemic manifestations of sarcoidosis such as kidney stones or cardiac arrhythmias?

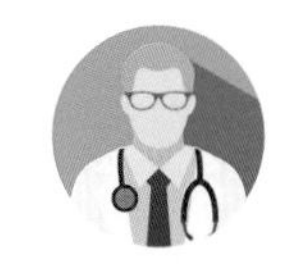

Pulmonologist A

No, but I'll ask for an electrocardiogram, an ultrasound of the heart and kidneys, as well as an ophthalmological visit.

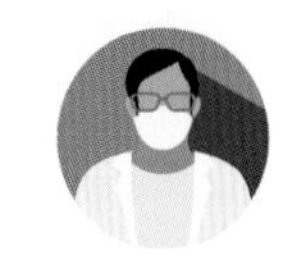

Pulmonologist B

Before starting a therapy, I'd like histological confirmation.
I thought back about the patient history and imaging. There are two mediastinal calcified lymph nodes on the CT scan, and their most common causes are granulomatous infections, especially tuberculosis and histoplasmosis. And what if intestinal granulomas were also expressions of TB? Pulmonary involvement of IBD is extremely rare.

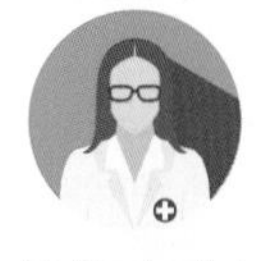

Pathologist

The diagnosis would be more probable if the patient had granulomas with caseous necrosis. But there was no necrosis on histological examination.

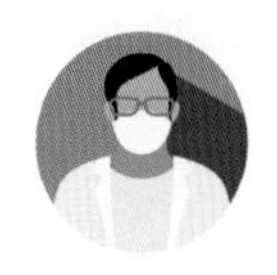

Pulmonologist B

We ran the QuantiFERON TB test; do you have any news of the result?

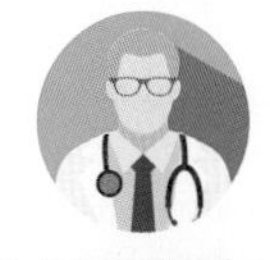

Pulmonologist A

It's not available yet.

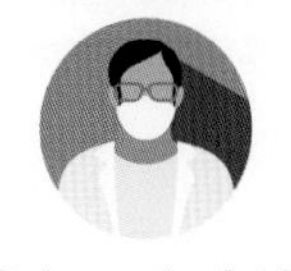

Pulmonologist B

I believe that further histology is appropriate. If we perform a surgical biopsy of the lung, we would certainly arrive at the
diagnosis.

Continued on following page

Discussion Topic 3 (Continued)

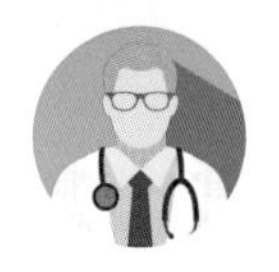

Pulmonologist A

Not the best choice in my opinion. Today you can get similar information with a pulmonary cryobiopsy, which is much less invasive.

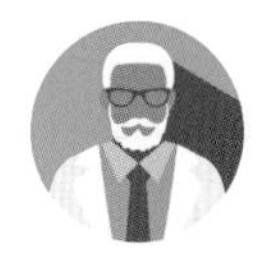

Radiologist

We can easily take tissue from one of the right laterocervical lymph nodes.

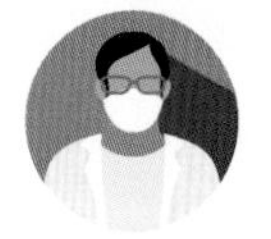

Pulmonologist B

For the diagnosis of sarcoidosis it would be fine. But isn't it better to seek information from the lung again and to repeat the TB diagnostic?

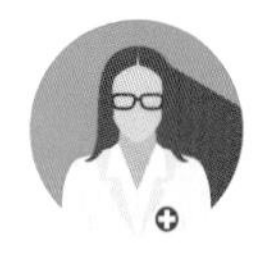

Pathologist

This is my proposal: let's do a biopsy of a cervical lymph node and do a polymerase chain reaction (PCR) to detect *M. tuberculosis* on the old colon specimens.

The patient underwent an ultrasound-guided needle biopsy of a right supraclavicular lymph node. Histology confirmed chronic non-necrotizing granulomatous lymphadenitis, strengthening the hypothesis of a diagnosis of sarcoidosis.

However, the interferon-γ release assay (QuantiFERON-TB Gold) turned very positive (29.75 UI/mL, normal values < 0.20), thus documenting that the patient had exposure to *M. tuberculosis*. A PCR for the detection of *M. tuberculosis* complex on lymph node biopsy was positive. PCR for *M. tuberculosis* complex was also positive in bowel specimens that had been stored after right colectomy.

Recommended Therapy and Further Indications

Both intestinal granulomas and those of the cervical lymph nodes were not attributed to sarcoidosis but rather to active TB. Glucocorticoid therapy was not initiated, and the patient was referred to the infectious disease department, where anti-TB therapy was set up with the four-drug regimen (rifampicin, isoniazid, pyrazinamide, and ethambutol) and concomitant administration of pyridoxine (vitamin B6). Monthly outpatient visits to the infectious disease clinic were scheduled. After a few weeks, cultures of lymph node specimens test turned positive for *M. tuberculosis*, and drug susceptibility testing did not show any drug resistance.

Follow-up and Outcomes

The patient always remained afebrile and with poor respiratory symptoms. Chest radiographs performed 1 and 2 months after initiation of anti-TB therapy showed a progressive reduction of opacities. After 2 months, the therapeutic regimen was reduced to only rifampicin and isoniazid for a further 4 months, then stopped without signs of relapse. A chest CT scan after a total of 6 months of anti-TB therapy documented the disappearance of the pulmonary lesions.

Focus on

Granulomatous Lung Diseases

Pulmonary granulomatosis includes a large and heterogeneous group of diseases characterized by different symptoms and evolutions (Table 11.1).

The diagnostic workup includes an accurate collection of the medical history, laboratory tests (e.g., cultures, specific serology, autoimmunity, precipitins), pulmonary function tests, imaging (chest radiography or high-resolution CT), multidisciplinary evaluation, and biopsies.

Infections are frequent causes of lung granulomatous diseases, especially mycobacteria and fungi such as *Aspergillus* spp. Thus, obtaining suitable biological samples (e.g., sputum, bronchial aspirate, BAL) is essential. In addition to cultures for common germs, direct microscopic examination with specific stains (Ziehl-Neelsen, Grocott methenamine silver, periodic acid–Schiff), culture for mycobacteria, and nucleic acid amplification test (NAAT) for *M. tuberculosis* complex should be performed.

Non-infectious causes include sarcoidosis (the most frequent in areas with a low incidence of tuberculosis), hypersensitivity pneumonitis (HP), dust inhalation (e.g., berylliosis), drug reactions, vasculitis (granulomatosis with polyangiitis [GPA], eosinophilic granulomatosis with polyangiitis [EGPA]), autoimmune diseases (rheumatoid arthritis, inflammatory bowel disease), and malignancies (e.g., lymphomatoid granulomatosis).

Granuloma results from a chronic inflammatory reaction with an accumulation of mononuclear inflammatory cells, mostly T cells and monocyte macrophages. This inflammatory response can occur at any age and in any body tissue.

Granuloma is a nonspecific finding. However, some features can help in the differential diagnosis. It is important to evaluate the distribution (e.g., it is mostly lymphatic in sarcoidosis, bronchocentric in infections and HP, random in miliary infections), histological characteristics (e.g., it is well formed in sarcoidosis, berylliosis, and infections; not well defined in HP, GPA, and the infectious forms of the immunocompromised; mainly non-necrotizing in sarcoidosis, necrotizing in infections, vasculitis, and malignancies), and the characteristics of the surrounding tissue (e.g., an inflammatory infiltrate is found in HP, infections, and connective tissue diseases).

TABLE 11.1 ■ **Main Causes of Granulomatous Lung Diseases**

Non-infectious		Infectious	
Inflammatory	• Sarcoidosis • Necrotizing sarcoid granulomatosis (NSG) • Inflammatory bowel disease	Mycobacterial	• *M. tuberculosis* • Non-tuberculous mycobacterial infection
Pulmonary lymphoid lesions	• Lymphomatoid granulomatosis (LYG) • Granulomatous-lymphocytic interstitial lung disease (GLILD)	Fungal	• Coccidioidomycosis • Cryptococcosis • Histoplasmosis • Blastomycosis • *Aspergillus* infection
Aspiration or exposure	• Aspiration pneumonia • Talcosis • Berylliosis • Hypersensitivity pneumonitis (HP)	Parasitic	• *Dirofilaria* infection
Vasculitis	• Granulomatosis with polyangiitis (GPA) (formerly Wegener granulomatosis) • Eosinophilic granulomatosis with polyangiitis (EGPA) (formerly Churg-Strauss syndrome)		
Collagen vascular disorders	• Rheumatoid lung nodules		

Focus on

Mediastinal Lymphadenopathy in Tuberculosis and Other Non-Malignant Conditions

Mediastinal lymphadenopathy can be due to inflammatory diseases, malignancies, and infections. It is best assessed by contrast-enhanced chest CT, which can reveal an increase in size of single nodes, loss of their normal ovoid shape, focal contour abnormalities, hypo- or hyperdensity in lymph nodes, invasion of surrounding mediastinal fat, coalescence of adjacent and enlarged nodes, and diffuse soft-tissue attenuation through the mediastinum with obliteration of the mediastinal fat. A mediastinal lymph node usually is considered enlarged when the short axis is > 10 mm.

The most common infectious causes of mediastinal lymphadenopathy are TB and fungal disease (mainly histoplasmosis and coccidioidomycosis). Sarcoidosis is a particularly frequent cause of this condition in young adults. Other causes include silicosis, drug reactions, amyloidosis, heart failure, Castleman disease, chronic obstructive pulmonary disease (COPD), and idiopathic pulmonary fibrosis (IPF).

Some characteristics can help in distinguishing benign from malignant nodes. Benign nodes usually are oval and exhibit a uniform appearance. Frequently (but not always), the presence of fat indicates benignity. Conversely, malignant nodes have irregular edges and tend to be more round than elongated. Heterogeneous enhancement of an enlarged node is another frequent feature of malignancies, even if it can be also found in benign diseases, such as TB.

Tuberculous lymphadenopathy is one of the most common forms of extrapulmonary TB. Lymphadenopathy is the main feature of primary TB, observed in 40% of adult cases and $> 90\%$ of pediatric cases. The most suggestive CT appearance of primary TB is enlarged unilateral hilar lymph nodes with hypodense centers due to caseous necrosis, and a peripheral denser and contrast-enhanced area, representing a rim of granulomatous inflammatory tissue.

The initial focus of pulmonary TB infection plus affected lymph nodes (the "Ghon complex") frequently undergoes a healing process, resulting in a visible parenchymal scar (sometimes calcified) and enlarged or calcified hilar or mediastinal nodes. Calcified lymph nodes are also common in fungal infections, pneumoconiosis, sarcoidosis, amyloidosis, or following a radio/chemotherapy treatment for leukemia. Some features can help in the differential diagnosis (Table 11.2), such as bilateral or unilateral involvement (the latter being more frequent in TB and viral infections) and the distribution of calcifications within the lymph node (e.g., eggshell in silicosis, icing sugar in sarcoidosis, and complete in TB).

Endosonography (transesophageal endoscopic ultrasound [with bronchoscope] fine needle aspiration, EUS-[B]-FNA and endobronchial ultrasound-guided transbronchial needle aspiration [EBUS-TBNA]), which is the diagnostic gold standard to detect malignant mediastinal lymph nodes, now represents the first test in the workup of mediastinal TB lymphadenopathy.

TABLE 11.2 ■ **Main Features of Benign Mediastinal Lymphadenopathy**

	Density	Bilateral	Asymmetrical	Calcification
Sarcoidosis	High	X		X
Silicosis, beryliosis	High	X		X
Tuberculosis	High or low		X	X
Amyloidosis	High	X		X
Castleman disease	High	X		
Fungal infection	Low	X		X
Heart failure	Normal			
Pulmonary fibrosis	Normal			
COPD	Normal			
Drug-induced	Normal	X		
Viral infection	Normal		X	

Focus on

The Reversed Halo Sign

The reversed halo (RH) sign, also known as the atoll sign, is a CT pattern seen on lung window settings, as a round area of ground-glass opacity (GGO) surrounded by a denser consolidation of crescentic shape (forming more than three-fourths of a circle) or complete ring. The consolidation should be at least 2 mm in thickness.

Usually, the central area of GGO is due to alveolar septal inflammation and cellular debris in alveolar spaces, while the peripheral consolidation corresponds to granulomatous lung tissue.

The RH sign was originally described in patients with cryptogenic organizing pneumonia (COP), although it is found in only about one-fifth of patients with COP. It was later observed in several other infectious diseases (e.g., tuberculosis, mucormycosis, aspergillosis, viral or bacterial pneumonia) and noninfectious diseases (e.g., sarcoidosis, pulmonary infarction, granulomatosis with polyangiitis).

In severely immunocompromised individuals, the RH sign is highly suggestive of early infection by an angioinvasive fungus. Such patients should be considered to have an infection until further analyses prove otherwise. The presence of nodules inside the RH or centrilobular nodules with a pattern of endobronchial spread ("tree-in-bud" sign) should rise the suspicion of active granulomatous disease (pulmonary tuberculosis or sarcoidosis) rather than COP.

The RH sign is the opposite of the halo sign, which is characterized by GGO surrounding a pulmonary consolidation (nodule or mass) and often represents alveolar hemorrhage. The halo sign is typically seen in invasive fungal infection (mainly aspergillosis), but it has also been described in primary tumors (mainly adenocarcinoma or adenocarcinoma in situ) or metastases.

LEARNING POINTS

- Granulomatous diseases with pulmonary involvement can have infectious and non-infectious causes.
- Benign causes of mediastinal calcified lymph nodes include tuberculosis and sarcoidosis.
- The reversed halo (RH) sign is commonly seen in cryptogenetic or secondary organizing pneumonia.
- Nodules inside the RH rise the suspicion of active granulomatous disease (tuberculosis or sarcoidosis).
- In BAL fluid, a $CD4^{+}$:$CD8^{+}$ ratio $>$ 3.5 suggests sarcoidosis but can also be found in tuberculosis and malignancies.

Further Reading

Imtiaz S, Batubara EM. Diagnostic value of bronchoscopy in sputum-negative pulmonary tuberculosis patients and its correlation with clinicoradiological features. *Ann Thorac Med.* 2022;17(2):124-131.

Lewinsohn DM, Leonard MK, LoBue PA, et al. Official American Thoracic Society/Infectious Diseases Society of America/Centers for Disease Control and Prevention clinical practice guidelines: diagnosis of tuberculosis in adults and children. *Clin Infect Dis.* 2017;64(2):e1-e33.

Maitre T, Ok V, Morel F, et al. Sampling strategy for bacteriological diagnosis of intrathoracic tuberculosis. *Respir Med Res.* 2021;79:100825.

Mondoni M, Repossi A, Carlucci P, et al. Bronchoscopic techniques in the management of patients with tuberculosis. *Int J Infect Dis.* 2017;64.

Nin CS, de Souza VV, do Amaral RH, et al. Thoracic lymphadenopathy in benign diseases: a state of the art review. *Respir Med.* 2016;112:10-17.

Ohshimo S, Guzman J, Costabel U, Bonella F. Differential diagnosis of granulomatous lung disease: clues and pitfalls: Number 4 in the series "Pathology for the clinician" Edited by Peter Dorfmüller and Alberto Cavazza. *Eur Respir Rev.* 2017;26(145):170012.

Park H, Kansara T, Victoria AM, et al. Intestinal tuberculosis: a diagnostic challenge. *Cureus.* 2021;13(2):e13058.

Sorino C, Cappelletti T. Tuberculosis Diagnostics: In Vivo and in Vitro Techniques. In: Sorino C, ed. *Diagnostic Evaluation of the Respiratory System.* New Delhi: Jaypee Brothers Medical Publishers; 2017:53-59.

PART IV

Connective Tissue Disease–Associated Lung Diseases

CHAPTER 12

Pulmonary Fibrosis and Solitary Pulmonary Nodule in Hidden Rheumatoid Arthritis

Riccardo Messina ■ Nunzia Cannizzaro ■ Roberto Marchese ■
Claudio Sorino ■ Sergio Agati ■ Nicola Scichilone

History of Present Illness

A 78-year-old Caucasian man underwent a visit at the outpatient pulmonology clinic complaining of persistent dry cough and dyspnea during moderate exertion in the last year. On the suggestion of his general practitioner, he had previously received a chest radiograph, which revealed an irregular reticulation in the lower zones, suspicious for interstitial lung disease (ILD).

Past Medical History

The patient was a never-smoker and previously an amusement park employee, with a family history negative for pulmonary disease. He declared to have an unspecified thyroid disease not requiring medical treatment, whereas he was on proton pump inhibitor therapy for gastroesophageal reflux disease and a sartan for hypertension. He denied home exposure to mold and parrots during the past few years. He reported no symptoms correlated with obstructive sleep apnea syndrome or asthma-related symptoms during his lifetime. Eight years earlier, he underwent radical bowel surgery for rectal cancer that had not required chemotherapy treatment.

Subsequently, he scrupulously complied with scheduled cancer follow-ups with no evidence of disease recurrence or extension.

Physical Examination and Early Clinical Findings

During the physical examination, the patient was alert and cooperative, apyretic, and eupneic at rest (respiratory rate 14 breaths/minute). Oxygen saturation (SpO_2) was 96% on room air, heart rate was 78 beats/min, and blood pressure was 120/65 mmHg. There were no current or previous signs and symptoms suggestive of a connective tissue disease (CTD) or systemic vasculitis. On chest auscultation, vesicular murmur appeared reduced in all lung areas with the presence of Velcro-like crackles at the bases bilaterally. He underwent a high-resolution computed tomography (HRCT) scan of the chest, which confirmed an ILD with reticulations, subpleural and basal honeycombing, and traction bronchiectasis, in the absence of features inconsistent with usual interstitial pneumonia (UIP) pattern (Figs. 12.1 and 12.2).

Pulmonary function tests (PFTs) revealed a restrictive ventilatory defect with a decreased diffusing capacity of the lung for carbon monoxide (DLCO): forced vital capacity (FVC) was 72% predicted, total lung capacity (TLC) 80% predicted, DLCO 55% predicted. He also performed a 6-minute walk test with no significant oxygen drop (distance covered 400 m, test not interrupted

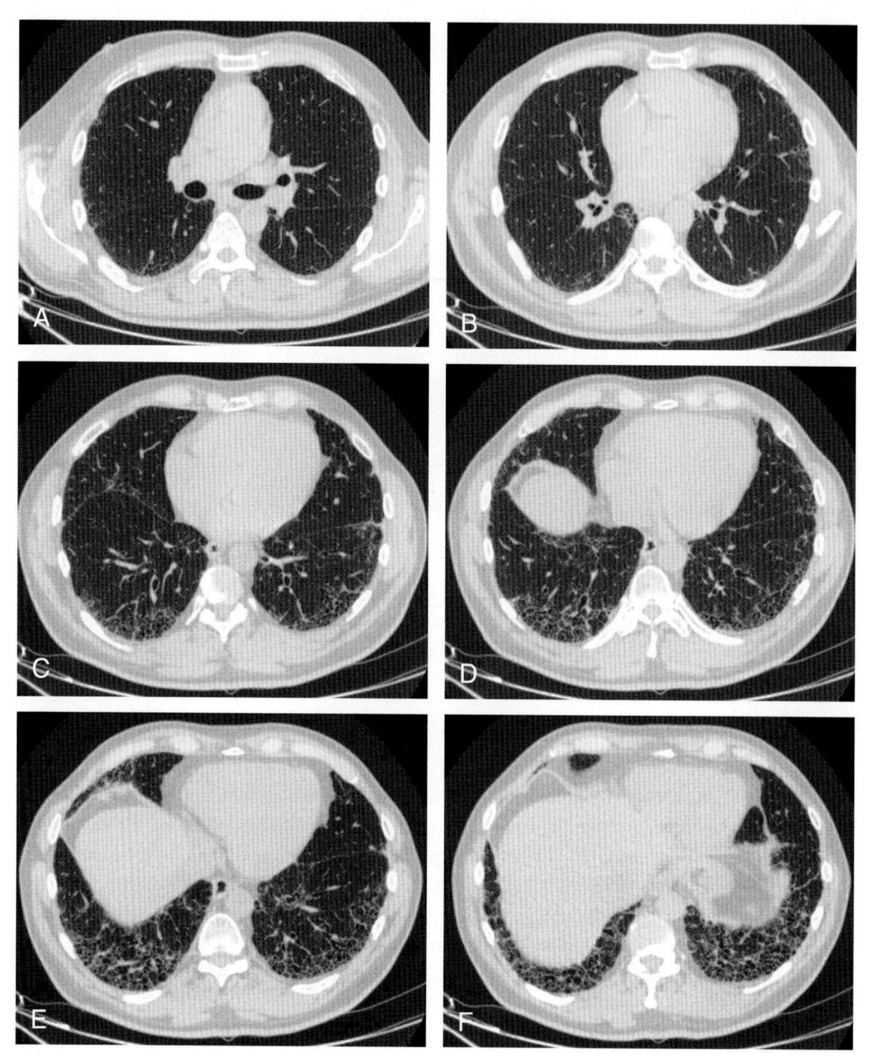

Fig. 12.1 High-resolution chest CT scan (axial view) showing a UIP pattern with reticular abnormalities, traction bronchiectasis, and subpleural/basal honeycombing.

early). During the second appointment, the screening for autoimmunity showed antinuclear antibodies (ANAs) positivity (titer 1:160) with negative extractable nuclear antigen (ENA) typing, negative myositis pattern, and no positive value was found for rheumatoid factor (RF), anti-cyclic citrullinated peptide antibodies (ACPAs), cytoplasmic antineutrophil cytoplasmic antibodies (c-ANCA), and perinuclear antineutrophil cytoplasmic antibodies (p-ANCA); inflammatory indexes and markers of acute viral hepatitis (hepatitis B and C virus) were also negative. Echocardiogram showed normal right heart sections, minimal tricuspid regurgitation, and preserved systolic function (left ventricular ejection fraction [LVEF] 65%).

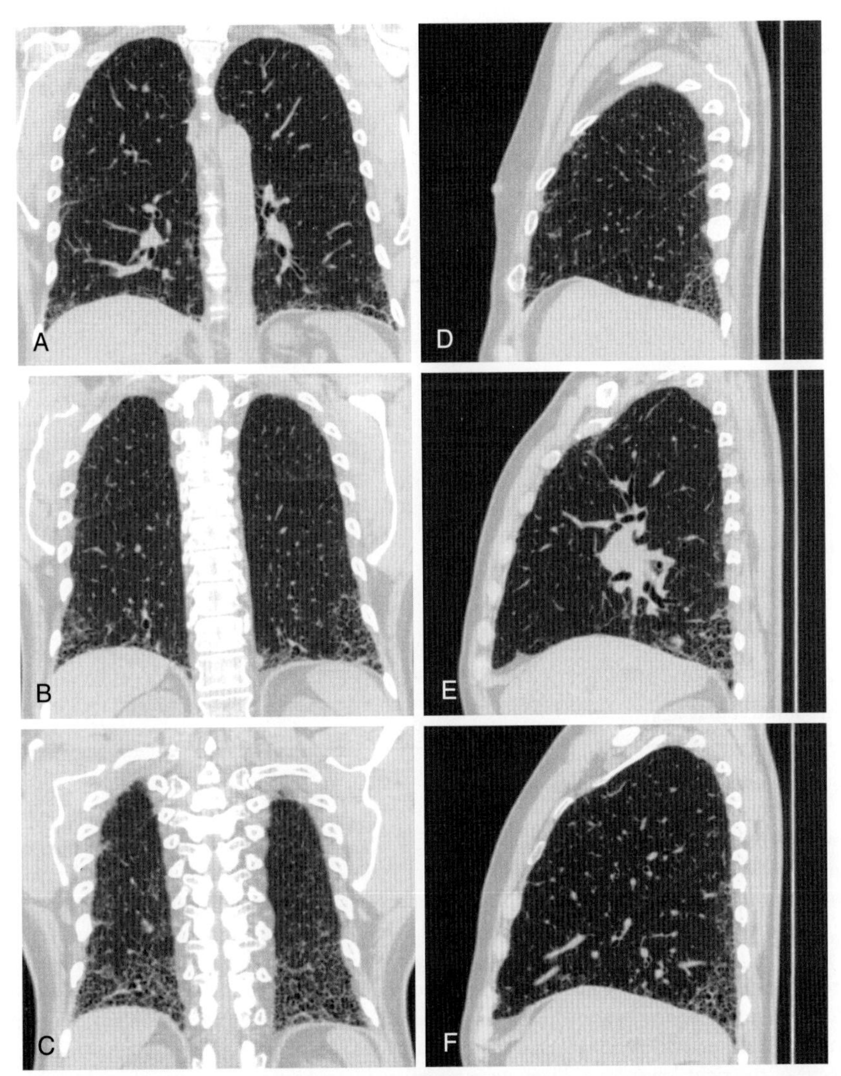

Fig. 12.2 UIP pattern at the coronal (A-C) and sagittal (D-F) reconstructions of the HRCT scan of the chest.

Discussion Topic 1

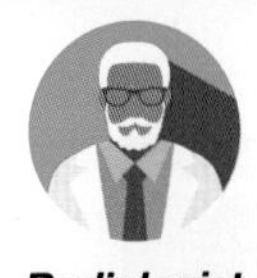

Radiologist

The chest HRCT of this patient leaves no doubts. There is a clear radiological pattern of usual interstitial pneumonia.

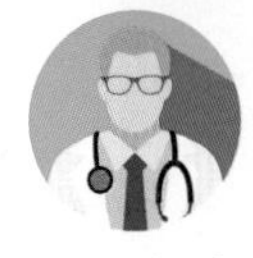

Pulmonologist A

Considering the clinical, functional, and radiological features, the most probable diagnosis is idiopathic pulmonary fibrosis (IPF).

Continued on following page

Discussion Topic 1 (Continued)

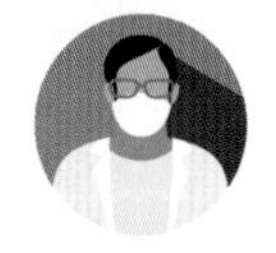

Pulmonologist B

Does the patient need a lung biopsy to confirm the diagnosis?

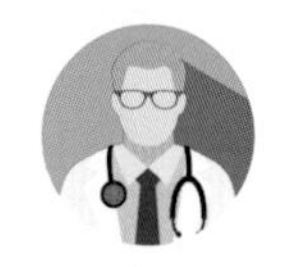

Pulmonologist A

No, he doesn't. In the appropriate epidemiological and clinical context, a radiological UIP pattern provides a highly confident diagnosis of IPF.

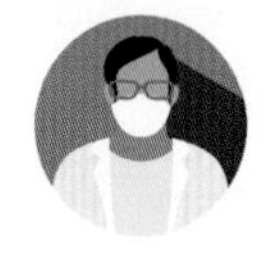

Pulmonologist B

We found an ANA positivity (1:160) on the blood tests. Would it raise the suspicion of ILD secondary to a CTD?

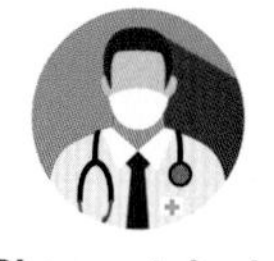

Rheumatologist

We don't have any signs or symptoms compatible with a diagnosis of CTD. Furthermore, ANA testing can be positive in IPF patients.

Clinical Course

A multidisciplinary team (MDT) reviewed lung CT scan images and confirmed the presence of a definite usual interstitial pneumonia (UIP) pattern. Based on clinical and radiological data, in the absence of evident underlying causes, a highly confident diagnosis of idiopathic pulmonary fibrosis (IPF) was made. Subsequently, the patient started an antifibrotic therapy with nintedanib, initially 150 mg twice daily for about 1 year, then 100 mg twice daily due to the occurrence of persistent gastrointestinal side effects. The patient remained stable on clinical, radiological, and functional aspects for the following 2 years. Then, a new chest CT scan performed for morphological reevaluation of the lung parenchyma revealed a solid nodule approximately 12 mm in diameter in the basal segment of the right lower lobe. There were no enlarged mediastinal or axillary lymph nodes. So, the case was discussed again by the MDT, including a thoracic surgeon with expertise in ILD, and a positron emission tomography (PET)-CT scan was proposed to add more information about the nodule. On the PET-CT scan, the lung lesion showed increased volume and mild metabolic activity, rising the suspicion of lung cancer at stage I (Fig. 12.3).

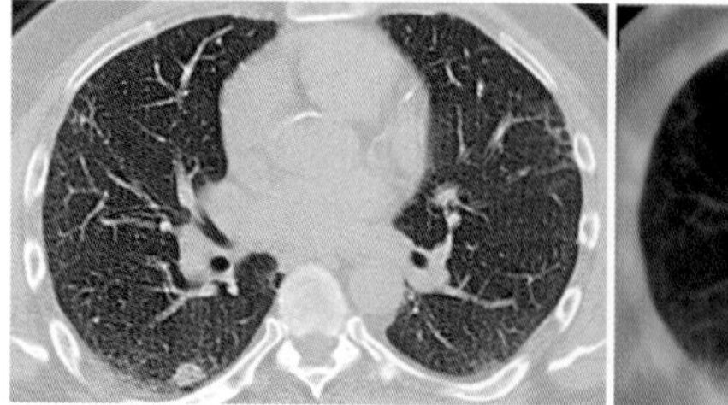

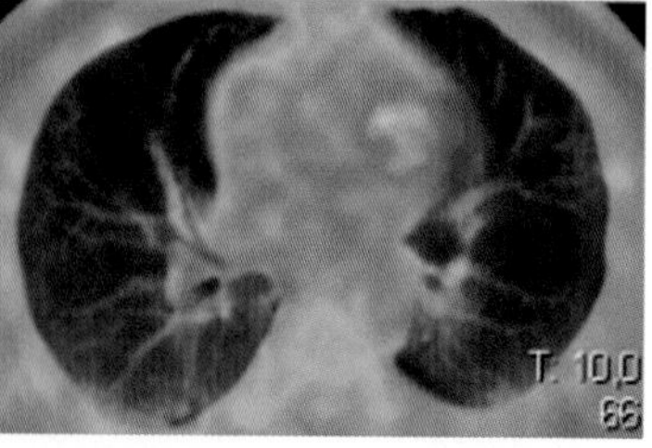

Fig. 12.3 Combined positron emission tomography (PET) and computed tomography (CT) scan showing fluorodeoxyglucose (FDG) uptake of the solitary pulmonary nodules in the right lower lobe.

Discussion Topic 2

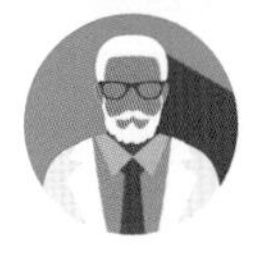

Radiologist

The nodule was not present on previous imaging, and PET-CT shows FDG uptake, albeit weak. The lesion is highly suspicious of malignancy.

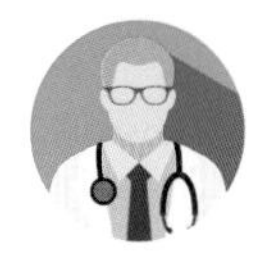

Pulmonologist A

Being an ex-smoker and having IPF make lung cancer even more likely.

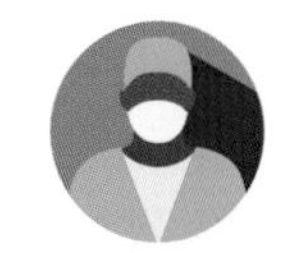

Thoracic Surgeon

There is no evidence of lymph node involvement or distant metastases. If it was lung cancer, it would be stage I, and we could propose a surgical approach to the patient.

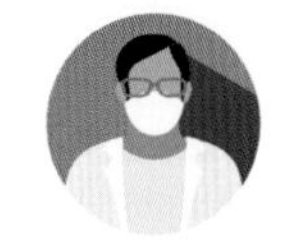

Pulmonologist B

Since the nodule is peripheral, a transthoracic needle biopsy (TTNB) could easily allow the diagnosis before performing thoracic surgery.

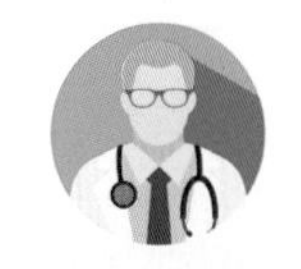

Pulmonologist A

I don't think this approach is the best. If a TTNB showed lung cancer, the patient would still have to undergo surgery, whereas if the TTNB were negative, I would still have some doubts as the procedure's sensitivity is not 100%.

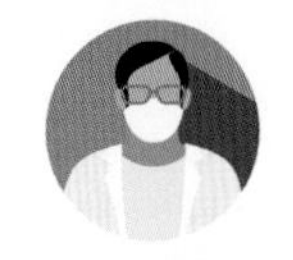

Pulmonologist B

What do you think about stereotactic body radiotherapy (SBRT)? When clinical suspicion is high and the patient is at high risk of complications after invasive procedures or surgery, it can be used to treat solitary lung nodules even without pathological confirmation.

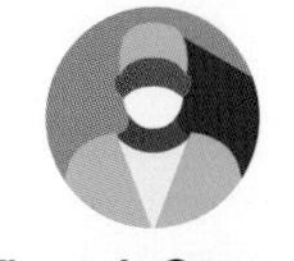

Thoracic Surgeon

There is less evidence of the efficacy of SBRT compared with radical surgery. It should be a second choice.

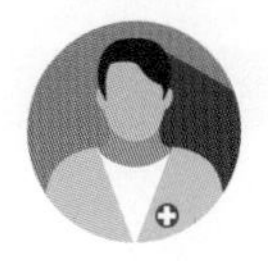

Oncologist

For correct management, we should take into consideration the patient's general clinical and functional condition.

Continued on following page

Discussion Topic 2 (Continued)

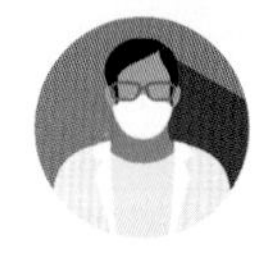

Pulmonologist B

Of course, a surgical procedure would be the best chance for the patient, but it can be too risky. It could lead to severe and life-threatening exacerbation of IPF.

Thoracic Surgeon

We could perform a wedge resection during a nonintubated video-assisted thoracic surgery (VATS) procedure. This could be less risky than other surgical procedures.

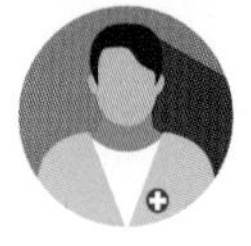

Oncologist

I agree. Moreover, the patient is able to carry out light or sedentary work, which corresponds to a World Health Organization performance status 1, and he has good nutritional status. These data, together with the results of the PFTs, would allow for the proposed approach.

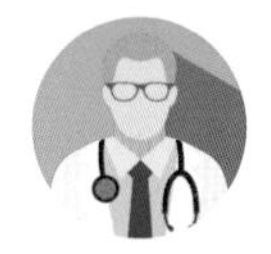

Pulmonologist A

We should complete the staging with a CT scan of the brain, as PET cannot detect metastases there, and then propose the surgical resection.

The patient was informed of the possible diagnostic-therapeutic choices, and he agreed to undergo a nonintubated VATS. The lung nodule in the basal segment of the right lower lobe was removed by wedge resection. A chest tube was kept for 4 days after the procedure. No acute lung exacerbations or additional severe side effects occurred, although oxygen supplementation via nasal cannulas was necessary for approximately 1 week.

The histological report of the lesion described a yellow nodule with a lung parenchyma free of neoplastic infiltration, characterized by an area of necrosis bordered by chronic inflammation. The surrounding lung parenchyma had a heterogeneous picture, characterized predominantly at the subpleural level of areas of extensive and marked interstitial fibrosis with adjacent alveolar ectasia (honeycombing), alternating with focal areas of regular architecture. Approximately 1 month after the lung surgery, the patient manifested the onset of acute articular hands pain with consensual appearance of swelling in the carpometacarpal joints bilaterally. An autoimmunity panel was repeated and showed a high titer of RF and ACPAs. Subsequently, the patient underwent a new rheumatology examination and received a diagnosis of rheumatoid arthritis on the basis of clinical and instrumental examinations.

Discussion Topic 3

Thoracic Surgeon

Despite the high risk of lung cancer, our patient's nodule was benign.

Discussion Topic 3 (Continued)

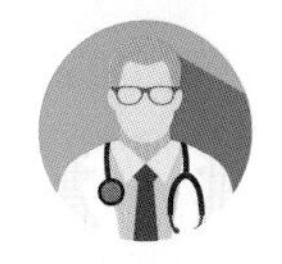

Pulmonologist A

I didn't expect it, but good for him.

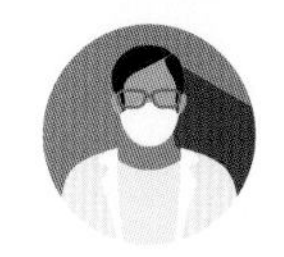

Pulmonologist B

He also developed rheumatoid arthritis symptoms.

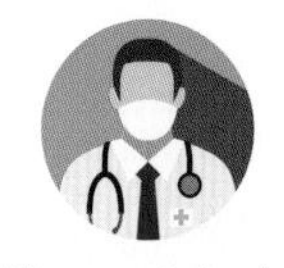

Rheumatologist

It is not often that they appear so late after lung involvement; however, the diagnosis of IPF would now be in doubt.

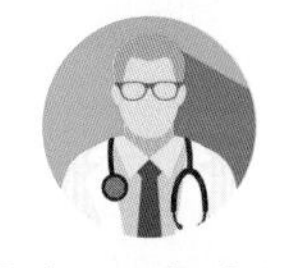

Pulmonologist A

I agree. Pulmonary involvement in rheumatoid arthritis often presents with a radiological and histological pattern of UIP that is indistinguishable from IPF unless there are other signs of CTD.

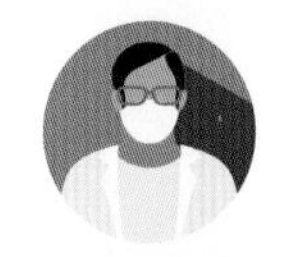

Pulmonologist B

What do we do with the antifibrotic treatment?

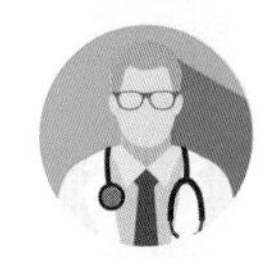

Pulmonologist A

There is robust evidence for the efficacy of nintedanib in cases of CTD-related ILD showing progressive fibrosis. Given his radiological picture and respiratory function, I would continue the treatment already started.

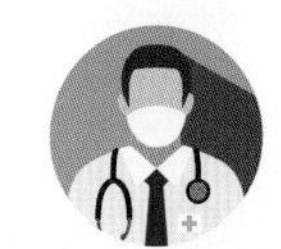

Rheumatologist

I'll also offer additional therapy to relieve the inflammation and pain in his joints.

Recommended Therapy and Further Indications at Discharge

The MDT recommended starting methotrexate, but after a few weeks of treatment joint pain remained poorly controlled. Therefore, an anti–tumor necrosis factor monoclonal antibody, abatacept, was added, and the patient achieved a good control of joint inflammation. A regular follow-up at the outpatient ILD clinic was scheduled, with lung function evaluation every 4 months, HRCT chest scan every 12 months, blood tests every 3 months, and regular rheumatological controls for the rheumatoid arthritis.

Follow-Up and Outcomes

The patient never interrupted the treatment for ILD based on antifibrotic therapy associated with the immunomodulating drugs, except for a transient (15 days) discontinuation of nintedanib, due to transitory onset of nausea, inappetence, and increased liver function tests. The patient never experienced severe lung infections; he was able to continue the treatment with the three drugs, maintaining stable lung function and a good quality of life during an entire year.

Focus on

Diagnosis Path and Treatment of RA-Associated ILD

Interstitial lung disease (ILD) is one of the most severe extra-articular manifestations of rheumatoid arthritis (RA-ILD). The prevalence of RA-associated ILD ranges from 1% to 58% according to the diagnostic technique used and to the population studied. The main risk factors for RA-ILD are older age, male sex, history of ever smoking, seropositivity for RF and ACPAs, late-onset RA, and longer disease duration. Several patients can develop ILD before joint manifestations. It has been hypothesized that the lung could play a central role in the development of AR through the local production of ACPAs. At an early stage of disease, pulmonary function tests may reveal a restrictive ventilatory defect with a decreased diffusing capacity of the lung for carbon monoxide even in the absence of respiratory symptoms.

Chest HRCT may confirm the diagnosis by showing a fibrotic pattern and provide information on the disease severity.

Differently from other CTD-related ILD, UIP is the most common radiological and pathological pattern of RA-ILD. The clinical course of RA-associated ILD is highly variable, with some patients having a progressive phenotype and others showing a stable disease. Other radiological patterns are nonspecific interstitial pneumonia (NSIP), obliterative bronchiolitis, and organizing pneumonia. Acute exacerbations of disease can occur with a quick worsening of lung function due to the disease itself or a lung infection. Immunosuppressants are the cornerstone of pharmacological therapy in RA. In patients with progressive ILD despite optimal treatment, it is possible to add antifibrotic therapy (nintedanib) on the basis of results of the INBUILD study.

Focus on

Solitary Pulmonary Nodules in IPF Patients

Patients with lung fibrosis are more likely to be found with a pulmonary nodule at the time of diagnosis or during the radiological follow-up. This finding is often challenging as IPF patients are at increased risk of developing lung cancer compared to the general population, although a lower prevalence is reported due the poor survival associated with IPF. Lung cancer in IPF occurs more frequently in patients with a smoking history ≥ 35 pack-years and emphysema and seems to be more commonly peripheral in location, predominantly in the lower lobes within areas of fibrosis.

The most commonly reported histology is squamous cell carcinoma. Current official guidelines are lacking about the most appropriate therapeutic approach to lung cancer in patients with IPF, and the physician evaluates the proper treatment case by case, influenced by the severity of the ILD and the lung cancer stage. Clinicians should take into consideration the higher treatment-related morbidity and mortality due to iatrogenic acute exacerbation of the underlying pulmonary fibrosis or pneumonia induced by intensive treatments such as surgery, radiation therapy, and chemotherapy.

Studies reported an increased detection of LC at an early stage in IPF patients due to the annual follow-up HRCT scan. This makes feasible a surgery approach, like sublobar resection, associated with good outcomes.

Rheumatoid nodules are a kind of lesion that can be found in the lungs of rheumatoid arthritis patients with or without ILD. Those nodules, usually detected by a CT scan and located in subpleural areas, can be solitary or multiple and solid, partially solid, or cavitary and can reach a size from a few millimeters to several centimeters. Differentiation of a rheumatoid nodule from a lung neoplasm can be challenging. Some features at the PET-CT scan can help distinguish rheumatoid nodules from malignancy, such as poor FDG uptake of the lesion or draining lymph nodes.

Focus on

Nonintubated Video-Assisted Thoracoscopic Surgery (VATS) in ILD

According to several studies, ILD patients who undergo intubated video-assisted surgical lung biopsy (VASLB) with the intent to collect lung tissue specimens are affected by an elevated rate of complications and mortality (up to 30% and 4%, respectively). Therefore, clinicians and thoracic surgeons rarely accept it in routine clinical practice for purely diagnostic purposes. On the other hand, awake-VASLB with single-lung ventilation seems to involve lower postoperative morbidities and mortality in frail patients such as those with ILD. This should be related to an anesthesiological approach that avoids neuromuscular blocking agents and allows maintaining a patient's spontaneous ventilation. This allows the patient to maintain spontaneous ventilation and reduces the risk of respiratory complications during mechanical ventilation, such as diaphragmatic dysfunctions, upper airway muscle weakness, and airway obstruction. For the same reason, in several studies, nonintubated VATS has proved to be a feasible technique for primary lung cancer surgery in patients with impaired pulmonary function and those considered at high risk for intubated general anesthesia.

On the other hand, deep anesthesia during VATS can induce hypecapnia, and this is easier to manage when the patient is intubated. Moreover, the occurrence of a complication during the procedure could require intubation, and this would be an emergent situation. Therefore, it is preferable to avoid awake-VATS in obese patients and those with a problematic oropharyngeal configuration.

LEARNING POINTS

- The diagnosis of IPF may be changed in favor of CDT-related ILD during follow-up due to the appearance of typical symptoms and changes in the autoimmunity profile.
- RA-ILD may occur with all radiological patterns of interstitial pneumonia, but the most common is the UIP, followed by the NSIP.
- Nonintubated VATS may allow for a wedge resection of a lung nodule in ILD patients with a lower risk for acute lung exacerbations or additional severe side effects compared with intubated techniques.
- Differentiating a rheumatoid nodule from lung cancer in a patient with RA-related ILD may require histological examination.
- Nintedanib is an effective antifibrotic in CTD-related ILDs with progressive fibrosis and can be combined with immunosuppressive drugs.

Further Reading

Jeganathan N, Cleland D, Sathananthan M. The association of lung cancer with pulmonary fibrosis. *ERJ Open Res*. 2022;8:00505-2021.

Kadura S, Raghu G. Rheumatoid arthritis-interstitial lung disease: manifestations and current concepts in pathogenesis and management. *Eur Respir Rev*. 2021;30(160):210011.

Koslow M, Young JR, Yi JES, et al. Rheumatoid pulmonary nodules: clinical and imaging features compared with malignancy. *Eur Radiol*. 2019;29(4):1684-1692.

Rabaneda EF, Atienza-Mateo B, Blanco R, et al. Efficacy and safety of abatacept in interstitial lung disease of rheumatoid arthritis: a systematic literature review. *Autoimmun Rev*. 2021;20(6):102830.

Raghu G, Remy-Jardin M, Myers JL, et al. American Thoracic Society, European Respiratory Society, Japanese Respiratory Society, and Latin American Thoracic Society. Diagnosis of idiopathic pulmonary fibrosis. An official ATS/ERS/JRS/ALAT clinical practice guideline. *Am J Respir Crit Care Med*. 2018;198(5): e44-e68.

Tomassetti S, Christian G, Ryu JH, et al. The impact of lung cancer on survival of idiopathic pulmonary fibrosis. *Chest*. 2015;147(1):157-164.

Wells AU. New insights into the treatment of CTD-ILD. *Nat Rev Rheumatol*. 2021;17:79-80.

Wells AU, Flaherty KR, Brown KK, et al. Nintedanib in patients with progressive fibrosing interstitial lung diseases—subgroup analyses by interstitial lung disease diagnosis in the INBUILD trial: a randomised, double-blind, placebo-controlled, parallel-group trial. *Lancet Respir Med*. 2020;8(5):453-460.

CHAPTER 13

Interstitial Lung Disease With High-Resolution Computed Tomography Pattern of Usual Interstitial Pneumonia in a Patient With Unknown Systemic Sclerosis

Carlo Vancheri ■ Gianluca Sambataro ■ Claudio Sorino

History of Present Illness

A 61-year-old Caucasian man presented to the outpatient pulmonology clinic due to dyspnea that had progressively worsened over the past 2 years.

He previously consulted his general practitioner, who suggested performing a chest radiograph and then a high-resolution computed tomography (HRCT) scan of the chest. This revealed an interstitial lung disease (ILD) characterized by diffuse honeycombing with subpleural and basal predominance, associated with traction bronchiectasis and areas of ground-glass opacities superimposed on reticulations (Fig. 13.1). The radiological findings were classified as a usual interstitial pneumonia (UIP) pattern.

For this reason, he was invited to undergo a consultation with a pulmonologist, who hypothesized a diagnosis of idiopathic pulmonary fibrosis (IPF) and sent the patient to the regional referral center for rare lung diseases in order to set the appropriate treatment.

Past Medical History

The patient was a tradesman, with no reported significant exposure to noxious agents. He was a mild former smoker (calculated 12 pack-years) who quit about 10 years before the visit. He took daily medication for slight systemic hypertension (ramipril 2.5 mg once a day). Recently, another pulmonologist introduced oral prednisone 37.5 mg/day and oxygen supplement at 2 L/min due to the evidence of respiratory failure already at rest.

Physical Examination and Early Clinical Findings

At the first assessment in the regional referral center for rare lung diseases, the patient showed severe dyspnea for minimal exertion. He was apyretic and had slightly increased blood pressure (140/85 mmHg). The heart rate was 111 beats/min, whereas the respiratory rate was 21 breaths/minute. Chronic type 1 respiratory failure was confirmed: oxygen saturation (SpO_2) at rest was 87% in room air, with pO_2 54.4 mmHg and pCO_2 36.8 mmHg at the arterial blood gas analysis. He reached SpO_2 of 92% with 2 L/min oxygen supplement. On chest examination, there were bilateral Velcro-like crackles in the mid-low lung fields. The patient complained of gastroesophageal reflux but no other symptoms compatible with connective tissue diseases (CTDs).

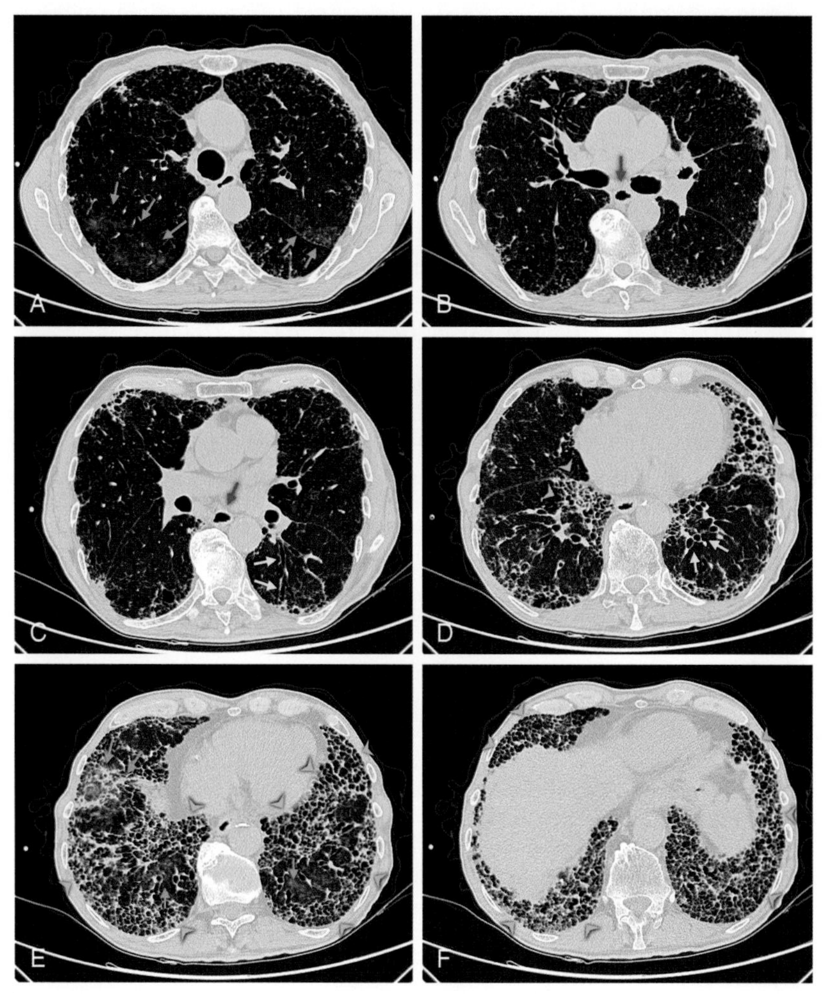

Fig. 13.1 High-resolution chest CT scan (lung parenchyma window) showing diffuse basal honeycombing (green arrowheads) and traction bronchiectasis (yellow arrows), which are both key radiological features of the usual interstitial pneumonia pattern. Some dilation of the esophagus (red arrows) and sporadic ground-glass opacities (light blue arrows) can also be noticed.

Discussion Topic 1

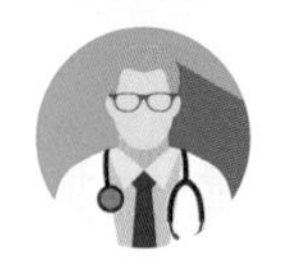

Pulmonologist A

Clinical and radiological findings all point to idiopathic pulmonary fibrosis (IPF).

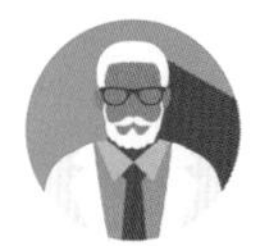

Radiologist

I agree. Honeycombing is a major high-resolution computed tomography (HRCT) criterion for usual interstitial pneumonia (UIP)-IPF when seen with a basal and peripheral predominance. A varying degree of ground-glass attenuation is common but, as in this case, should not predominate.

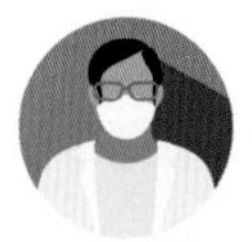

Pulmonologist B

However, it's important to exclude other interstitial lung diseases (ILDs) that may occur with a radiological UIP pattern.

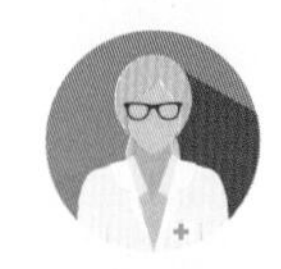

Pulmonologist C

In my opinion, a CTD-associated ILD should be considered because honeycomb cysts are extensive. A honeycombing occupying > 70% of the fibrotic portions of the lung is called an "exuberant honeycombing sign," which raises the suspicion of CTD.

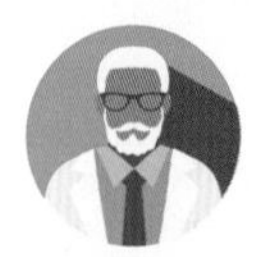

Radiologist

Also, there's some dilation of the esophagus, which is a sign compatible with systemic sclerosis (SSc). It occurs in about three-quarters of patients and appears to be related to the development of ILD.

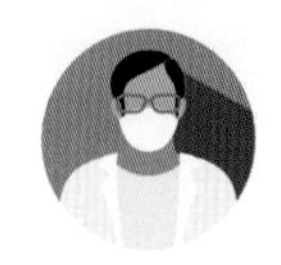

Pulmonologist B

We will have our rheumatologist visit the patient.

The patient was evaluated by a rheumatologist who used to work alongside the pulmonologists as part of the unit's multidisciplinary team. During the physical examination, the rheumatologist found a microstomia (i.e., limited mouth opening due to tightening and hardening of the skin around the mouth) and thickening of the skin on the hands proximal to the metacarpophalangeal joints, as well as proximal to the elbows and knees, without any sign of acral ulcers or pitting scars (Fig. 13.2). The rheumatologist suspected an SSc in a diffuse subset; he subjected the patient to a nailfold videocapillaroscopy (NVC) directly at the first assessment. NVC was positive for a "late" scleroderma pattern, characterized by a low number of giant capillaries and extensive avascular areas (Fig. 13.3). Considering that the patient did not refer symptoms compatible with Raynaud phenomenon (RP), he underwent a provoking test, clearly showing a complete RP. Therefore, the patient was invited to gradually reduce corticosteroids and to have blood tests including autoimmunity. A week later, the diagnosis of SSc was further confirmed by the presence of antinuclear antibodies (ANA) 1:640 with nucleolar staining and anti-Scl70 positivity at a high titer.

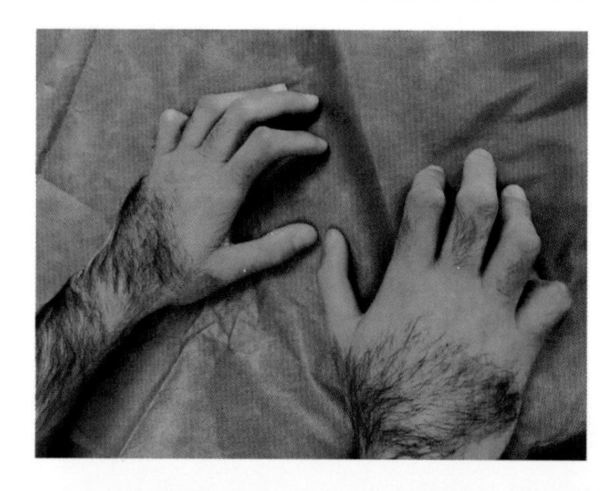

Fig. 13.2 Skin thickening proximal to metacarpophalangeal joints.

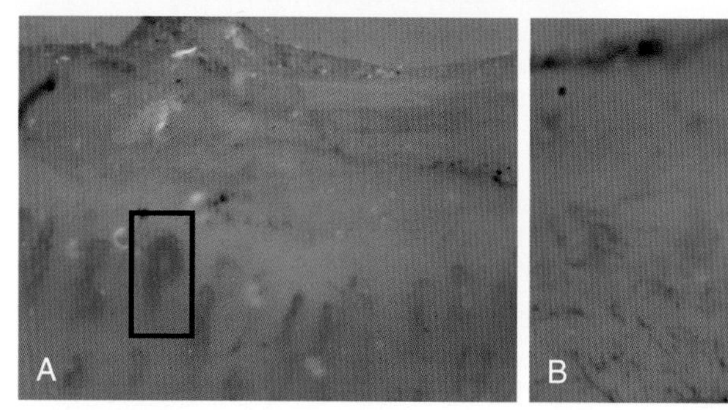

Fig. 13.3 Nailfold videocapillaroscopy (NVC) showing a single giant capillary (A) and a large avascular area due to severe capillary loss (B). The presence of giant capillaries on NVC has a specificity for SSc > 95%. They are the hallmark of the "early" and "active" scleroderma patterns, whereas the "late" scleroderma pattern is characterized by the combination of severe loss of capillaries combined with abnormal shapes.

Discussion Topic 2

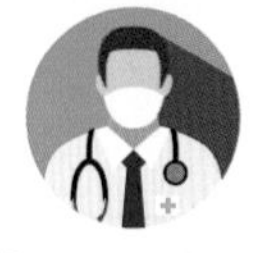

Rheumatologist

The clinical picture, together with the instrumental and laboratory findings, is pathognomonic for SSc.

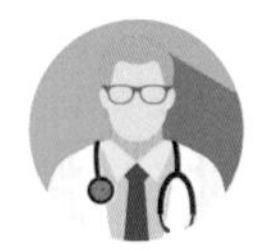

Pulmonologist A

So is the ILD secondary to the SSc? I believed it was IPF as HRCT shows a UIP pattern.

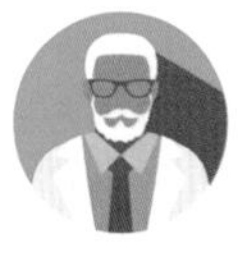

Radiologist

Indeed, nonspecific interstitial pneumonia (NSIP) is the most common interstitial pattern of SSc-ILD, found in more than two-thirds of patients. However, ILD in advanced CTDs may occur with a radiological UIP pattern.

Discussion Topic 2 (Continued)

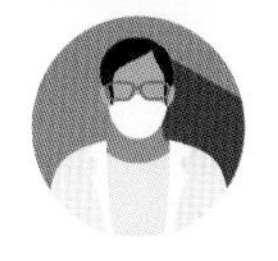

Pulmonologist B

Unlike this case, ILD is more commonly found in an individual with a previous diagnosis of SSc.

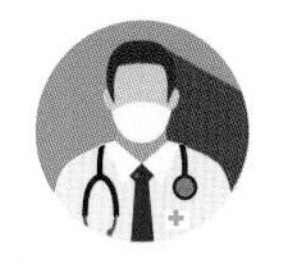

Rheumatologist

Sometimes the patient barely notices the symptoms, as they come on gradually. We cannot accurately estimate the disease duration of the patient, but, based on the extension of the skin involvement, probably SSc started > 3 years before our assessment.

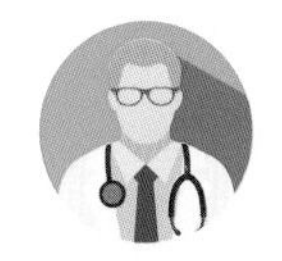

Pulmonologist A

Could a lung biopsy give us additional information?

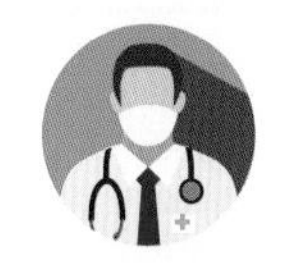

Rheumatologist

The diagnosis is confident. I believe that the risk of acute exacerbation could exceed the utility of the information we could obtain.

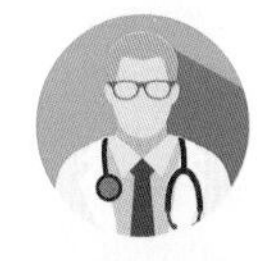

Pulmonologist A

I get it. And what for treatment?

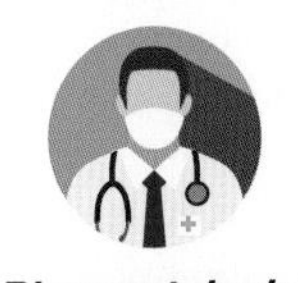

Rheumatologist

High doses of corticosteroids in SSc put the patient at risk for scleroderma renal crisis, which is a rare but life-threatening complication. As our patient is stable, we should significantly reduce steroids and start immunosuppression therapy.

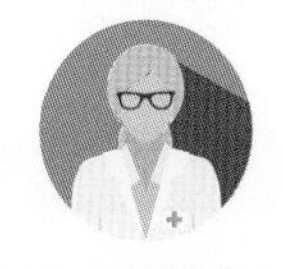

Pulmonologist C

The radiological pattern is mainly fibrotic rather than inflammatory. Why do you think that immunosuppressants can be effective in this patient?

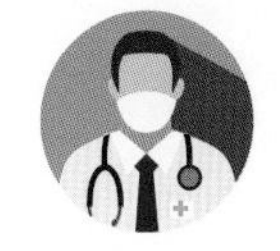

Rheumatologist

The pathogenesis of the disease is inflammatory, and it's associated with a high risk for different visceral involvement. Immunosuppressive drugs can prevent or reduce other systemic manifestations. Despite the fibrotic pattern, we can assume effectiveness anyway.

Continued on following page

Discussion Topic 2 (Continued)

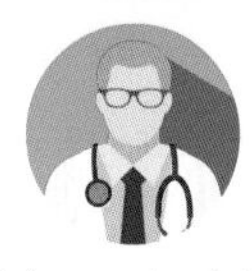

Pulmonologist A

I'll schedule pulmonary function tests (PFTs) including measurement of lung diffusion. Will the patient need any more tests?

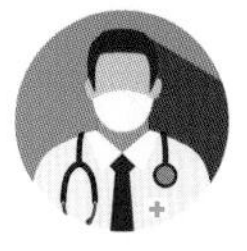

Rheumatologist

He should undergo transthoracic echocardiography to estimate pulmonary arterial hypertension and evaluate the presence of pericardial effusions, although there is no trace of the latter on the chest CT.
Additionally, electrocardiography and Holter monitor could be useful in detecting arrhythmias.

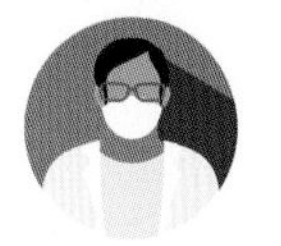

Pulmonologist B

We should establish a follow-up with periodic clinic visits, blood tests, and pulmonary function evaluation.

Clinical Course

At the confirmation of the diagnosis, the patient underwent PFTs, which showed a restrictive pattern with forced vital capacity (FVC) of 55% predicted and total lung capacity (TLC) of 59% predicted. Diffusion lung capacity for carbon monoxide (DLCO) was also reduced to 42% of predicted. For the treatment of SSc with lung involvement, the patient was put on oral prednisone 7.5 mg daily and mycophenolate mofetil (MMF) 2 g daily. Acetylsalicylic acid 100 mg/day, nifedipine 60 mg/day, and esomeprazole 20 mg/day were also introduced. The patient showed persistent 3-year disease stabilization in terms of symptoms, lung function, and imaging. He tolerated the treatment well, without significant side effects, and the sole new clinical change was the onset of anxiety requiring therapy.

After this period of time, the patient complained of worsening dyspnea without a fever and needed a higher oxygen supplement at rest. Significant functional deterioration was found on PFTs with FVC 44% predicted (11% decline) and DLCO 28% predicted. The patient performed a new chest HRCT scan that showed a reduction of ground-glass opacity with no other signs of acute infection and a more evident UIP pattern (Fig. 13.4). Although the quantitative involvement of the lung was substantially similar to what was observed in the first HRCT, its quality showed a clear fibrotic evolution.

Discussion Topic 3

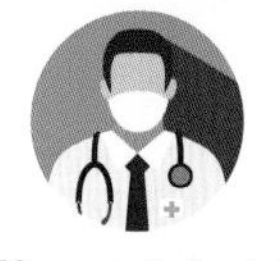

Rheumatologist

After several years of stability, the dyspnea worsened. However, chest HRCT findings are reported as relatively stable. Can you take a look?

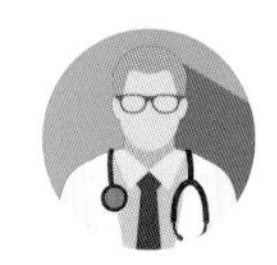

Pulmonologist A

Yes, sure. I agree with the radiologist: the total amount of lung involvement is similar, and the images are not suggestive of infection or acute exacerbation. Nevertheless, the disease most likely progressed.

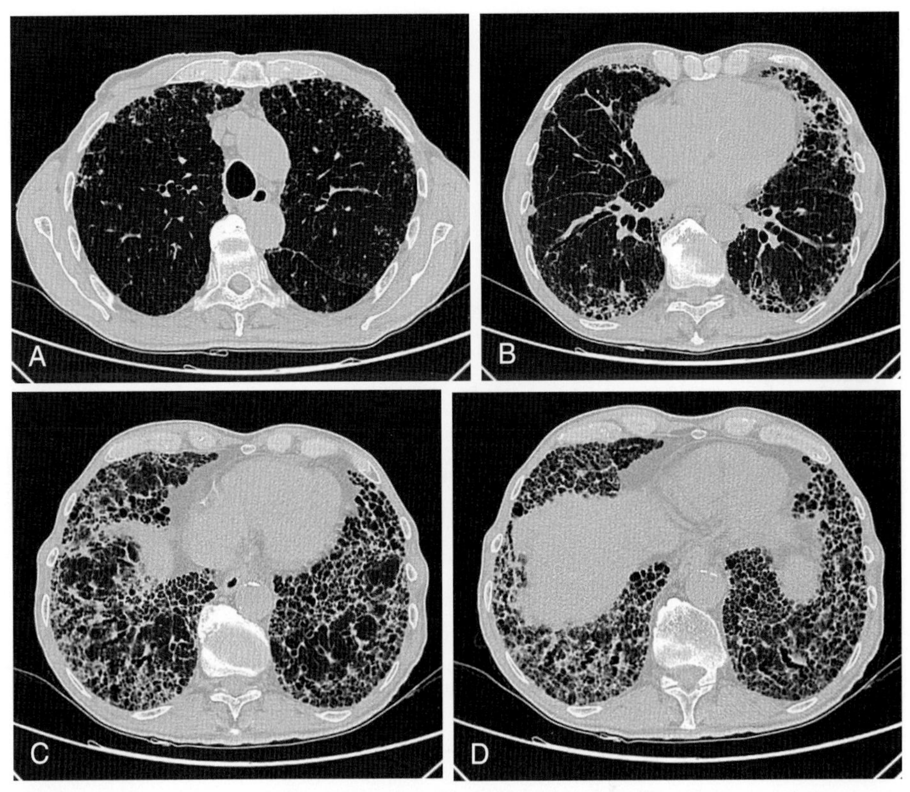

Fig. 13.4 Follow-up HRTC of the chest showing substantially stable UIP pattern without ground-glass superimposed opacities.

Discussion Topic 3 (Continued)

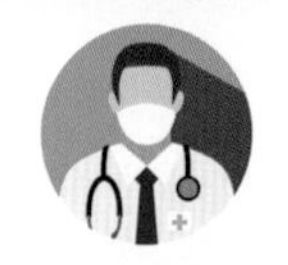

Rheumatologist

What makes you think so?

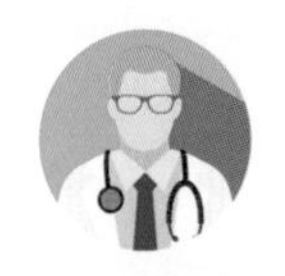

Pulmonologist A

The patient has no clinical or radiological signs of acute exacerbation, yet he is increasingly dyspneic, his oxygen requirement is increased, and lung function is deteriorating.

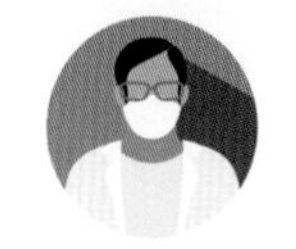

Pulmonologist B

We should do something. In patients with SSc-ILD, a relative decline in FVC of > 10% in 1 year or a decline in FVC of 5% to 10% plus a decline in DLCO of > 15% is a predictor of mortality.

Continued on following page

Discussion Topic 3 (Continued)

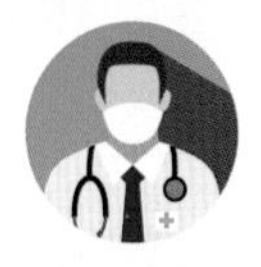

Rheumatologist

Is superimposed pulmonary artery hypertension (PAH) possible?

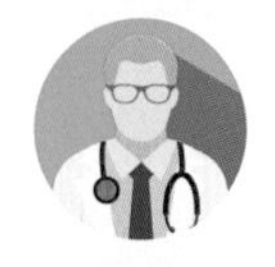

Pulmonologist A

Yes, it can be a cause of worsening dyspnea. However, a new transthoracic echocardiogram showed no parameters suggesting PAH.

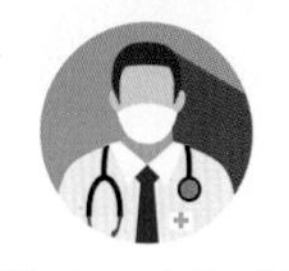

Rheumatologist

I would prescribe a short cycle of intravenous steroids and increase the dosage of mycophenolate mofetil to 3 g/day. What else?

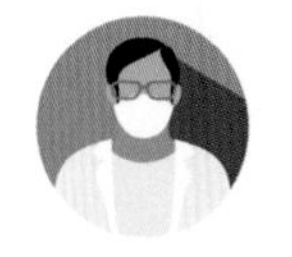

Pulmonologist B

We can also add antifibrotic drugs to slow the disease progression. The patient should be carefully monitored. In case of further worsening, hospitalization and further examinations could be needed.

Recommended Therapy and Further Indications

The new clinical picture was interpreted as a progression of the disease. Therefore, the patient was treated with a high dosage of methylprednisolone (100 mg/day for 3 days), and he started antifibrotic therapy with oral nintedanib 150 mg twice daily, in add-on with MMF that was increased to 3 g/day. The patient acquired new stabilization in 2 months.

Follow-up and Outcomes

After 6 years of follow-up, the patient was in poor, but stable, condition. Interestingly, throughout this period, the patient's RP was responsive to nifedipine without requiring second-line treatment. Despite the diffuse subset of SSc, the patient did not develop any other visceral involvement. Sporadically, he had some traction ulcers on the anterior surface of proximal interphalangeal joints but with relatively rapid healing and very small pitting scars. He had no acral ulcers, calcifications, or pulmonary artery hypertension.

Focus on

Overview of Systemic Sclerosis

SSc is an autoimmune disorder characterized by parallel fibrotic and vascular damage in the skin and internal organs. It is about 4 times more common in women than in men.

Antinuclear antibodies (ANA) may be present in > 90% of cases of SSc, and at least one of the more specific autoantibodies (anti-centromere, anti-SCL70, and anti-RNA polymerase III) is present in up to 70% of the cases. Based on the skin involvement, SSc can be classified as diffuse, limited, or sine scleroderma.

The *diffuse* subset is characterized by a rapid onset and severe fibrotic damage in multiple organs (most frequently, skin, gastrointestinal tract, lungs, kidneys, skeletal muscle, and pericardium).

The *limited* subset was formerly known as the CREST syndrome (due to its main features: calcinosis, Raynaud phenomenon, esophageal dysmotility, sclerodactyly, and telangiectasia). This shows a slower progression but with prevalent vascular damage, acral ulcers, and pulmonary artery hypertension.

In *sine scleroderma* SSc, the patient has SSc-related antibodies and visceral manifestations without skin tightening.

Table 13.1 shows the most used criteria for the diagnosis of SSc.

A skin thickening proximal to the metacarpophalangeal joints can be considered pathognomonic for SSc. Skin involvement and, above all, Raynaud phenomenon (RP) are usually present years before the development of other signs of the disease, although patients often could not pay significant attention to them. As mild RP can be not reported, or even not noted by the patients, provoking test is a useful diagnostic tool in suspected cases. Nailfold videocapillaroscopy is commonly positive in SSc and, in some conditions, such as idiopathic inflammatory myopathies, could be positive regardless of the presence of RP.

Three major categories of capillaroscopic findings are described: “early,” “active,” and “late” patterns.

Currently, lung involvement is the most common cause of death among SSc patients, whereas renal crisis, characterized by malignant hypertension and oligo/anuric acute renal failure, was the leading cause of mortality before the discovery of the angiotensin-converting enzyme (ACE) inhibitors.

TABLE 13.1 ■ **Criteria for the Classification of Systemic Sclerosis According to the European League Against Rheumatism and the American College of Rheumatology. Patients With a Score ≥ 9 Are Considered to Have Definite Systemic Sclerosis (Sensitivity 91%, Specificity 92%)**

	Score
Skin thickening of the fingers of both hands extending proximally to the metacarpophalangeal joints	9
Telangiectasia	2
Abnormal nailfold capillaries	2
Pulmonary arterial hypertension or interstitial lung disease, or both	2
Raynaud phenomenon	3
Skin thickening of the fingers (only count highest score)	
Puffy fingers	2
Sclerodactyly of the fingers	4
Fingertip lesions (only count highest score)	
Digital tip ulcers	2
Fingertip pitting scars	3
Scleroderma-related autoantibodies (e.g., anti-centromere, anti-topoisomerase 1, or anti-RNA polymerase 3)	3

Focus on

Pulmonary Involvement in SSc

Pulmonary involvement in SSc includes interstitial lung disease (ILD) and pulmonary arterial hypertension (PAH). SSc-ILD is more common in the diffuse form of SSc (about half of patients) but can occur in all three subsets and remains a major cause of morbidity and mortality.

Respiratory symptoms are initially nonspecific and comprise dyspnea on exertion and nonproductive cough. Physical examination typically reveals Velcro-like crackles on auscultation in addition to the typical fibrotic changes of the skin.

Pulmonary function tests can be normal in early SSc-ILD. In advanced stages, they reveal restriction, even if some patients may develop a small airway disease with possible additional obstruction.

The diffusing capacity for carbon monoxide (DLCO) is usually reduced, although volume-adjusted values (DLCO/VA) often lie within the normal limits unless there is a vasculopathy such as PAH. A rapid decline in DLCO is the most significant marker of poor outcome.

HRCT of the chest is the gold standard for the diagnosis of SSc-ILD. A nonspecific interstitial pneumonia (NSIP) pattern, with a greater proportion of ground-glass opacities and a less-represented coarse reticulation, can suggest the presence of a CTD and occurs in $>$ 80% of patients with SSc-ILD. However, all the HRCT patterns can be found in SSc-ILD and other CTD-related ILD, being the UIP pattern prevalent in rheumatoid arthritis and longstanding SSc.

Recently, lung ultrasound has been proposed as a screening tool to detect lung involvement in SSc, suggested by the finding of B-lines (lung comet tail signs) that originate from thickened interlobular septa.

Because ILD could be the first or even the sole clinical manifestation of SSc, a first-line panel of autoantibodies including ANA, rheumatoid factors, anti-citrullinated protein antibodies, and anti-extractable nuclear antigens should be performed in all patients diagnosed with ILD.

A complete clinical visit, the search for autoantibodies, and appropriate instrumental assessments with NVC, HRTC, and transthoracic echocardiogram are generally sufficient to assess the diagnosis.

A right heart catheterization is indicated when PAH is suspected, while bronchoalveolar lavage can help to exclude other differential diagnoses, mainly superinfections. The necessity of lung biopsy is rare and should be correctly assessed, balancing the risk for the patient and the diagnostic yield.

Focus on

Comprehensive Management of SSc and Treatment of SSc-ILD

The management of SSc should take into account that it is a systemic disease that often severely affects different organs. Corticosteroids raise the risk for scleroderma renal crisis, reported in about 5% to 25% of patients during clinical history. Disease duration of $<$ 4 years, diffuse and rapidly progressive skin thickening, anemia, urinary casts, increased serum levels of creatinine, and seropositivity are other well-known risk factors. Angiotensin-converting enzyme (ACE) antagonists are useful for the management of this life-threatening manifestation.

Severe dyspnea can be also associated with PAH. The presence of this complication should be considered in any patient, and in particular in those with significant dyspnea not associated with severe ILD. The DETECT algorithm is useful for the identification of patients at risk of PAH. It can be suspected in the presence of high serum levels of NT-proBNP, urate, anti-centromere antibodies, telangiectasias (currently or formerly), FVC%/DLCO% $<$ 1.6, longstanding disease, and RP. Possible treatment includes prostaglandins, endothelin receptor antagonists, and phosphodiesterase inhibitors, alone or in combination.

Gastroesophageal reflux is one of the most common clinical signs of SSc; it is also associated with almost all other kinds of ILDs. Proton pump inhibitors can be useful, at least to improve the quality of life of these patients.

The infusion of iloprost can be useful to treat and prevent severe RP and ulcers. Bosentan, an endothelin receptor antagonist, also has been proved to prevent new digital ulcers.

In the past decades, ILD became the main cause of mortality in SSc. The prognosis seems to be not associated with the HRCT pattern, mortality in UIP patients in several reports was similar to NSIP patients. Despite the common presence of an NSIP pattern associated with SSc, a long-term high dosage of steroids (15–20 mg/day) should be avoided for the above-mentioned risk of renal crisis.

Pulse cyclophosphamide and mycophenolate mofetil (MMF) are the first-line treatment, but generally the latter is preferred due to the better safety profile. Cyclophosphamide should be considered as a potentially useful treatment for progressive ILD-SSc. Azathioprine could be used in mild forms; however,

Focus on (Continued)

Comprehensive Management of SSc and Treatment of SSc-ILD

MMF proved to be superior. Some evidence of efficacy has been reported for rituximab, an anti-CD20 monoclonal antibody, also improving FVC. The blockage of the interleukin-6 pathway through tocilizumab also proved to stabilize FVC in early SSc with elevated C-reactive protein. Recently, nintedanib was approved for the treatment of progressive fibrosing SSc-ILD, proving to reduce the decline of FVC by about 50% in this subset of patients. Subgroup analysis proved that antifibrotic treatment with nintedanib could be useful mainly when associated with conventional immunosuppressive treatment. In patients with ILD other than IPF and radiological evidence of pulmonary fibrosis, progressive pulmonary fibrosis (PPF) is currently defined as at least two of the following three criteria occurring within the past year with no alternative explanation: (1) worsening respiratory symptoms, (2) physiological evidence of disease progression, and (3) radiological evidence of disease progression. Details on the current criteria suggested to define PPF are shown in Table 13.2

Finally, it should be highlighted that significant immunosuppression was associated with acute exacerbation of UIP pattern secondary to idiopathic pulmonary fibrosis but not SSc-ILD; therefore, the correct diagnostic assessment is crucial to establish the appropriate treatment.

LEARNING POINTS

- Interstitial lung disease (ILD) is a frequent complication of systemic sclerosis (SSc) both in the limited and diffuse form.
- SSc-ILD is often progressive and has a poor prognosis.
- Nonspecific interstitial pneumonia (NSIP) is the most common HRCT pattern in CTD-related ILD, although usual interstitial pneumonia (UIP) can also be found, especially in rheumatoid arthritis and longstanding SSc.
- When chest HRCT shows an NSIP or a UIP pattern in a patient with SSc, confirmatory lung biopsy is usually not required for the diagnosis of SSc-ILD.
- Long-term high-dose corticosteroids in SSc should be avoided as they raise the risk of renal crisis.
- Randomized placebo-controlled trials demonstrated that nintedanib reduces the rate of FVC decline in patients with SSc-ILD as well as chronic fibrosing ILDs with a progressive phenotype.

TABLE 13.2 ■ **Suggested Criteria for the Definition of Progressive Pulmonary Fibrosis (PPF)**

1. Worsening respiratory symptoms
2. Physiological evidence of disease progression (either of the following): a. Absolute decline in FVC ≥ 5% predicted within 1 year of follow-up b. Absolute decline in DLCO (corrected for hemoglobin) ≥ 10% predicted within 1 year of follow-up
3. Radiological evidence of disease progression (one or more of the following): a. Increased extent or severity of traction bronchiectasis and bronchiolectasis b. New ground-glass opacity with traction bronchiectasis c. New fine reticulation d. Increased extent or increased coarseness of reticular abnormality e. New or increased honeycombing f. Increased lobar volume loss

The exclusion of alternative explanations of worsening features in patients with suspected progression is crucial. Particular attention should be paid to those without clear evidence of worsened HRCT chest findings.

Reprinted with permission of the American Thoracic Society. Raghu G, Remy-Jardin M, Richeldi L, et al. Idiopathic Pulmonary Fibrosis (an Update) and Progressive Pulmonary Fibrosis in Adults: An Official ATS/ERS/JRS/ALAT Clinical Practice Guideline. *Am J Respir Crit Care Med.* 2022 May 1;205(9):e18-e47. The American Journal of Respiratory and Critical Care Medicine is an official journal of the American Thoracic Society.

Further Reading

Coghlan JG, Denton CP, Grunig E, et al. Evidence-based detection of pulmonary arterial hypertension systemic sclerosis: the DETECT study. *Ann Rheum Dis.* 2014;73:1340-1349.

Gabrielli A, Avvedimento EV, Krieg T. Scleroderma. *N Engl J Med.* 2009;360:1989-2003.

Hoffmann-Vold AM, Allanore Y, Alves M, et al; EUSTAR collaborators. Progressive interstitial lung disease in patients with systemic sclerosis-associated interstitial lung disease in the EUSTAR database. *Ann Rheum Dis.* 2021;80(2):219-227.

Konopka KE, Myers JL. Interstitial lung disease pathology in systemic sclerosis. *Ther Adv Musculoskelet Dis.* 2021;13:1759720X211032437.

Kowal-Bielecka O, Fransen J, Avouac J, et al. Update of EULAR recommendations fot the treatment of systemic sclerosis. *Ann Rheum Dis.* 2017;76:1327-1339.

Mouthon L, Bussone G, Bereznè A, et al. Scleroderma renal crisis. *J Rheumatol.* 2014;41:1040-1048.

Raghu G, Remy-Jardin M, Richeldi L, et al. Idiopathic pulmonary fibrosis (an update) and progressive pulmonary fibrosis in adults: an official ATS/ERS/JRS/ALAT clinical practice guideline. *Am J Respir Crit Care Med.* 2022;205(9):e18-e47.

Roofeh D, Jaafar S, Vummi D, Khanna D. Management of systemic sclerosis-associated interstitial lung disease. *Curr Opin Rheumatol.* 2019;31:241-249.

Sambataro D, Sambataro G, Libra A, et al. Nailfold videocapillaroscopy is a useful tool to recognize definite forms of systemic sclerosis and idiopathic inflammatory myositis in interstitial lung disease patients. *Diagnostics (Basel).* 2020;10:523.

Sambataro D, Sambataro G, Pignataro F, et al. Patients with interstitial lung disease secondary to autoimmune diseases: how to recognize them? *Diagnostics (Basel).* 2020;10:208.

Steen VD, Medsger TA. Changes in causes of death in systemic sclerosis, 1972–2002. *Ann Rheum Dis.* 2007;66:940-944.

Van Den Hoogen F, Khanna D, Fransen J, et al. 2013 Classification Criteria for Systemic Sclerosis: an American College of Rheumatology/European League Against Rheumatism collaborative initiative. *Ann Rheum Dis.* 2013;72:1747-1755.

CHAPTER 14

Interstitial Lung Disease Associated With the Antisynthetase Syndrome

Sonye Karen Danoff ■ Claudio Sorino ■ Stacey-Anne Brown

History of Present Illness

A 40-year-old woman presented to the outpatient interstitial lung disease (ILD) clinic for a second opinion due to progressive dyspnea and cough for the past year. She was first noted to have symptoms 1 year prior to presentation, and a high-resolution computed tomography (HRCT) scan of the chest demonstrated a reticular interstitial pattern in the lower zones. An initial autoimmune serology was negative, and a lung biopsy was suggested but the patient declined and was lost to follow-up.

Shortly before being seen in the ILD clinic, she re-presented to her local pulmonologist with morning stiffness without obvious joint swelling, worsening cough, and exertional dyspnea. Pulmonary function tests at that time demonstrated moderate restrictive impairment and moderate gas transfer defect (Fig 14.1). A new chest HRCT (Fig 14.2) showed lower lobe predominant peripheral reticulation with extensive ground-glass opacities, traction bronchiectasis, and areas of subpleural sparing. An autoimmune workup was repeated, and a low-titer (1:40) antinuclear antibody (ANA) level with cytoplasmic pattern was found. A surgical lung biopsy was performed, and histology was interpreted as unclassifiable pattern of fibrosis with lymphocytic inflammation and occasional giant cells. She was placed empirically on prednisone 0.5 mg/kg per day and referred to the ILD clinic for further evaluation.

Past Medical History

The patient was a never smoker, and she worked as a veterinary technician, with intermittent exposure to pet birds and rodents. The only pertinent past medical history was obesity, acid reflux controlled on proton pump inhibitor and lifestyle modification, and postnasal drip. She had no family history of rheumatological or pulmonary disease.

Physical Examination and Early Clinical Findings

Physical examination was notable for a pleasant woman in no acute distress, who was morbidly obese (body mass index 38.92 kg/m^2), hypertensive (blood pressure 150/90 mmHg), afebrile, and with an oxygen saturation of 99% on room air. She had a normal cardiopulmonary examination but with digital fissuring and hyperkeratosis of the medial surfaces of her second digits bilaterally, so-called "mechanic's hands" (Fig 14.3). She had no joint swelling or tenosynovitis.

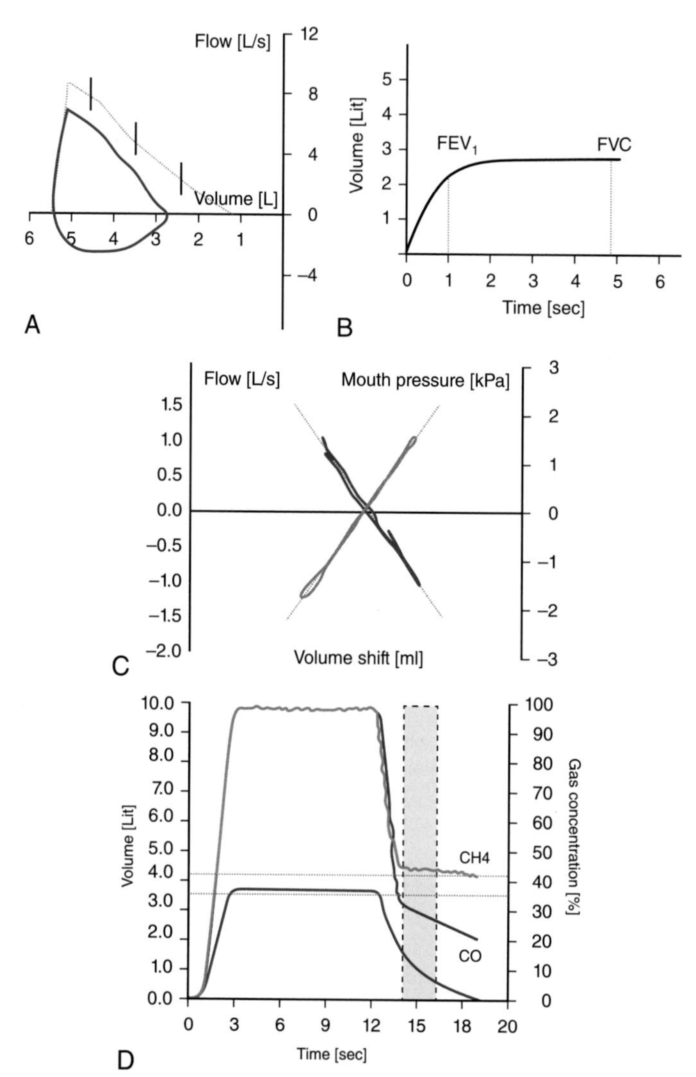

Index	Measured	Predicted	Z-Score	LLN	ULN	% Predicted
FEV_1 (Lit)	2,28	2,995	-1,925	2,386	3,586	76,12
FVC (Lit)	2,85	3,654	-1,792	2,914	4,421	78
FEV_1/FVC	0,8	0,824	-0,389	0,713	0,915	97,09
TLC (Lit)	4,10	5,187	-1,927	4,251	6,224	79,05
RV (Lit)	0,8	1,285	-1,376	0,72	2,046	62,26
RV/TLC	19,51	24,618	-0,852	14,986	35,071	79,26
DLCO	12,54	21,355		16,9	26,649	58,72

E FEV_1, forced expiratory volume in 1 second; LLN, lower limit of normal; LLN, upper limit of normal; FVC, forced vital capacity; RV, residual volume; TLC, total lung capacity; DLCO, diffusing capacity of the lungs for carbon monoxide.

Fig 14.1 Pulmonary function tests at clinical presentation. (A) Flow-volume curve; (B) volume-time curve; (C) plethysmography; (D) single-breath diffusing capacity of the lung for CO; (E) measured parameters. There is a moderate restriction with $FEV_1/FVC > LLN$, $TLC < LLN$, $FEV_1 < 80\%$ predicted (z-score between –2 and –2.5) and a moderate reduction in diffusing capacity.

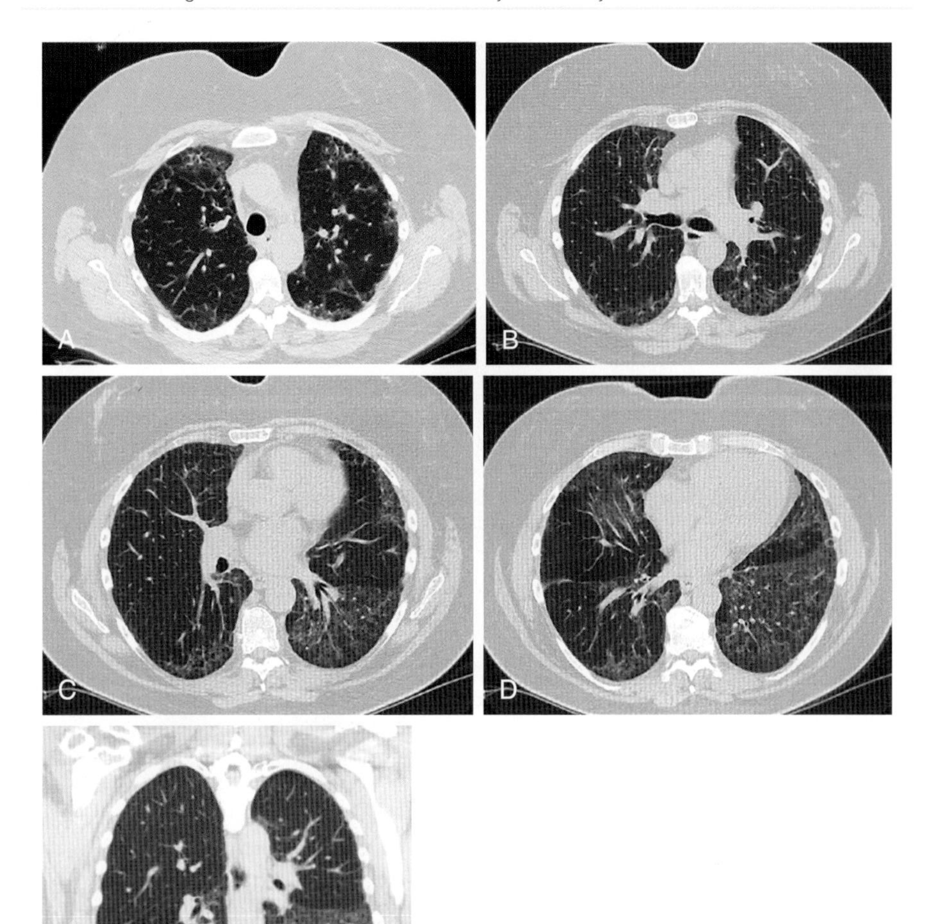

Fig 14.2 Chest CT scan (lung window setting) in the axial (A–D) and coronal (E) plane showing an ILD with lower lobe predominant peripheral reticulation, ground-glass opacities, traction bronchiectasis, and areas of subpleural sparing.

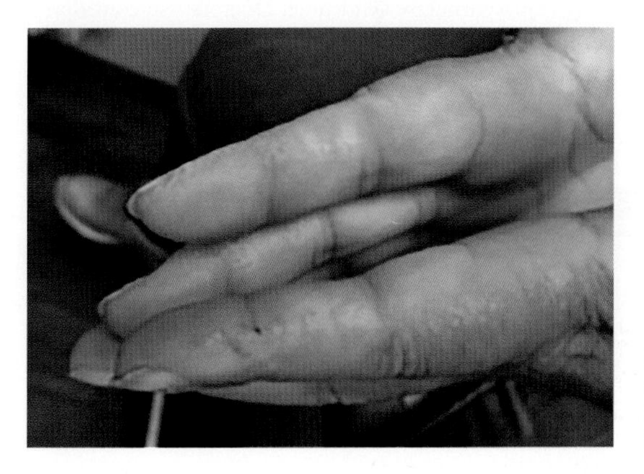

Fig 14.3 Photo of the patient's hands showing digital fissuring and hyperkeratosis of the medial surfaces of her second fingers ("mechanic's hands").

Discussion Topic 1

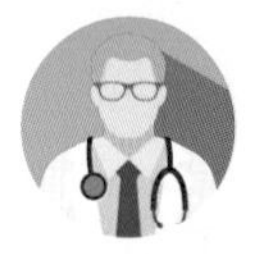

Pulmonologist A

Our patient has an ILD with a reticular interstitial pattern in the lower lung zones. There is no honeycombing and she is a young woman who never smoked, so there is no element pointing toward idiopathic pulmonary fibrosis (IPF).

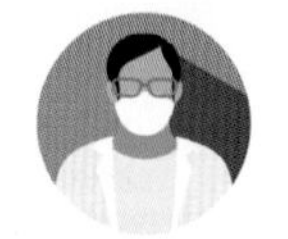

Pulmonologist B

It's probably the worsening of a chronic disease. The patient began having symptoms at least a year ago.

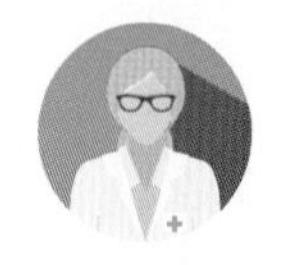

Pulmonologist C

Imaging doesn't have the appearance of postinfectious scarring, nor the distribution of chronic interstitial edema. What about ILD associated with connective tissue disease?

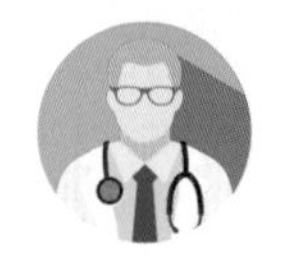

Pulmonologist A

I think it's very likely. Her mechanic's hands make me think of an ILD associated with antisynthetase syndrome or dermatomyositis.

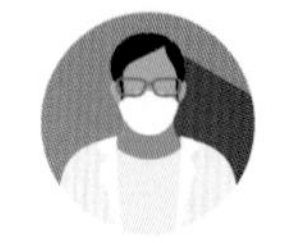

Pulmonologist B

She has exposure to birds. Hypersensitivity pneumonitis should also be considered in the differential diagnosis.

Clinical Course

Given the patient's examination findings of mechanic's hands, joint pain with morning stiffness, and ILD, the leading differential diagnosis was antisynthetase syndrome. Doctors also considered hypersensitivity pneumonitis, given her occupational exposure to birds. Further testing involved laboratory evaluation of myositis-specific and myositis-associated antibodies to complete the autoimmune workup. Her myositis autoantibody panel showed a positive anti–PL-12 antibody.

Discussion Topic 2

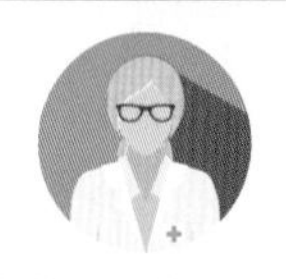

Pulmonologist C

Can myositis present without any evidence of typical skin rash or muscle weakness?

Discussion Topic 2 (Continued)

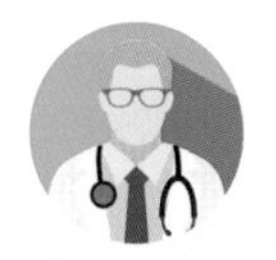

Pulmonologist A

The antisynthetase syndrome is characterized by the presence of one of eight currently known autoantibodies against the aminoacyl transfer RNA (tRNA) synthetases, the most common being anti–Jo-1. Symptoms may include myositis, skin findings (including mechanic's hands), inflammatory arthritis, fever, Raynaud phenomenon, and ILD. ILD may be the first, only, or most prominent feature of antisynthetase syndrome.

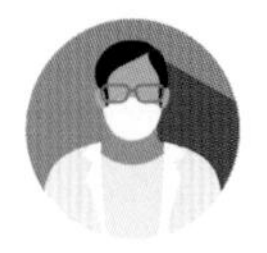

Pulmonologist B

Would you have expected a higher ANA titer with antisynthetase syndrome?

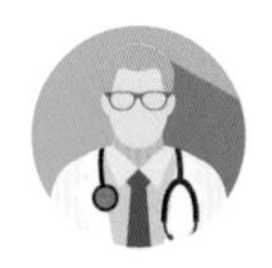

Pulmonologist A

ANA may be negative in antisynthetase syndrome, but when positive, the pattern is typically cytoplasmic since the aminoacyl tRNA synthetases are cytoplasmic proteins.

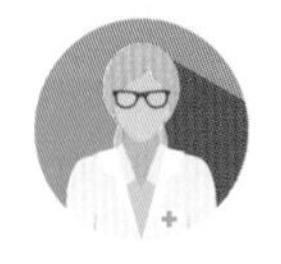

Pulmonologist C

Why was her surgical pathology so ambiguous?

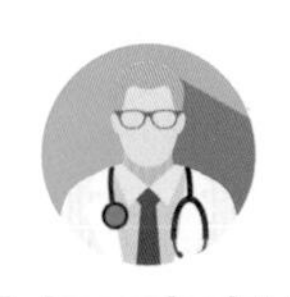

Pulmonologist A

Pathologic findings in ILD associated with myositis may be broad and include nonspecific interstitial pneumonia, usual interstitial pneumonia, unclassifiable fibrosis, and organizing pneumonia. Diffuse alveolar damage can be seen when ILD presents acutely. Histopathology is typically not needed when a connective tissue disorder (CTD) is present at diagnosis. In this case, a surgical biopsy may not have been needed had further serologic testing been performed initially. Many features of her presentation were suggestive of a CTD-associated ILD, including her age, sex, imaging findings, and reported symptoms.

Recommended Therapy and Further Indications

Doctors confirmed the diagnosis of antisynthetase syndrome; the patient was initiated on steroid-sparing therapy (in this case, mycophenolate mofetil), and her prednisone was slowly weaned over several months. She was referred for co-management with rheumatology for other organ surveillance.

Discussion Topic 3

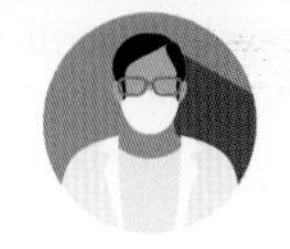

Pulmonologist B

What autoantibodies are typically tested if there is a concern for antisynthetase syndrome?

Continued on following page

Discussion Topic 3 (Continued)

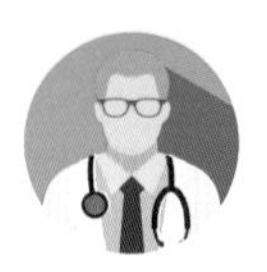

Pulmonologist A

The antisynthetase antibodies include Jo-1 (His-RS), PL-7 (Thr-RS), PL-12 (Ala-RS), OJ (Ile-RS), EJ (Gly-RS), and KS (Asn-RS). In addition to these autoantibodies, we often test for anti-MDA5, which is another myositis-specific antibody, as well as Ro52, a myositis-associated antibody.

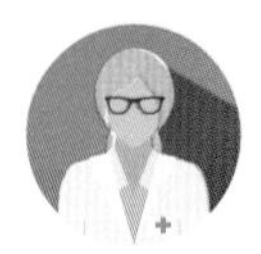

Pulmonologist C

What other features can be seen in patients with antisynthetase syndrome?

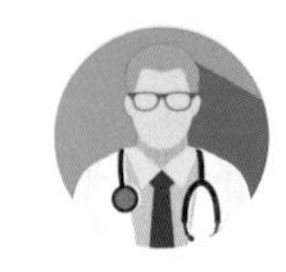

Pulmonologist A

Patients with antisynthetase syndrome can present with a broad spectrum of systemic symptoms including fever as well as the skin findings typical for dermatomyositis including Gottron papules and a heliotrope, as well as mechanic's hands. Calcinosis may also be present. Hair loss is also a common presenting complaint. Finally, muscle pain or weakness can be present.

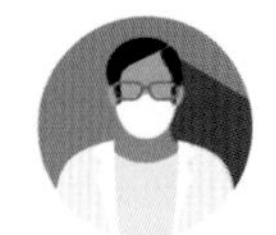

Pulmonologist B

Do all patients with antisynthetase present in the subacute fashion that this patient did?

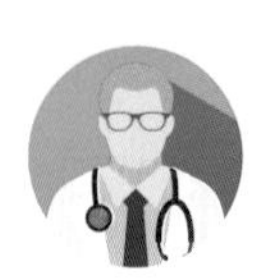

Pulmonologist A

The presentation of ILD in antisynthetase syndrome can vary from subclinical (present on imaging but with no apparent symptoms) to fulminant disease with rapid respiratory failure. The initial treatment of the ILD should be matched to the symptom burden and acuity of disease progression. Very rapid progression often will necessitate hospital admission and treatment with intravenous pulse steroids. In this case, while the patient had progressive symptoms, the rate of progression was over weeks to months and she had relatively preserved pulmonary function tests, so she was started on a steroid-sparing agent as an outpatient and her steroids were tapered.

Follow-up and Outcomes

Fortunately, this patient improved with the institution of a steroid-sparing agent and was able to taper off prednisone. She had monitoring safety labs to limit the risk from her immunosuppressive therapy. Pulmonary function tests were evaluated every 3 months for the first year and demonstrated improving lung function, which correlated with her improved functional capacity. She also participated in pulmonary rehabilitation, which contributed to improved strength and endurance. She was counseled on weight loss to achieve a healthier BMI. She underwent age-appropriate cancer screening. She was also encouraged to remain up to date on her vaccinations. After 1 year from her ILD consultation, she was continuing on mycophenolate.

TABLE 14.1 ■ **Myositis Subtypes by Association With Interstitial Lung Disease**

Myositis subtypes associated with ILD
• Dermatomyositis
• Clinically amyopathic dermatomyositis
• Polymyositis
• Myositis overlap syndromes
• Antisynthetase syndrome
Myositis not typically associated with ILD
• Inclusion body myositis
• Immune-mediated necrotizing myositis

Focus on

Overview of Idiopathic Inflammatory Myopathies and Associated ILD

Idiopathic inflammatory myopathies (IIMs) are a diverse group of autoimmune disorders usually characterized by muscle weakness and inflammation; however, extramuscular manifestations are often present. Historically, the three major subgroups were polymyositis, dermatomyositis (DM), and inclusion body myositis. However, the discovery of several myositis-specific and myositis-associated antibodies has expanded the existing subgroups to include clinically amyopathic dermatomyositis (CADM), overlap myositis syndrome, the antisynthetase syndrome, and immune-mediated necrotizing myopathy. Of these subgroups, the following are associated with ILD (Table 14.1): the antisynthetase syndrome, CADM, DM, polymyositis, and myositis-overlap syndromes (with features of other rheumatological diseases).

DM involves characteristic skin manifestations and proximal muscle involvement and may present in juvenile and adult forms. Notable skin findings include periorbital heliotrope rash, facial erythema, V-shaped rash on anterior trunk (V-sign) or back (shawl sign), and Gottron papules, which are erythematous papules on the joints of the dorsal surface of the hands that may also be seen on the knees and elbows. Myositis-specific antibodies include anti-melanoma differentiation–associated gene 5 (*MDA5*), anti-transcriptional intermediary factor 1 (TIF1), anti-nuclear matrix protein 2 (NXP2), anti–small ubiquitin–like modifier activating enzyme (SAE), and anti–Mi-2, although 20% of cases are seronegative. CADM is an important subtype characterized by skin and/or extramuscular manifestations only; muscle involvement is often minimal or absent. *MDA5* is associated with CADM as well as rapidly progressive ILD.

Polymyositis was previously defined as the subtype of IIM with chronic muscle weakness without skin findings. Immune-mediated necrotizing myopathy, myositis-overlap syndromes, and the antisynthetase syndrome were often described as polymyositis but are now described as separate entities. Polymyositis now exists as a designation of clinical myositis not involving these subgroups.

IIMs are rare diseases, but the exact epidemiology is difficult to characterize given inconsistencies of subgroup classifications across studies, as well as ascertainment bias (in subsets of patients who underwent muscle biopsies or were seen in specialized centers).

ILD is a significant cause of morbidity and mortality in IIMs and occurs in 23% to 53% of patients, with a higher prevalence in Asian individuals with IIMs than in American and European populations. There was a temporal trend with an increasing prevalence reported since 2010, although this may be a result of greater recognition among clinicians and wider availability of clinical myositis autoantibody testing.

Risk factors for developing ILD in IIM include older age, fever, arthralgias, elevated inflammatory markers, and the presence of antisynthetase antibodies and *MDA5* antibodies.

Focus on

Pathobiology of ILD in IIMs

The mechanism by which ILD develops in IIMs is poorly understood. The most common hypothesis is an unidentified environmental trigger leading to autoimmunity in the setting of genetic predisposition. Viral infections have been posited as an inciting event in the development of myositis. Preceding viral infections have been associated with dermatomyositis and polymyositis in a large Swedish nationwide registry. Recently, COVID-19 infection has been associated with the development of dermatomyositis-associated antibodies. Other environmental exposures have been explored. Smoking is an important

Continued on following page

Focus on (Continued)

Pathobiology of ILD in IIMs

exposure associated with anti–Jo-1 positivity and the antisynthetase syndrome in Caucasians but negatively associated with the anti–transcriptional intermediary factor 1 (TIF1) antibody associated with DM. Ultraviolet radiation density and lower latitudes are associated with dermatomyositis. However, the reported associations are weak and not clearly associated with the development of ILD.

Studies have implicated genes of the major histocompatibility complex in the pathogenesis of IIMs. Two landmark genomewide association studies in European populations found that alleles of the MHC 8.1 ancestral haplotype convey the strongest risk of DM/PM. *HLA-DRB1*03-DQA1*05-DQB1*02* was strongly associated with ILD in a UK case-control study of 225 patients with myositis and 527 control subjects. Importantly, while the single nucleotide polymorphism in the promoter region of the mucin 5B *(MUC5B)* gene is associated with sporadic and familial cases of idiopathic pulmonary fibrosis, it has not been shown to be significantly associated with ILD in myositis.

Activated macrophages and $CD8^{+}$ T cells are present in lung specimens of patients with myositis-associated ILD. Several histological patterns of ILD may be present, including nonspecific interstitial pneumonia (NSIP), organizing pneumonia (OP), usual interstitial pneumonia (UIP), lymphocytic interstitial pneumonia (LIP), and an unclassifiable pattern. An NSIP–OP overlap may be observed as well. Data are sparse, as lung biopsies are not routinely performed. NSIP is the most common pattern observed in two case series of patients with DM/polymyositis. In a cohort of 17 patients who underwent surgical lung biopsies, NSIP was observed in 65%, UIP in 12%, OP in 12%, LIP in 6%, and unclassifiable in 6%. Findings were similar in a cohort of 41 biopsy specimens, in which NSIP was observed in 61%, OP in 22%, and UIP in 17%. For patients with respiratory failure or rapidly progressive ILD, the most common histological subtype is diffuse alveolar damage.

Focus on

Clinical Manifestation of ILD in Subgroups of IIMs

The presentation has been summarized as (1) rapidly progressive ILD (RP-ILD), (2) slowly progressive ILD, and (3) asymptomatic disease. Symptomatically, patients may present with progressive dyspnea and cough. Patients may present with ILD without muscle involvement. On physical examination, crackles may be auscultated. For patients with myositis, symmetrical proximal weakness may be observed, and characteristic skin findings based on the subtype of myositis may be observed as outlined here. Radiographically, patients present with interstitial abnormalities or consolidations on HRCT scan. Patients are often restricted on pulmonary function tests, with a reduction in diffusion capacity. We describe the following clinical scenarios based on antibody positivity.

THE ANTISYNTHETASE SYNDROME

The antisynthetase syndrome involves the presence of one of eight autoantibodies against the amino-acyl transfer RNA (tRNA) synthetases, which are cytoplasmic enzymes that connect amino acids to their corresponding tRNA during protein synthesis (Table 14.2).

The classic triad of antisynthetase syndrome includes myositis, interstitial lung disease, and arthritis. Other symptoms include rash, unexplained fever, and Raynaud phenomenon. However, it is less common for patients to experience the complete triad, and symptoms may not occur contemporaneously. Criteria for the antisynthetase syndrome are not well established, but two often-cited proposed criteria are those published by Connors et al. and Solomon et al. (Table 14.3).

The authors favor the Connors criteria, as a recent analysis found the sensitivity of the Solomon criteria to be low. As aforementioned, symptoms may not all be present at the time of initial presentation, and a delay in diagnosis may be detrimental, particularly for patients presenting with respiratory failure.

Polyarthralgias and arthritis are seen in 50% to 70% of patients, though joint erosions are less common. Myositis is seen in 45% to 100% of patients, depending on the antibody profile and selection criteria used. Muscle involvement, when present, ranges from asymptomatic elevation in muscle enzymes to myalgias and severe proximal muscle weakness. Mechanic's hands are often described in 19% to 55% and represent hyperkeratosis of the tips and lateral aspects of the fingers; the feet may also be involved. Fever and Raynaud's are present in approximately 30% to 40%.

ILD is seen in 69% to 100% of patients, may be isolated on initial presentation, and represents a major source of morbidity. A pooled analysis of 309 cases of antisynthetase syndrome–associated

TABLE 14.2 ■ **Antibodies Present in the Antisynthetase Syndrome and Their Target Antigen***

Antibody	Target Antigen
Anti–Jo-1	Histidyl-tRNA synthetase
Anti –PL-7*	Threonyl-tRNA synthetase
Anti–PL-12*	Alanyl-tRNA synthetase
Anti-OJ	Isoleucyl-tRNA synthetase
Anti-EJ	Glycyl-tRNA synthetase
Anti-Zo	Phenylalanyl-tRNA synthetase
Anti-KS	Asparaginyl-tRNA synthetase
Anti-YRS	Tyrosyl-tRNA synthetase

Antibodies anti–PL-7 and antiyPL-12 are most associated with ILD.

TABLE 14.3 ■ **Proposed Criteria for the Antisynthetase Syndrome**

Connor et al. Criteria	Solomon et al. Criteria
Positive for an antisynthetase antibody AND one or more of the following: • Myositis • ILD • Arthritis • Unexplained persistent fever • Raynaud's • Mechanic's hands	Positive for an antisynthetase antibody AND two major criteria OR one major and two minor criteria Major criteria • ILD • Myositis Minor criteria • Fever • Arthritis • Mechanic's hands

Focus on (Continued)

Clinical Manifestation of ILD in Subgroups of IIMs

ILD found that NSIP was the most prevalent radiological pattern (41%), followed by UIP (24%) and OP (19%). Acute lung injury was present in 15% of cases.

The antibody profile in the antisynthetase syndrome is partially associated with certain clinical manifestations. The most common antisynthetase antibody is anti–Jo-1 (seen in 10–30% of IIMs), followed by PL-7 (5–10%) and PL-7 (5%). ILD is more prevalent in PL-7 and PL-12 antibody-positive antisynthetase syndromes. Arthritis is a common feature of anti-Jo–positive antisynthetase syndrome, with 24% presenting with isolated arthritis. A pooled analysis of 11 studies (72 patients) with PL-7–positive antisynthetase syndrome noted ILD was prevalent in 77%, with myositis in 75% and arthritis in 56%. Importantly, pericarditis was reported in 20% to 50% of cases in European cohorts with PL-7 positivity. One of the largest multicenter cohort studies of PL-12 antibody–positive antisynthetase revealed the presence of ILD in 90% of cases. Notably, the majority of this cohort was African American (52%).

Regarding treatment, there are no clear consensus guidelines on how to approach therapy. Glucocorticoids remain the first line, although in a large series patients achieved stability with rituximab as induction and maintenance and azathioprine with and without corticosteroids. Additional steroid-sparing agents include mycophenolate, calcineurin inhibitors, and methotrexate.

Prognostically, clinical improvement is observed in approximately 60% of patients with therapy. A poor DLCO (<45%) and a radiographic UIP are predictors of deterioration.

Continued on following page

Focus on (Continued)

Clinical Manifestation of ILD in Subgroups of IIMs

MDA5-POSITIVE DERMATOMYOSITIS

ILD associated with MDA5-DM was first described by Sato et al. in 2005, in which a cohort of Japanese patients with a rapid-progressive ILD and CADM were found to have antibodies to a polypeptide that was approximately 140 kDa, which was labeled CADM-140. Sato et al. later found the CADM-140 autoantigen to be identical to the RNA helicase encoded by melanoma differentiation–associated gene 5 (*MDA5*), which is a cytoplasmic pattern recognition receptor expressed by cells of the innate immune system. Activation of MDA5 helicase leads to the release of proinflammatory cytokines, thereby playing a vital role in the host adaptive immune response to viruses. Given this role, preceding viral infection is hypothesized to be an important disease trigger.

There are no accepted diagnostic criteria; therefore, the authors use a clinical diagnosis of DM or ILD and MDA5 positivity to support the diagnosis. The gold standard test is immunoprecipitation.

MDA5 positivity is less associated with muscle weakness (and is seen in approximately 30%); most patients are amyopathic. The skin manifestations are notable for the classic skin manifestations of dermatomyositis: periorbital heliotrope rash, V and shawl signs, and Gottron papules. In addition, more specific to MDA5-DM are skin ulcerations that are thought to be due to an underlying vasculopathy and painful palmar papules, which may ulcerate as well. Other cutaneous manifestations include panniculitis, digital gangrene, oral ulcers, and alopecia.

ILD is present in 76%, and arthralgias in 69%. The most distinct radiologic pattern is an acute alveolitis with lower lobe predominant consolidation and ground glass seen in 50% in a cohort of MDA5-DM patients; an additional 33% had diffuse ground-glass opacities. Whereas UIP is a significant risk factor in progressive ILDs seen in other IIMs, radiographic fibrosis does not appear to be common in MDA5-associated ILD. Spontaneous pneumomediastinum is a rare complication and is associated with a worse prognosis.

While combination therapy with corticosteroids and calcineurin inhibitors with or without cyclophosphamide is usually used at the onset, we favor the use of intravenous immunoglobulin over cyclophosphamide. Triple therapy has been shown to improve survival compared to an incremental or step-up regimen for patients with rapid-progressive ILD; survival at 12 months was 85% compared to 33% of historical controls who started off with prednisone monotherapy. The combination of prednisone and calcineurin inhibitor has been examined prospectively without cyclophosphamide; a similar 12-month survival exceeding 80% was observed for tacrolimus. Alternative therapies include intravenous immunoglobulin, plasma exchange, rituximab, and tofacitinib.

Selected patients with a rapidly progressive course despite therapy may benefit from lung transplantation.

While the presence of rapidly progressive ILD can be catastrophic, some patients have a milder, more treatment-responsive phenotype very similar to the antisynthetase syndrome. Recently, three distinct phenotypes have been observed with varying prognoses. In an analysis of 83 patients, 18% presented with rapidly progressive ILD, with 86% requiring intensive care unit (ICU) admission and 80% dying within 3 months of diagnosis. However, a second cluster (55% of the cohort) presented with skin and joint symptoms and had a favorable prognosis (all were alive at 3 months). The third cluster presented with skin vasculopathy and myositis; 36% required ICU admission and 5% experienced premature death within 3 months.

DM/PM AND OVERLAP SYNDROMES

Historical cases of PM-associated ILD are likely to be now classified as the antisynthetase syndrome or an overlap. The overlap syndrome is defined as an IIM along with another connective tissue disease (or features thereof) and is present in approximately 25% of cases of IIMs. The clinical presentation is heterogenous, and associated antibodies include anti-Ku, anti–PM-Scl, anti-U1RNP, and anti-Ro52. Anti-Ro52 positivity when present with MDA5 and anti–Jo-1 portends a worse prognosis and more aggressive ILD course.

The most common overlap syndromes are systemic sclerosis (accounting for one-third of OM in a large cohort) followed by rheumatoid arthritis, Sjogren's, and systemic lupus erythematosus (SLE). The OM most associated with ILD is the scleroderma–myositis overlap. Scleroderma–myositis overlap is more commonly manifested as limited cutaneous disease and polymyositis. In a study of 39 patients with scleroderma–myositis overlap, 56% had limited skin disease and 92% had PM (as opposed to 8% with DM). ILD was present in 72% of cases, and overlap patients had higher inflammatory markers, and a greater prevalence of Raynaud's and dysphagia. Historically, important antibodies seen in this overlap include the PM–scleroderma complex, anti-Ku, and anti-U1RNP. However, these antibodies were not highly present in this and other cohorts so as to define the syndrome.

Focus on (Continued)

Clinical Manifestation of ILD in Subgroups of IIMs

In a cohort of patients with SLE-myositis overlap, ILD was observed in 26% of patients, but this was modified by the presence of scleroderma overlap (ILD seen in 50% of patients with SLE–scleroderma–myositis compared to 4% with just SLE–myositis).

There are no established guidelines on how to treat overlap myositis-associated ILD. Glucocorticoids remain first line; however, frequently used steroid-sparing agents include azathioprine, mycophenolate, and methotrexate. The authors favor the use of mycophenolate for scleroderma overlap given its proven efficacy in scleroderma ILD, with salvage therapies including rituximab and intravenous immunoglobulin.

Patients with scleroderma–myositis have a higher incidence of ILD (83%), compared to 49% with scleroderma alone. Mortality was reported at 32%, with cardiac involvement accounting for half the deaths.

LEARNING POINTS

- Antisynthetase syndrome is an autoimmune condition characterized by antibodies directed against an aminoacyl transfer RNA synthetase, which manifests clinically through signs and symptoms including ILD, myositis, Raynaud phenomenon, fever, hyperkeratotic fingertips (mechanic's hands), and arthritis.
- There is a higher prevalence and increased severity of ILD in patients with antisynthetase syndrome, compared to other inflammatory myopathies such as dermatomyositis and polymyositis.
- Diagnosis of antisynthetase syndrome requires a multidisciplinary approach with rheumatology and pulmonary evaluations, serology, imaging, and occasionally muscle and/or lung biopsy.
- ILD is a major source of morbidity and mortality for patients with myositis. Its presentation may be varied in tempo, severity, and histology.
- All patients with a new diagnosis of ILD should be screened for amyopathic forms. Given the limitations in serologic testing particularly in overlap syndromes and MDA5 disease, a high index of suspicion is required to ensure timely therapy.
- Patients with antisynthetase syndrome often require multimodality immunosuppressive therapy to control the muscle and/or pulmonary manifestations of their disease.
- The follow-up of patients with antisynthetase syndrome mandates careful attention to the adverse effects of chronic immunosuppressive therapy, as well as disease-related sequelae including progressive ILD necessitating lung transplantation, pulmonary hypertension, and malignancy.

Further Readings

Allenbach Y, Benveniste O, Stenzel W, Boyer O. Immune-mediated necrotizing myopathy: clinical features and pathogenesis. *Nat Rev Rheumatol.* 2020;16(12):689-701.

Connors GR, Christopher-Stine L, Oddis CV, Danoff SK. Interstitial lung disease associated with the idiopathic inflammatory myopathies: what progress has been made in the past 35 years? *Chest.* 2010;138(6):1464-1474.

Cottin V, Thivolet-Béjui F, Reynaud-Gaubert M, et al. Interstitial lung disease in amyopathic dermatomyositis, dermatomyositis and polymyositis. *Eur Respir J.* 2003;22(2):245-250.

De Santis M, Isailovic N, Motta F, et al. Environmental triggers for connective tissue disease: the case of COVID-19 associated with dermatomyositis-specific autoantibodies. *Curr Opin Rheumatol.* 2021;33(6):514-521.

Flashner BM, VanderLaan PA, Nurhussien L, et al. Pulmonary histopathology of interstitial lung disease associated with antisynthetase antibodies. *Respir Med.* 2022;191:106697.

Fujisawa T, Hozumi H, Kamiya Y, et al. Prednisolone and tacrolimus versus prednisolone and cyclosporin A to treat polymyositis/dermatomyositis-associated ILD: a randomized, open-label trial. *Respirology.* 2021;26(4):370-377.

Gasparotto M, Gatto M, Saccon F, et al. Pulmonary involvement in antisynthetase syndrome. *Curr Opin Rheumatol.* 2019;31(6):603-610.

González-Pérez MI, Mejía-Hurtado JG, Pérez-Román DI, et al. Evolution of pulmonary function in a cohort of patients with interstitial lung disease and positive for antisynthetase antibodies. *J Rheumatol.* 2020;47(3):415-423.

Gui X, Shenyun S, Ding H, et al. Anti-Ro52 antibodies are associated with the prognosis of adult idiopathic inflammatory myopathy-associated interstitial lung disease. *Rheumatology (Oxford).* 2022;61(11): 4570-4578.

Hallowell RW, Ascherman DP, Danoff SK. Pulmonary manifestations of polymyositis/dermatomyositis. *Semin Respir Crit Care Med.* 2014;35(2):239-248.

Hervier B, Uzunhan Y, Hachulla E, et al. Antisynthetase syndrome positive for anti-threonyl-tRNA synthetase (anti-PL7) antibodies. *Eur Respir J.* 2011;37(3):714.

Jensen ML, Løkke A, Hilberg O, et al. Clinical characteristics and outcome in patients with antisynthetase syndrome associated interstitial lung disease: a retrospective cohort study. *Eur Clin Respir J.* 2019;6(1): 1583516.

Johnson C, Pinal-Fernandez I, Parikh R, et al. Assessment of mortality in autoimmune myositis with and without associated interstitial lung disease. *Lung.* 2016;194(5):733-737.

Long K, Danoff SK. Interstitial lung disease in polymyositis and dermatomyositis. *Clin Chest Med.* 2019;40(3):561-572.

Lundberg IE, Fujimoto M, Vencovsky J, et al. Idiopathic inflammatory myopathies. *Nat Rev Dis Primers.* 2021;7(1):86.

Marie I, Hachulla E, Chérin P, et al. Interstitial lung disease in polymyositis and dermatomyositis. *Arthritis Rheum.* 2002;47(6):614-622.

Marie I, Hatron PY, Dominique S, et al. Short-term and long-term outcomes of interstitial lung disease in polymyositis and dermatomyositis: a series of 107 patients. *Arthritis Rheum.* 2011;63(11):3439-3447.

McPherson M, Economidou S, Liampas A, Zis P, Parperis K. Management of MDA-5 antibody positive clinically amyopathic dermatomyositis associated interstitial lung disease: a systematic review. *Semin Arthritis Rheum.* 2022;53:151959.

Opinc AH, Makowska JS. Antisynthetase syndrome: much more than just a myopathy. *Semin Arthritis Rheum.* 2021;51(1):72-83.

Sun KY, Fan Y, Wang YX, et al. Prevalence of interstitial lung disease in polymyositis and dermatomyositis: a meta-analysis from 2000 to 2020. *Semin Arthritis Rheum.* 2021;51(1):175-191.

Svensson J, Holmqvist M, Lundberg IE, Arkema EV. Infections and respiratory tract disease as risk factors for idiopathic inflammatory myopathies: a population-based case-control study. *Ann Rheum Dis.* 2017;76(11):1803-1808.

Tanizawa K, Handa T, Nakashima R, et al. HRCT features of interstitial lung disease in dermatomyositis with anti-CADM-140 antibody. *Respir Med.* 2011;105(9):1380-1387.

Wu W, Guo L, Fu Y, et al. Interstitial lung disease in anti-MDA5 positive dermatomyositis. *Clin Rev Allergy Immunol.* 2021;60(2):293-304.

Yanagihara T, Inoue Y. Insights into pathogenesis and clinical implications in myositis-associated interstitial lung diseases. *Curr Opin Pulm Med.* 2020;26(5):507-517.

Zamora AC, Hoskote SS, Abascal-Bolado B, et al. Clinical features and outcomes of interstitial lung disease in anti-Jo-1 positive antisynthetase syndrome. *Respir Med.* 2016;118:39-45.

Zhang L, Wu G, Gao D, et al. Factors associated with interstitial lung disease in patients with polymyositis and dermatomyositis: a systematic review and meta-analysis. *PLoS One.* 2016;11(5):e0155381.

PART V

Rare and Ultra-Rare Interstitial Lung Diseases

CHAPTER 15

Pulmonary Alveolar Microlithiasis: An Ultra-Rare Disease

Eda Boerner ■ Francesco Bonella

History of Present Illness

A 47-year-old woman complained of dry cough and dyspnea on exertion for > 10 years. Due to these symptoms, the general practitioner sent her to a primary respiratory physician. A chest radiograph was performed and showed an uncommon interstitial pattern with diffuse micronodular opacities. Consequently, the patient was referred to the center for interstitial and rare lung diseases and was hospitalized for further diagnostic procedures and treatment options.

Past Medical History

The patient had no smoking history, known allergies, malignancies, or autoimmune diseases. She had hypertension, chronic renal failure, hypothyroidism, and anemia. There was no significant occupational exposure as a housewife, but she admitted contact with birds in her house. She was living in a small village in Syri, and had five children. Consanguinity was reported in the family history. Fourteen years before the admission, unspecified parenchymal lung disease had been diagnosed. She took daily medications for hypertension and hypothyroidism, as well as vitamin D supplements.

Physical Examination and Early Clinical Findings

At the admission, the patient was alert, cooperative, and afebrile (body temperature 36.8°C [98.24°F]). Oxygen saturation was 95% at room air on pulse oximetry. Her heart rate was 75 beats/min, and respiratory rate was 16 breaths/minute.

On the physical examination, skin color was pale but there was no sign of cyanosis or peripheral oedema. The chest sound was vesicular in the apical zones and diminished in the basal zones. At percussion, apical zones were resonant and lower zones were dull.

The chest radiograph findings were confirmed: there were multiple small sandlike calcific micronodular opacities (microliths, calcipherites, or calcospherites) predominantly in the basal lobes, configuring the "sandstorm lung." A black pleural sign, which describes the vertical strip of peripheral hyperlucency between the ribs and the adjacent diffusely dense calcified lung parenchyma, was also detected. The mediastinal heart contour and diaphragm were blurred due to intensive microliths (Fig. 15.1A, B).

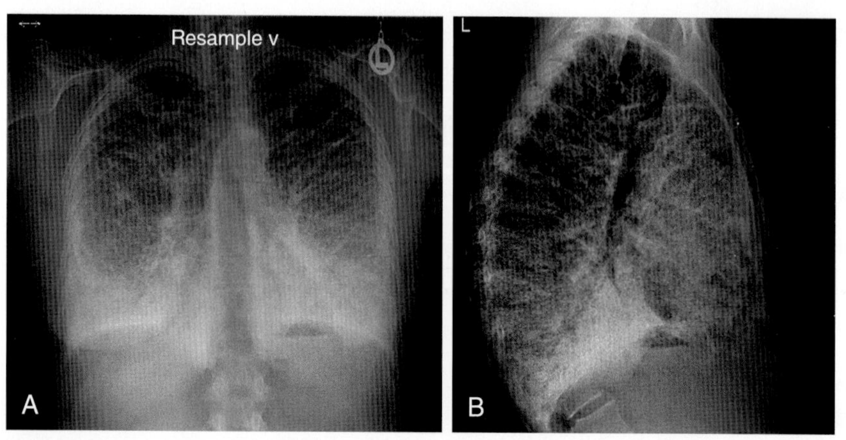

Fig. 15.1 (A) Posteroanterior chest radiograph showing diffuse bilateral small sandlike calcific micronodular opacities ("sandstorm lung"). (B) Lateral view showing multiple micronodules with linear radiolucency at the pleural boundaries around the diaphragm.

Discussion Topic 1

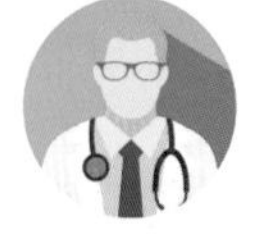

Pulmonologist A

Chest radiograph shows diffuse pulmonary micronodules, as in interstitial or airspaces diseases.

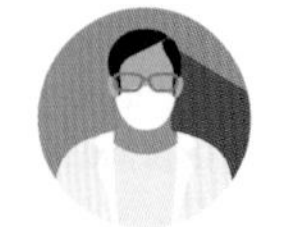

Pulmonologist B

I did not expect such extensive alterations, given that the patient's respiratory symptoms are not so striking.

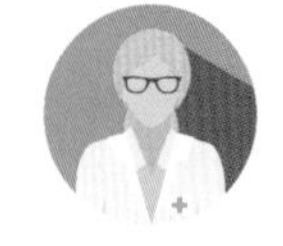

Pulmonologist C

Does she have signs of acute or chronic infection?

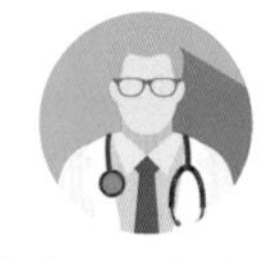

Pulmonologist A

No recent episodes of fever. Not even weight loss.

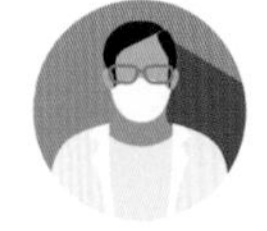

Pulmonologist B

It is essential to carry out further investigations: blood tests, pulmonary function tests, and chest computed tomography (CT).

Clinical Course

Blood tests showed mild renal failure (serum creatinine 1.79 mg/dL, urea 95 mg/dL) and mild microcytic anemia (hemoglobin 10.8 g/dL, mean corpuscular volume 77 fL, normal range 80–95 fL). There was no leukocytosis (white blood cell count 7210/mm^3) or increase of systemic inflammation markers (C-reactive protein < 5 mg/L). The platelet count was 125.000 cells/μL, international normalized ratio was 1.09. Brain-type natriuretic peptide was within the normal range (186 pg/mL). Both tuberculin skin test and QuantiFERON-TB test turned out negative.

Pulmonary function test showed mild pulmonary restriction with forced vital capacity at 73% of predicted and severe impairment of diffusing capacity of the lungs for carbon monoxide (DLCO, 27% of predicted) (Table 15.1). Arterial blood gas analysis showed hypoxemia and hypocapnia with PaO_2 76 mmHg, $PaCO_2$ 36 mmHg, and increased alveolar-arterial oxygen gradient, 31 mmHg.

Doctors decided to perform a high-resolution computed tomography (HRCT) of the chest to better define the diffuse abnormalities detected on chest radiograph.

Chest HRCT confirmed sandstorm-like diffuse calcifications with subpleural and peribronchial distribution, particularly affecting the lower lobes and the paracardiac region. There were also ground-grass opacities with thickening of interlobular septa in both lungs and a linear radiolucency at the pleural boundaries around the heart and diaphragm (Fig. 15.2, A, B).

TABLE 15.1 ■ **Pulmonary Function Tests at Admission and in Follow-Up.**

	FVC (% predicted)	FEV_1 (% predicted)	DLCO (% predicted)	Room air PaO_2 (mmHg)
At admission	66	71	27	76
At 1 year	71	67	24	65
At 2 years	73	67	26	61
At 3 years	66	69	24	59
At 4 years	65	70	22	55

FEV_1, forced expiratory volume in 1 second; FVC, forced vital capacity; DLCO, diffusing capacity of the lungs for carbon monoxide; PaO_2, arterial partial pressure of oxygen.

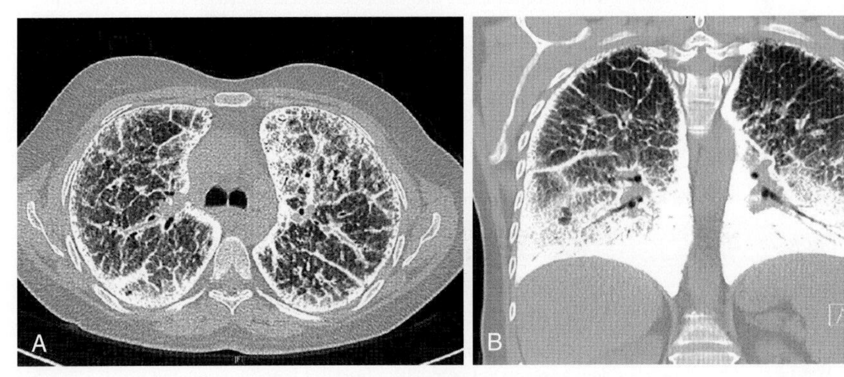

Fig. 15.2 Axial (A) and coronal (B) chest CT scan showing pleural thickening of interlobular septa in both lungs, ground-glass opacities, calcifications in the lower lobes, and a linear radiolucency at the pleural boundaries around the heart and diaphragm.

Discussion Topic 2

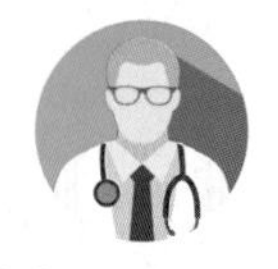

Pulmonologist A

Chest HRCT confirmed the presence of widespread sandlike intra-alveolar calcifications.

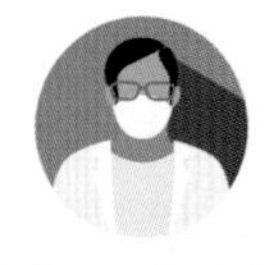

Pulmonologist B

It looks just like a "sandstorm lung," a sign of pulmonary alveolar microlithiasis!

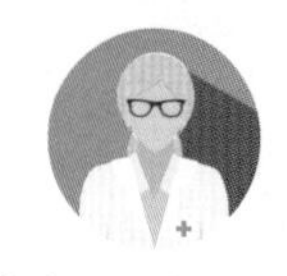

Pulmonologist C

Ground-glass opacities due to alveolar filling and thickening of interlobular septa may also be seen in pulmonary alveolar proteinosis (PAP). Bone scintigraphy of the lungs with technetium-99m methylene diphosphonate is recommended to demonstrate that lung micronodules are avid for the tracer and consistent with bone.

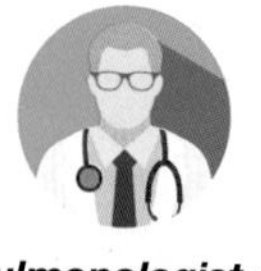

Pulmonologist A

We shouldn't overlook other possible differential diagnoses: pulmonary microcalcifications can occur with miliary tuberculosis, sarcoidosis, pneumoconiosis, varicella pneumonia.

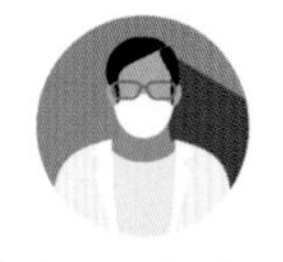

Pulmonologist B

In my opinion, the HRCT findings are highly suggestive of PAM. However, as this is an ultra-rare disease, I agree to ask for a scintigraphy to establish a definitive diagnosis.

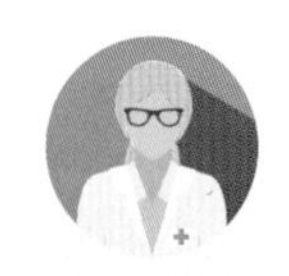

Pulmonologist C

Another way to confirm the diagnosis could be a bronchoscopy, as microliths may be seen in bronchoalveolar lavage (BAL) samples. This is also useful for exclusion of other possible differential diagnoses.

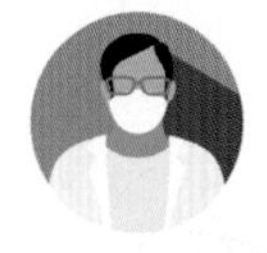

Pulmonologist B

Do we need further invasive procedures such as cryobiopsies?

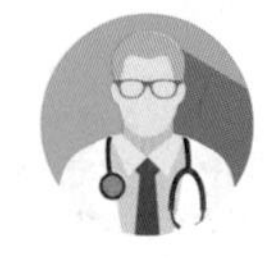

Pulmonologist A

Cryobiopsy can be helpful, but given the possible complications, it should be considered only in patients with preserved lung function and no contraindications such as pulmonary hypertension.

Bone scintigraphy showed increased tracer activity in both lungs, but no changes in the bones were detected (Fig. 15.3).

Bronchoscopy with bronchoalveolar lavage (BAL) was performed for further analysis of differential diagnosis. BAL fluid showed moderate neutrophilia and mild eosinophilia.

At light microscopy, anthracotic changes were observed in the macrophages. There were no acellular globules and debris, which are hallmarks of PAP, nor lamellar microliths, which are typical findings of PAM (Fig. 15.4).

Physicians decided not to perform cyrobiopsy due to severe impairment of lung diffusion capacity with raised risk of complications and unfavorable risk/benefit ratio of the procedure.

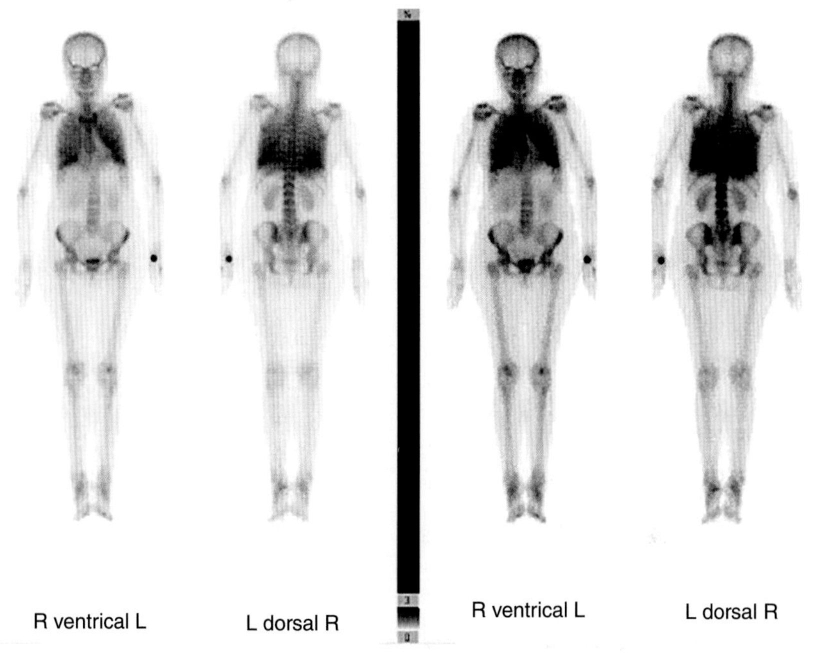

Fig. 15.3 Technetium-99m methylene diphosphonate (Tc-99m MDP) whole-body bone scintigraphy revealing lung uptake and no relevant bone uptake.

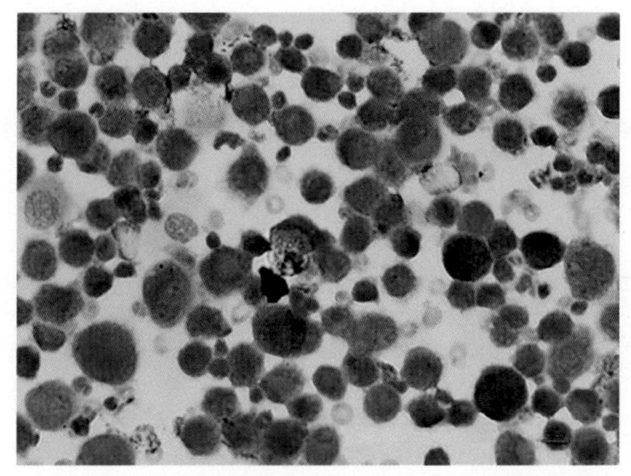

Fig. 15.4 Black anthracotic depositions in the alveolar macrophages with moderate neutrophilia and slight eosinophilia at light microscopy of BAL fluid (original magnification ×60, Giemsa stain).

Discussion Topic 3

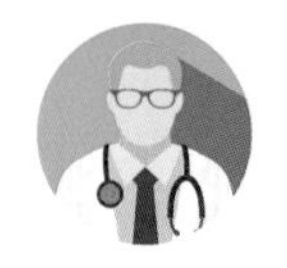

Pulmonologist A

Is there any technical, biochemical, or molecular diagnostic method available to detect the disease less invasively than histological assessment?

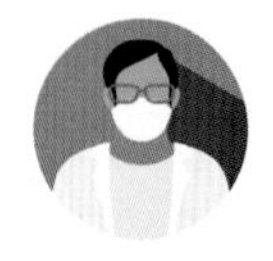

Pulmonologist B

Genetic testing should be performed, if a PAM is suspected. A *SLC34A2* gene mutation causes a defect in the uptake of phosphate by type II pneumocytes and a deposition of calcium phosphate stones in the alveoli.

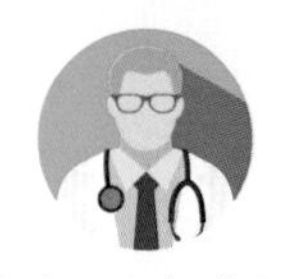

Pulmonologist A

Is the disease autosomal dominant or recessive? Should we test the children or siblings?

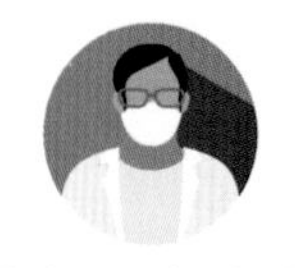

Pulmonologist B

PAM is an autosomal recessive disease. It's commonly detected in patients with history of consanguinity in the family. Therefore, genetic counseling should be offered to the family members.

Physicians decided to perform genetic testing of the mother and all five children to confirm the suspected diagnosis of PAM. The results from the direct DNA sequence analysis of the coding regions of the *SLC34A2* gene have shown a c.1328del [p.(Leu443Argfs*6)] variant in homozygous form on the patient. The variant causes a shift of the translational reading frame leading to a premature stop-codon in exon 12 and is predicted to interfere with the structure and function of the protein. The same mutation in heterozygous form was shown in all five of her children, which were all healthy.

Recommended Therapy and Further Indications

The patient was not prescribed any drug therapy. She was given recommendations to reduce the risk of respiratory infections, including influenza and pneumococcal vaccinations.

Follow-Up and Outcomes

The patient and her children were followed at the center for interstitial and rare lung diseases. Lung function tests remained stable over 4 years (Table 15.1), but increased calcific micronodular opacities and reduced translucency were detected in the apical lobes (Fig. 15.5). Moreover, the patient developed a respiratory insufficiency under effort, so oxygen supplementation was started and she was referred for lung transplantation.

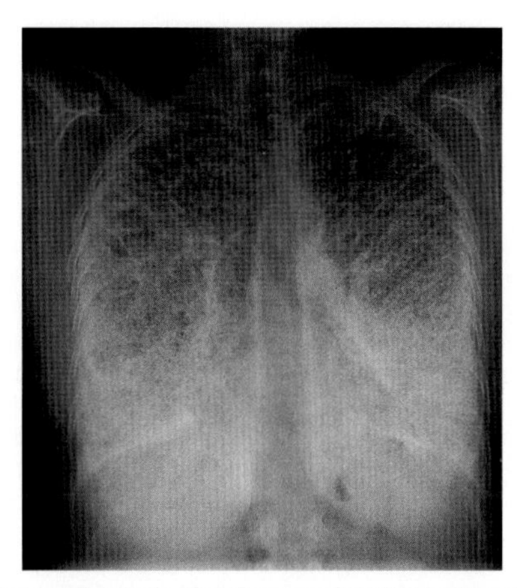

Fig. 15.5 Posteroanterior chest radiograph after 3 years showing increased calcific micronodular opacities and reduced translucency in the apical lobes after 3 years.

Focus on

Pulmonary Alveolar Microlithiasis (PAM): Disease Overview

PAM is an ultra-rare disease, with almost 1,100 cases reported in the literature. PAM has been described in Turkey, Japan, India, China, the United States, and Italy, but case distribution is not uniform. The trend to a familial occurrence of PAM is frequent. The disease affects both sexes, with a slight predominance among males, especially among sporadic cases. Disease onset occurs mostly in the third and fourth age decades with a progressive decline thereafter and very few cases in the elderly. Due to the unspecific clinical presentation and the extremely low awareness even among specialists, it is almost impossible to consider this disorder early in the differential diagnostic flow of diffuse parenchymal lung diseases. This translates into a diagnostic delay and referral to an expert center. Although there is paucity of data regarding long-term prognosis, the disease is mostly slowly progressive with reduced survival. The longest reported follow-up period is about 60 years.

Environmental factors like smoking, cold weather, inhalational exposure, and recurring lung infections may accelerate the disease course, but further confirmation of these observations is needed. Death seems to occur in the fifth decade of life, resulting from respiratory and right heart failure.

Focus on

Diagnostic Approach of PAM

At the presentation, most of the patients are asymptomatic. There is a remarkable discrepancy between radiological findings and symptoms. It is usually an incidental finding on chest radiograph, which is obtained due to preoperative or other screening reasons. The symptoms usually appear at the third or fourth decade of life. The most common symptom is dyspnea, followed by cough, sputum, hemoptysis, and fatigue. At the physical examination of patients in advanced stage, clubbing, cyanosis, and basilar rales might be detected. However, a typical clinicoradiological discrepancy exists in an early phase of the disease, when, despite a massive lung parenchymal involvement at chest radiograph or HRCT, symptoms and functional impairment are slight. Patients can remain clinically stable over years. Radiological findings on both chest radiograph (sandstorm lung) and HRCT (sandstorm-like diffuse calcifications, ground-grass opacity with thickening of interlobular septa, linear radiolucency at the pleural boundaries around the heart and diaphragm) are pathognomonic. A definitive diagnosis can generally be achieved through BAL fluid light microscopy analysis or lung biopsy with demonstration of intra-alveolar microliths.

Because technetium-99m methylene diphosphonate compounds have a natural affinity for calcification foci at the soft tissue level, whole body scintigraphy can be used as an ancillary examination.

Continued on following page

Focus on (Continued)

Diagnostic Approach of PAM

Differential diagnoses of PAM on imaging are metastatic calcification in chronic renal failure, pulmonary alveolar proteinosis, pulmonary amyloidosis, miliary tuberculosis, sarcoidosis, pneumoconiosis, and varicella pneumonia. It is important to differentiate PAM from such other diseases for the sake of appropriate treatment: PAM has on HRCT much more dense calcifications, and the clinical symptoms of other diseases are more severe. Recently, four stages have been proposed for the radiological severity.

In patients with PAM, extrapulmonary calcifications have been described in kidneys, prostate, testicles, seminal vesicles, periurethral and epididymis, aorta and mitral valves, pericardium, the gastric wall, and in the lumbar sympathetic chain, causing infertility, hematuria, and gallstones. Positron emission tomography might be useful for the detection of extrapulmonary involvement.

Due to the autosomal recessive nature of disease, PAM is detected commonly in patients with consanguineous marriage history. In the literature, most of the cases are reported from Turkey, Italy, China, India, Japan, and the United States. Because of the autosomal recessive inheritance, the children of the patients should be tested for a mutation in the *SLC34A2* gene, and genetic counseling should be advised.

The *SLC34A2* gene encodes sodium-dependent phosphate co-transporter, found in surfactant-secreting type II pneumocytes. This defect causes reduced uptake of phosphate by these cells and deposition of calcium phosphate stones in the alveoli. The microliths are round or ovoid and have a concentric laminated appearance of 0.01 to 2.8 mm in diameter. At the early phase of disease, the lung tissue remains normal; however, over time with the expansion of the microliths, alveolar walls become compressed and damaged, and lung parenchyma is replaced by fibrosis.The decision about performing interventional procedure depends on the severity of functional impairment and the clinical condition of the patient. Therefore, a decision to obtain a tissue sample should be carefully taken based on a multidisciplinary team discussion, since cryo- and surgical biopsies have higher risk of complications.

Focus on

Treatment of PAM

For now, there is no evidence-based or approved treatment for PAM available; data originate from the cases documented in the literature. Treatment with whole lung lavage (WLL) has been applied with the intent to remove microliths from the alveoli, but it has been shown to be ineffective in terms of stopping disease progression. Biphosphonates use has been proposed as a disease-modifying treatment, but its efficacy on radiological and clinical evolution is scarce.

A certain degree of symptom relief has been reached with corticosteroids, but their use does not seem to affect prognosis.

Treatment with sodium thiosulfate and a low-phosphate diet are also reported, but their efficacy is limited.

Long-term oxygen treatment should be timely considered in hypoxemic PAM patients, and pulmonary rehabilitation offered even in early disease phases. Prevention of respiratory infection is crucial to avoid rapid deterioration or accelerated disease progression. Bilateral lung transplantation remains the only curative option. To date, no recurrence after transplantation has been reported.

LEARNING POINTS

- PAM is an ultra-rare monogenic lung disorder, with accumulation of calcium microliths in the alveoli.
- Clinical presentation is not specific, and diagnosis can be suspected only through chest radiograph or HRCT, with the typical sandstorm aspect.
- BAL fluid analysis or biopsy samples show the accumulation of the characteristic microliths in the alveoli, whereas whole-body scintigraphy is a complementary examination.
- Genetic test for the pathogenic autosomal recessive *SLC34A2* mutation is considered confirmatory of a PAM diagnosis. Genetic counseling can be offered to asymptomatic first-degree family members.
- Lung transplantation is the only curative option at present; patients should be timely referred to specialized interstitial lung disease centers.

Further Readings

Bendstrup E, Jönsson ÅLM. Pulmonary alveolar microlithiasis: no longer in the stone age. *ERJ Open Res.* 2020;6(3).

Castellana G, Castellana G, Gentile M, Castellana R, Resta O. Pulmonary alveolar microlithiasis: review of the 1022 cases reported worldwide. *Eur Respir Rev.* 2015;24(138):607-620.

Chan ED, Morales DV, Welsh CH, McDermott MT, Schwarz MI. Calcium deposition with or without bone formation in the lung. *Am J Respir Crit Care Med.* 2002:165(12):1654-1669.

Delic JA, Fuhrman CR, Trejo Bittar HE. Pulmonary alveolar microlithiasis: AIRP best cases in radiologic-pathologic correlation. *Radiographic.* 2016:36(5):1334-1338.

Huqun IS, Miyazawa H, Ishii K, Uchiyama B, Ishida T, Hagiwara K. Mutations in the SLC34A2 gene are associated with pulmonary alveolar microlithiasis. *Am J Respir Crit Care Med.* 2007:175(3):263-268.

Klikovits T, Slama A, Hoetzenecker K, et al. A rare indication for lung transplantation-pulmonary alveolar microlithiasis: institutional experience of five consecutive cases. *Clin Transplant.* 2016:30(4):429-434.

CHAPTER 16

Pulmonary Alveolar Proteinosis in a Woman With Respiratory Failure and Crazy-Paving Pattern on Chest Computed Tomography

Sara Lettieri ■ Davide Piloni ■ Francesca Mariani ■
Angelo Guido Corsico ■ Ilaria Campo

History of Present Illness

A 47-year-old Philippine woman was referred to the pulmonology clinic due to progressively worsening exertional dyspnea. She also complained of a 6-month dry cough with occasional production of whitish sputum. She reported no fever, chest pain, hemoptysis, or weight loss.

Past Medical History

The patient was a caretaker without any exposure to pneumotoxic agents and had no smoking habit. No familial history of respiratory diseases was reported. Her medical history included systemic arterial hypertension in treatment with a β-blocker and hypercholesterolemia that was not pharmacologically treated.

Physical Examination and Early Clinical Findings

At the first evaluation, the patient was apyretic, with severe dyspnea at rest. Oxygen saturation measured by pulse oximetry (SpO_2) was 87% on room air, heart rate was 96 beats/min, and blood pressure was 130/90 mmHg. Chest auscultation revealed fine bibasilar end-inspiratory fixed crackles. Cardiac and abdominal physical examinations were normal, and there was no peripheral edema or jugular vein distention. Chest radiograph showed bilateral parenchymal infiltrates in the mid- and lower-lung fields (Fig. 16.1). Blood tests were unremarkable as hemoglobin, leukocytes, and renal and hepatic function indexes were in the normal range; serum procalcitonin was negative, C-reactive protein was 6 mg/dL (normal value: <0.5 mg/dL), and lactate dehydrogenase (LDH) was 348 mU/mL (normal range: 125-220 mU/mL). No significant antinuclear antibody (ANA) titer was detected (1:80). Extractable nuclear antigens (ENA) were negative. Arterial blood gas analysis (ABGA) confirmed acute hypoxemic respiratory failure with PaO_2 51 mmHg, $PaCO_2$ 33.1 mmHg, pH 7.45, and HCO_3^- 28.5 mmol/L. Alveolar-arterial oxygen gradient (A-aDO_2) was 59.2 (expected normal value <12). Oxygen supplementation was necessary to improve gas exchange. Pulmonary function tests (PFTs) showed severe restrictive ventilatory defect, with forced expiratory volume in 1 second (FEV_1) 43%, forced vital capacity (FVC) 47%, and total lung capacity (TLC) 65% of the predicted value. The diffusing capacity of the lungs for carbon monoxide (DLCO) was severely impaired with a percentage of predicted values of 19%.

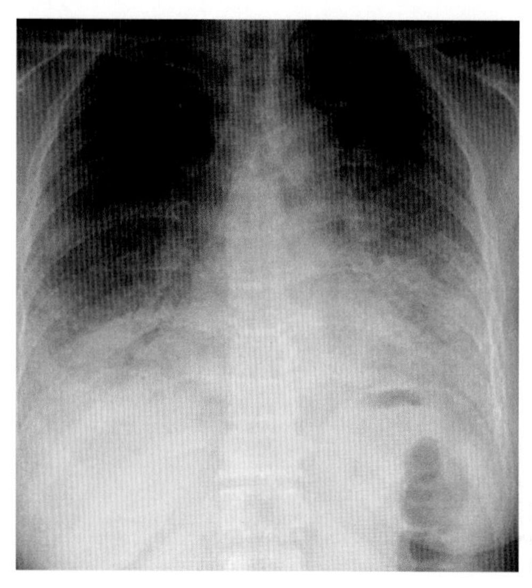

Fig. 16.1 Chest X-ray at first clinical presentation showing an interstitial reticular pattern in the mid- and lower lung fields.

Discussion Topic 1

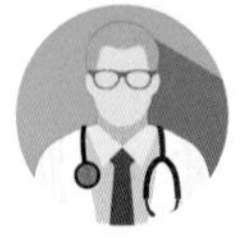

Pulmonologist A

Our patient complains of cough and dyspnea with acute hypoxemic-hypocapnic respiratory failure. We must hospitalize her.

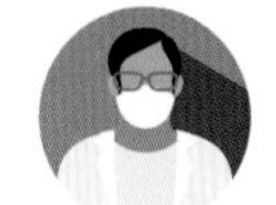

Pulmonologist B

She needs a high oxygen supplement to get sufficient saturation. Do you think she may have pulmonary embolism?

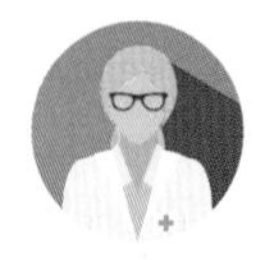

Pulmonologist C

The symptoms began several months ago, and the chest radiograph shows bilateral parenchymal infiltrates. An interstitial lung disease seems more likely to me.

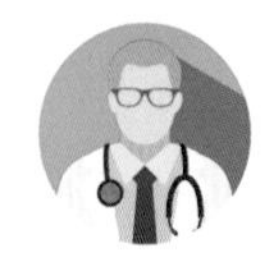

Pulmonologist A

We certainly should do a computed tomography (CT) scan of the chest. Administration of contrast medium will allow us to exclude a pulmonary embolism.

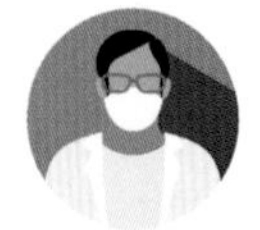

Pulmonologist B

No signs of heart failure?

Discussion Topic 1 (Continued)

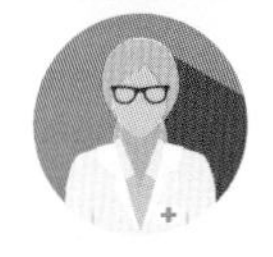

Pulmonologist C

She has no peripheral edema or jugular vein distention. The ECG shows sinus tachycardia. Anyway, I'd ask for echocardiography.

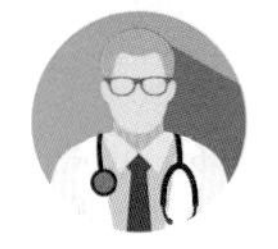

Pulmonologist A

Should we give her antibiotics? The patient may have a lower respiratory tract infection. And what about intravenous glucocorticoids; do you think they could help?

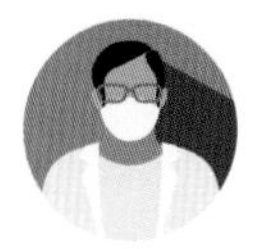

Pulmonologist B

The patient has no leukocytosis and low indexes of inflammation. We don't know the cause. I'd wait to see the chest CT before starting any therapy.

Clinical Course

Due to worsening of respiratory conditions, the patient was admitted to the pulmonology unit. The supplement of 50% oxygen through the Venturi mask, allowed the patient to obtain an SpO_2 of 96%. She underwent CT scan of the chest (Fig. 16.2), which revealed a bilateral, symmetrical

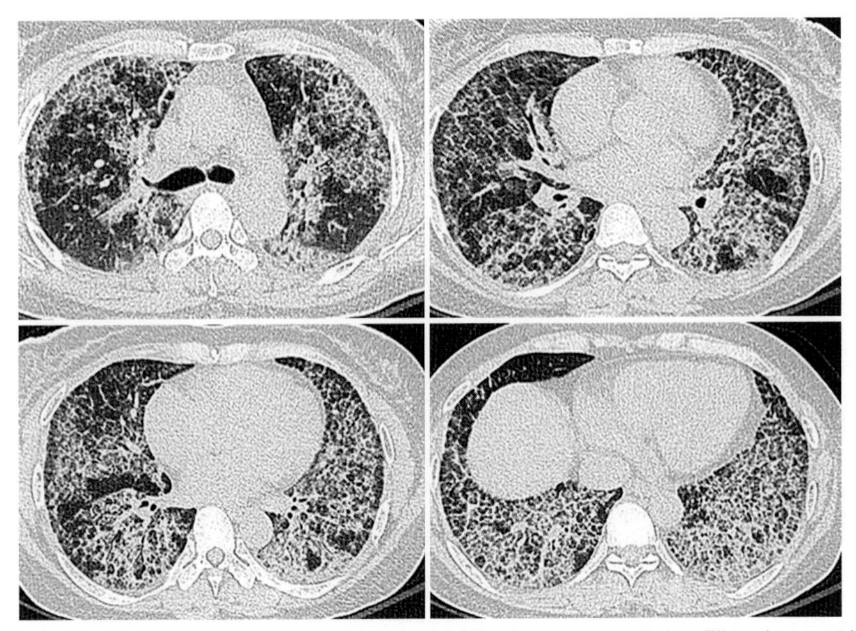

Fig. 16.2 Chest high-resolution computed tomography (HRCT) scans at admission. Bilateral symmetrical alveolar opacities with typical "crazy paving" pattern involving all five lobes are detectable. Few pulmonary lobules at the upper lobes are partially spared by the disease.

"crazy paving" pattern, due to ground-glass opacities delimited by interlobular septal thickening, with craniocaudal gradient.

No signs of pulmonary embolism were found.

Discussion Topic 2

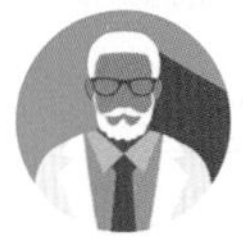

Radiologist

Chest CT scan showed ground-glass opacities and septal thickening with "crazy-paving" pattern. It is strongly suggestive for pulmonary alveolar proteinosis.
In many cases, the radiological findings are more severe than the clinical symptoms would suggest.

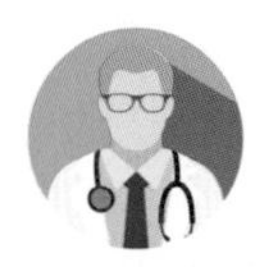

Pulmonologist A

Indeed, the hematocrit is at the upper limits. This may indicate that the patient has been hypoxemic for some time.

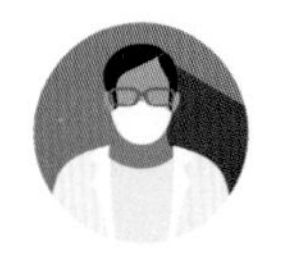

Pulmonologist B

However, other conditions should be considered in differential diagnosis, mainly *Pneumocystis jirovecii* pneumonia but also pulmonary edema, alveolar hemorrhage, and lepidic lung carcinoma. Bronchoscopy with bronchoalveolar lavage (BAL) should be recommended.

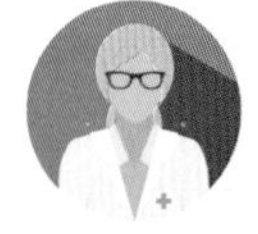

Pulmonologist C

If possible, we'd also need a transbronchial lung biopsy.

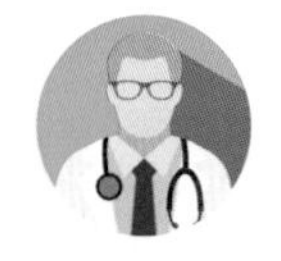

Pulmonologist A

The procedure could be dangerous. The patient already has severe respiratory failure. We will have to do it with the assistance of the anesthetist.

A bronchoscopy was performed: opaque, milky, periodic acid–Schiff (PAS)-positive lipoproteinaceous BAL fluid was collected. Transbronchial lung biopsies revealed well-preserved alveoli filled with eosinophilic, granular, and PAS-positive material and foamy alveolar macrophages. CT scan, BAL fluid appearance, and histology were compatible with pulmonary alveolar proteinosis (PAP) (Fig. 16.3). Serum granulocyte-macrophage colony stimulating factor (GM-CSF) autoantibody concentration was abnormal (44 μg/mL) (normal range: ≤3.1 μg/mL), thus supporting a diagnosis of autoimmune PAP.

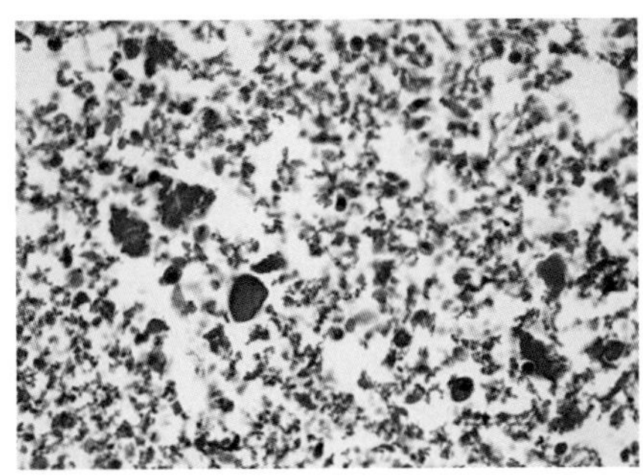
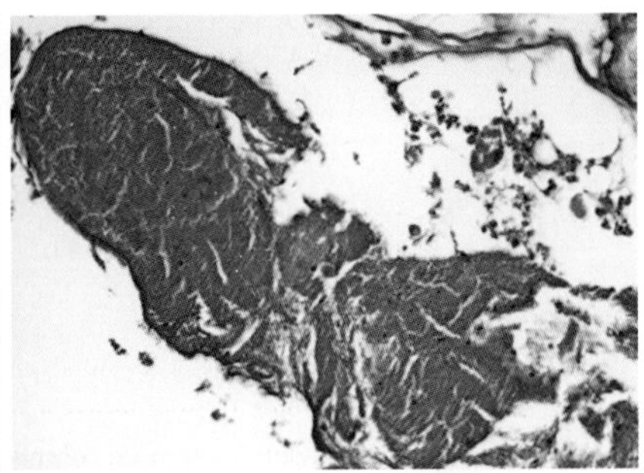

Fig. 16.3 BAL histopathology. Periodic acid–Schiff (PAS)-positive amorphous material encompassing alveolar macrophages is a relevant feature of PAP BAL at light microscopy (a, magnification ~×40; b, magnification ~×200).

Discussion Topic 3

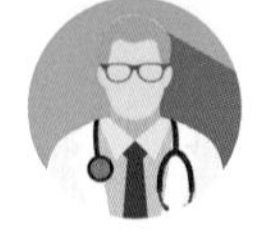

Pulmonologist A

BAL fluid was opaque, milky, and PAS positive. Although we are still waiting for histological confirmation, PAP diagnosis is highly probable.

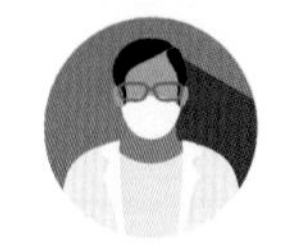

Pulmonologist B

Once the histology confirms the diagnosis, we have to dose anti–GM-CSF autoantibody levels to confirm the autoimmune etiology, representing the 90% of cases of PAP. If in the normal range, we have to consider secondary causes of PAP.

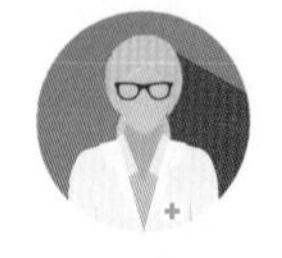

Pulmonologist C

The patient has severe acute respiratory failure and significant disease extent on CT scan of the chest. A whole lung lavage (WLL) is necessary to remove excessive surfactant filling alveoli and relieve symptoms.

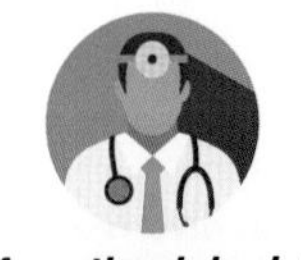

Anesthesiologist

Certainly, there is indication for WLL execution. We will perform it in the intensive care unit (ICU). We will use a double endotracheal tube and lateral decubitus position. We will treat first the left lung, which is smaller than the right one.

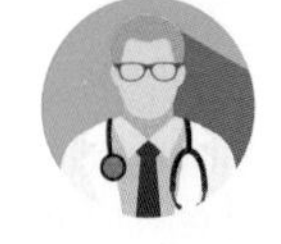

Pulmonologist A

Enterobacter aerogenes was isolated on BAL cultural exam. We will treat lung infection prior to performing WLL.

Continued on following page

Discussion Topic 3 (Continued)

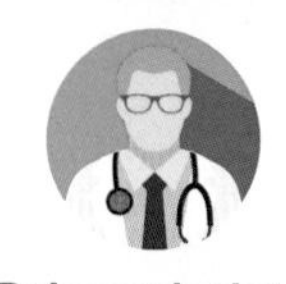

Pulmonologist A

How long will the WLL procedure be?

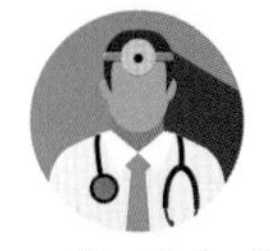

Anesthesiologist

Assuming that no complications arise, we will perform a one-session sequential bilateral WLL. The lavage duration of a single lung is about 3 to 4 hours. The entire procedure may require 7 to 8 hours. The patient will return to the pulmonology unit within 48 hours.

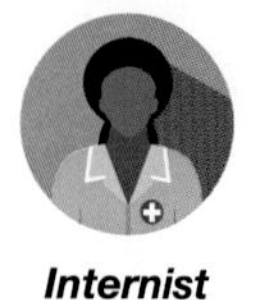

Internist

Which are the possible complications of WLL? What is the rate?

Anesthesiologist

Complications are rare when WLL is performed in expert centers and includes hypoxemia, pneumothorax, fluid leakage, pleural effusion, superimposed infection, and acute respiratory distress syndrome.

Recommended Therapy and Further Indications

Due to severely impaired respiratory conditions, the patient underwent WLL. As *Enterobacter aerogenes* was isolated from BALF culture, targeted antibiotic therapy was administered before the lavage. The patient was transferred to the ICU and intubated with a double-lumen endotracheal tube. The left lung was lavaged first: 15 L of warmed saline solution (37°C = 98.6°F), divided in aliquots of 500 mL, was instilled and drained by gravity. Concurrently, the other lung was mechanically ventilated. When the collected fluid began to be clear, manual chest percussions were added to improve drainage. The patient was in lateral decubitus, which offers some advantages: 1) more effective manual percussions on the lung and 2) blood perfusion diverted toward the ventilated lung, with subsequent reduction of ventilation-perfusion mismatch and hypoxemia. The entire procedure continued until the effluent fluid was completely clear. Sequentially, the right lung was lavaged with 17 L of saline solution. Fig. 16.4 shows the typical milky appearance of collected effluent fluid.

After WLL, the patient returned to the pulmonology unit, where she underwent a course of wide-spectrum antibiotic (intravenous piperacillin/tazobactam 4.5 gr every 8 hours) and low-dose diuretic (intravenous furosemid 20 mg once daily) for 5 to 6 days. Dyspnea, cough, and oxygen saturation improved, resulting in 95% to 96% on room air, and the patient could be weaned from oxygen. Chest radiograph at discharge showed a reduction of bilateral, interstitial thickening (Fig. 16.5). After 3 months, PFTs were repeated: lung volumes recovered to the normal range (FEV_1 92%, FVC 89%, and TLC 76% of the predicted value) and DLCO

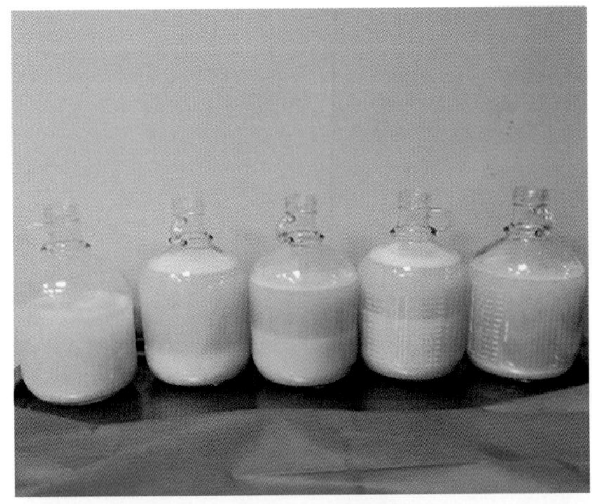

Fig. 16.4 Effluent fluid collected during WLL. The typical milky, opaque gross appearance can be observed. A cellular, dense sediment is settled to the bottom of the bottles.

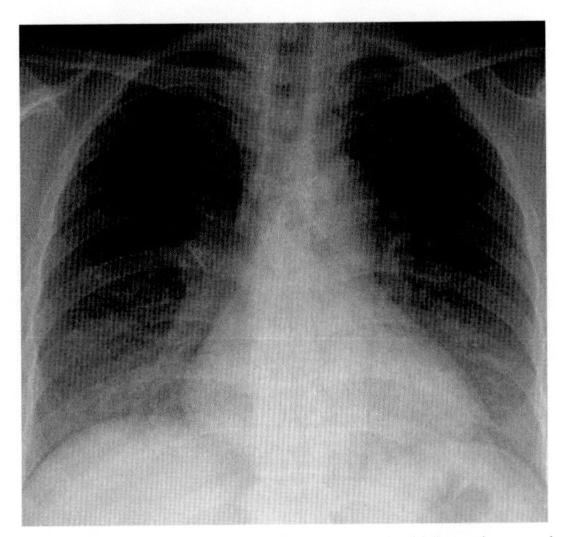

Fig. 16.5 Chest radiograph after WLL treatment. An improvement of bilateral parenchymal transparency is appreciable.

improved (72% of the predicted value). The 6-minute walk test was successfully completed without oxygen desaturation.

Follow-Up and Outcomes

After 1 year, the patient reported worsening dyspnea and mucous cough: radiographic examinations showed PAP recurrence, and blood gas analysis revealed hypoxemic acute respiratory failure. The patient underwent a second WLL with about 8 L of saline solution used for both lungs. Although the treatment was effective, the clinical benefit lasted a limited time. During the following 3 years, the patient underwent an additional four WLL treatments due to PAP worsening. Afterward,

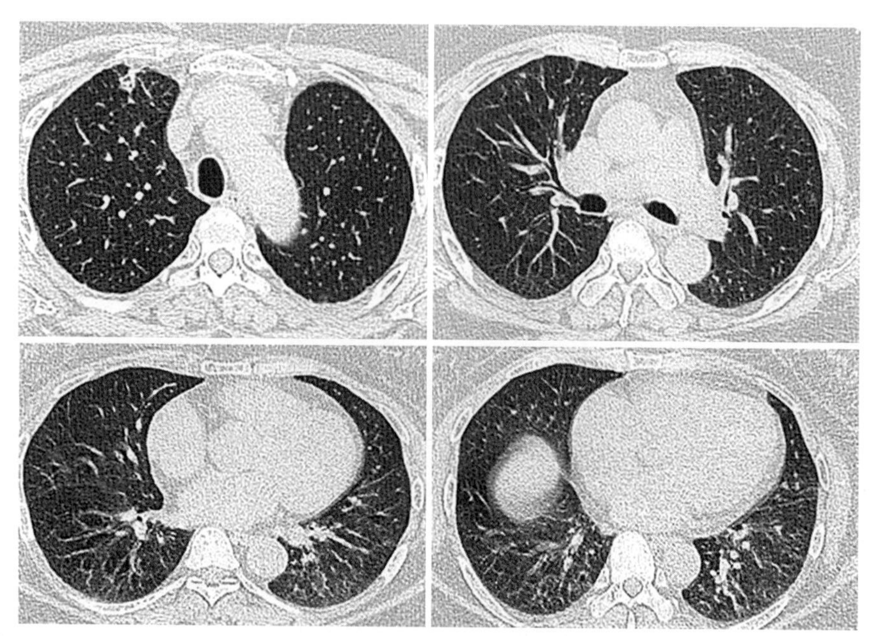

Fig. 16.6 Chest high-resolution scan on PAP remission. No more ground-glass opacities are valuable. Mild residual septal thickening is present at lower lobes.

considering the frequent recurrence of the pulmonary infiltrates, the patient was enrolled in a phase 3, multicenter randomized clinical trial evaluating the efficacy of inhaled recombinant GM-CSF (rGM-CSF) and received rGM-CSF nebulizer solution (300 μg) administered once daily, for a year. Treatment was well tolerated, and no adverse effects were reported. She completed the treatment and follow-up period, with planned monthly visits, and held good clinical, radiological, and functional conditions. Subsequent clinical course was characterized by stable remission of PAP, confirmed by high-resolution CT of the chest, which showed progressive resolution of ground-glass opacities and septal thickening and residual small patches of alveolar flooding (Fig. 16.6). The patient was scheduled for follow-up with annual visits of comprehensive physical examination, PFTs and DLCO evaluation, 6-minute walk test, and chest radiograph or CT scan.

Focus on

Classification of PAP

Pulmonary alveolar proteinosis (PAP) is an ultra-rare syndrome with an estimated prevalence of 6.87 per million in the general population. The progressive accumulation of surfactant within the alveoli leads to a variable impairment of respiratory function, ranging from asymptomatic form to severe hypoxemic respiratory failure and death. In accordance with the underlying pathogenetic mechanism, PAP is currently classified as primary, secondary, or congenital. Primary PAP is caused by the disruption of granulocyte-macrophage colony stimulating factor (GM-CSF), which is responsible for impaired surfactant catabolism in the alveolar macrophages. It includes autoimmune PAP and hereditary PAP. Autoimmune PAP represents the most common clinical form, accounting for 90% of cases, and is caused by the presence of a high level of neutralizing antibodies targeting GM-CSF. Hereditary PAP, accounting for <1% of cases, is due to autosomal recessive mutations in the genes encoding for the α or β chain of the GMCSF receptor (*CSF2RA* and *CSF2RB*, respectively) and is clinically, physiologically, and histologically indistinguishable from the autoimmune form. Secondary PAP is associated with underlying conditions reducing alveolar macrophages number or functions, included surfactant clearance, such

Focus on (Continued)

Classification of PAP

as hematological disorders, malignancies, immunodeficiency syndromes, chronic inflammatory syndromes, chronic infections, inhalation of fumes, and organic or inorganic dust. Hematological disorders (especially mielodysplastic syndromes) are responsible of >75% of cases with adult-onset secondary PAP. Congenital PAP is determined by mutations in genes encoding for proteins involved in surfactant production, such as *SFTPB, SFTPC, ABCA3*, or *Nkx2.1*. It occurs in neonates, children, and adults and causes respiratory disease invariably associated with pulmonary fibrosis and various levels of dysfunctional surfactant accumulation. Rarely, the etiology of PAP is indefinable (unclassified PAP).

Focus on

Diagnostic Algorithm of PAP

PAP should be suspected in the presence of symptoms, like slowly progressive dyspnea with or without cough and fatigue, associated with the characteristic high-resolution CT findings, represented by interlobular septal thickening and interspersed patchy ground-glass opacities with "crazy paving" appearance. BAL fluid analysis can confirm the diagnosis of PAP since it appears characteristically milky and opaque. The microscopic examination demonstrates basophilic and periodic acid–Schiff (PAS) acellular globules, as well as foamy alveolar macrophages positive to oil-red-O staining and a substantial amount of weakly PAS-positive cell debris. Transbronchial or surgical lung biopsy should be limited to selected cases when PAP diagnosis cannot be suspected from tomographic and BAL appearance.

Once PAP is confirmed, serum GM-CSF autoantibody measurement allows differentiation of autoimmune PAP from other PAP-causing diseases. If normal levels of GM-CSF autoantibodies (<5 μg/mL) are detected, the autoimmune form is excluded and further investigations are necessary: accurate research for possible secondary PAP-causing disease, serum GM-CSF measurement, and GM-CSF signaling test. High levels of serum GM-CSF indicate GM-CSF receptor dysfunction, highlighting hereditary PAP, which can be confirmed by the GM-CSF signaling test and specific gene analysis. Normal levels of serum GM-CSF and a GM-CSF signaling test within normality suggest the presence of congenital PAP that should be assessed with a specific genetic test. For diagnostic assessment, pulmonary function tests can be performed. Spirometry is generally within normal limits in the early stages of the disease, whereas a decreased forced vital capacity and total lung capacity, consistent with a restrictive pattern, can be found in the case of more severe disease. Frequently, the diffusion capacity of the lung for carbon monoxide is reduced and correlates with disease severity. Laboratory exams are usually within the normal range, except lactate dehydrogenase, whose levels are frequently high and reflect the A-aDO_2 gradient. Several biomarkers have been studied to identify disease severity, such as serum tumor antigens (CEA, CYFRA 21-1, and NSE) and lung-epithelium–derived proteins (KL6, SP-A, SP-B, and SP-D). However, none of them have been proved specific or diagnostic for PAP.

Focus on

Management of PAP

Whole lung lavage (WLL) is the current standard therapy for primary PAP and some cases of secondary PAP. WLL is an invasive procedure performed under general anesthesia, in the intensive care unit, using a double-lumen endotracheal tube: while one lung is mechanically ventilated, the other is repeatedly filled with warm saline (from 5 up to 40 L) per lung, to physically remove the surfactant. Manual clapping can be added to improve sediment removal. Although technical improvements have occurred since its first execution in the 1960s, WLL remains a nonstandardized procedure, is highly operator dependent, and is performed in a limited number of specialized centers. Common indications to WLL are 1) presence of persistent or progressive respiratory failure; 2) presence of exercise desaturation (5% points); and 3) significant limitation in daily or sports activities, especially in young patients. Complications are rare and include hypoxia, pneumothorax, hydrothorax, minor bleeding from airway injury, balloon rupture, superimposed infection, and acute respiratory distress syndrome. Segmental and lobar lavage practiced during bronchoscopy have also been reported. GM-CSF augmentation is a novel therapy emerging as a possible alternative to WLL in patients with autoimmune PAP. The treatment permits the

Continued on following page

Focus on (Continued)

Management of PAP

neutralization of autoantibodies and the reactivation of GM-CSF pathway, thus restoring macrophage maturation and surfactant catabolism. The inhalation route has shown a higher response rate than subcutaneous, with no serious adverse events. Aerosolized recombinant GM-CSF improves gas transfer (A-aDO_2 gradient, DLCO), exercise tolerance, quality of life, and reduces ground-glass opacities. Currently, phase 3 randomized clinical trials are ongoing to better define the safety and efficacy of GM-CSF. Based on the evidence of increased cholesterol content in surfactant of PAP patients, novel therapeutic strategies targeting cholesterol homeostasis have been studyed, including statins and PPAR γ-agonists. Other treatments, such as plasmapheresis to remove the autoantibodies and rituximab (an anti–B-cell monoclonal antibody) to induce B-lymphocyte depletion, have been attempted in autoimmune PAP, but their efficacy and safety remain controversial. Corticosteroids are not effective, since they can increase surfactant production and suppress alveolar macrophages function. In secondary PAP, the therapeutic approach is often dictated by the underlying disease. However, WLL can be successfully associated. Therapy for congenital PAP is supportive, although lung and hematopoietic stem cell transplantation has been reported.

LEARNING POINTS

- PAP is a rare syndrome caused by progressive accumulation of surfactant within pulmonary alveoli leading to variable gas exchange impairment.
- PAP includes different diseases currently classified as primary, secondary, or congenital according to the pathogenesis.
- Diagnosis of PAP should be highly suspected in presence of a compatible clinical picture, typical chest high-resolution CT findings, and a milky BAL fluid appearance.
- Autoantibodies targeting GM-CSF are pathognomonic for autoimmune PAP, which accounts for 90% of cases of PAP.
- WLL remains the gold standard therapy. Nebulized recombinant GM-CSF is a promising novel pathogenesis-based approach.

Further Readings

Campo I, Luisetti M, Griese M, et al; WLL International Study Group. Whole lung lavage therapy for pulmonary alveolar proteinosis: a global survey of current practices and procedures. *Orphanet J Rare Dis.* 2016;11(1):115.

Campo I, Mariani F, Rodi G, et al. Assessment and management of pulmonary alveolar proteinosis in a reference center. *Orphanet J Rare Dis.* 2013;8:40.

McCarthy C, Lee E, Bridges JP, et al. Statin as a novel pharmacotherapy of pulmonary alveolar proteinosis. *Nat Commun.* 2018;9(1):3127.

Sakagami T, Beck D, Uchida K, et al. Patient-derived granulocyte/macrophage colony-stimulating factor autoantibodies reproduce pulmonary alveolar proteinosis in nonhuman primates. *Am J Respir Crit Care Med.* 2010;182(1):49-61.

Suzuki T, Sakagami T, Young LR, et al. Hereditary pulmonary alveolar proteinosis: pathogenesis, presentation, diagnosis, and therapy. *Am J Respir Crit Care Med.* 2010;182(10):1292-1304.

Trapnell BC, Inoue Y, Bonella F, et al; IMPALA Trial Investigators. Inhaled molgramostim therapy in autoimmune pulmonary alveolar proteinosis. *N Engl J Med.* 2020;383(17):1635-1644.

Trapnell BC, Nakata K, Bonella F, et al. Pulmonary alveolar proteinosis. *Nat Rev Dis Primers.* 2019;5(1):16.

Uchida K, Beck DC, Yamamoto T, et al. GM-CSF autoantibodies and neutrophil dysfunction in pulmonary alveolar proteinosis. *N Engl J Med.* 2007;356(6):567-579.

CHAPTER 17

Idiopathic Pleuroparenchymal Fibroelastosis in a Never-Smoker Woman With a History of Hypersensitivity Pneumonitis

Jannik Ruwisch ■ Claudio Sorino ■ Antje Prasse

History of Present Illness

A never-smoker, 57-year-old woman complained of increasing shortness of breath and a persistent cough, producing only sporadically white-gray sputum, without hemoptysis and without a specific circadian rhythm. Moreover, she had a considerable weight loss exceeding 4 kg in the last 6 months in combination with a compromised quality of life (7/10 on a visual analogue scale) related to limited exercise tolerance. Manifest shortness of breath only occurred upon high-intensity physical exercise (Modified Medical Research Council [mMRC] dyspnea scale = 0) but was reported as progressively increased over the past 2 years. The patient denied chest pain when resting or taking deep breaths. She had no fever or other signs of infection, no symptoms in organs or systems other than the respiratory, and no recent hospital admissions.

Past Medical History

The patient worked as a travel consultant in a regional travel office. Her familial history was negative for interstitial lung diseases (ILDs) or other chronic respiratory diseases. She had no prior exposition to either radiation or chemotherapy. Twenty years before the current presentation, the patient was diagnosed with hypersensitivity pneumonitis (HP), following manifestation of a dry persistent cough. In this context, exposure to avian dust was identified back then, as the patient held two budgerigars (*Melopsittacus undulatus*) in her flat. Corresponding precipitins against avian antigens turned positive, and an immunosuppressive treatment with corticosteroids had been initiated. The respiratory symptoms were largely resolved, and the patient had a good quality of life for many years. However, 2 years before the current presentation, the symptoms recurred. She denied recent long-distance travels or contact to dust or mold or continued exposure to birds. An antigen screening questionnaire revealed no ongoing exposure to known relevant pulmonary antigens. Chest computed tomography (CT) imaging findings were interpreted as a nonspecific ILD, whereas a bronchoscopy with bronchoalveolar lavage (BAL) and transbronchial biopsies showed a marginal lymphocytosis and a nonspecific fibroelastic remodeling of the parabronchial parenchyma. Her pulmonologist prescribed a second course of prednisolone in suspicion of relapsed HP. However, this had no significant effects on either shortness of breath or cough, and she was also prescribed long-term oxygen therapy during exertion. Physical tolerance further deteriorated in the following months, when the patient was finally referred to the outpatient clinic for ILD for further differential diagnostics.

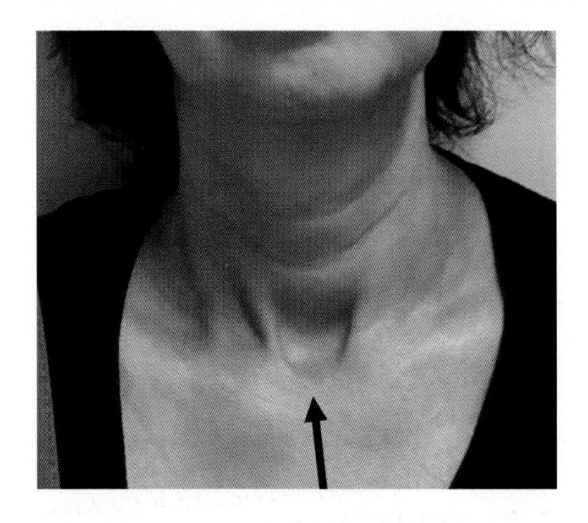

Fig. 17.1 Inspection of the patient's thoracic cage. A deepened suprasternal notch is evident (arrow).

Physical Examination and Early Clinical Findings

At presentation, the patient had a body mass index (BMI) of 21.5 kg/m^2. A flat chest and a prominent suprasternal notch (Fig. 17.1) were noticed. Fine crackles were absent upon auscultation as was no wheezing; percussion was damped over the upper lung lobes. She was able to climb two flights of stairs with the use of oxygen 2 L/min with mild shortness of breath (New York Heart Association class II), while the resting pulse oximetry values were sufficient without supplemental oxygen. The screening for fatigue (Fatigue Assessment Scale [FAS]), major depression (Patient Health Questionnaire-9 [PHQ]), and anxiety (Generalized Anxiety Disorder 2-item [GAD-2]) remained negative. The remainder of the physical examination and particularly the evaluation of the ankles, joints, and skin revealed no signs suggestive of rheumatological disease.

On chest radiograph, a pronounced bilateral reticulation pattern, predominating in the upper lobes, with no signs of pleural effusions became evident. A reduction in the anteroposterior chest diameter (platythorax) was also noticed.

Discussion Topic 1

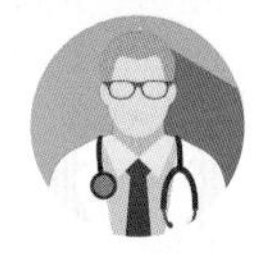

Pulmonologist A

The patient has a persistent cough and dyspnea. Her symptoms recently became very disabling. We need a prompt pulmonary diagnostic workup.

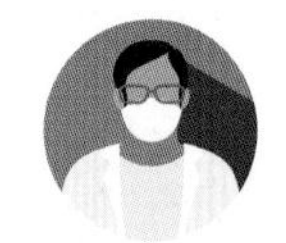

Pulmonologist B

She had a significant weight loss. A malignant process should be included in the differentials.

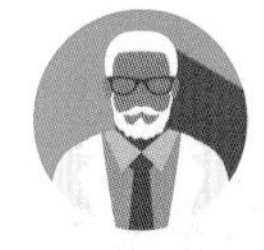

Radiologist

No masses are evident on chest radiograph, while there appears to be interstitial involvement predominantly of the upper lobes.

Discussion Topic 1 (Continued)

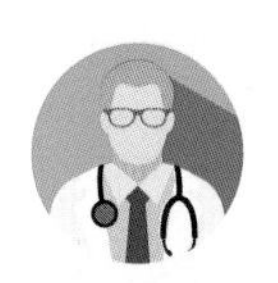

Pulmonologist A

This could be compatible with the evolution of her hypersensitivity pneumonitis toward a fibrosing form.

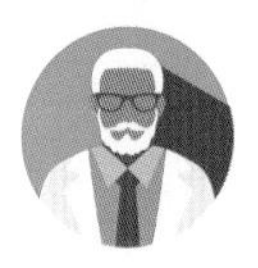

Radiologist

There is also a reduction in the anteroposterior diameter of the chest, usually indicating marked volume contraction of the upper lobes in combination with decreased chest wall elastance.

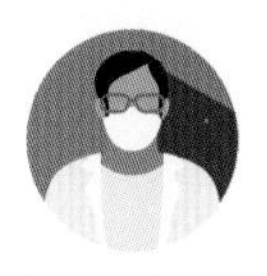

Pulmonologist B

We should perform a comprehensive diagnostic process for ILDs, again including pulmonary function tests, thoracic high-resolution computed tomography (HRCT), and autoantibody panel.

Clinical Course

The patient underwent pulmonary function tests (PFTs) that depicted a restrictive ventilation pattern with preserved Tiffeneau index, forced expiratory volume in 1 second (FEV_1) of 1.52 L = 54% predicted, vital capacity. (VC) of 1.74 L = 51% predicted, total lung capacity (TLC) of 2.87 L = 53% predicted, and a compromised gas transfer factor (DLCO 4.49 mmol = 50% predicted). Of note, CO uptake after correction for the alveolar volume remained preserved with 1.8 mmol (112% predicted), indicating an additional feature of extrapulmonary restriction. The 6-minute walk test (6MWT) revealed a slight exercise-induced limited oxygenation (Fig. 17.2).

Antinuclear antibody (ANA) screening showed a slight speckled staining pattern (titer 1:640). A subsequently performed extractable nuclear antigen screening (ENA-Screen) remained negative. Since the preexisting diagnosis of hypersensitivity pneumonitis with sensitization against birds, antigen-specific IgG against avian and mold antigens were tested (Table 17.1). While IgG anti dove and budgerigar tested only marginally positive, IgG anti aspergillus antigens tested positive. Further laboratory workup depicted no signs of lymphocytic or neutrophilic inflammation. Rheuma factor and anticitrullinated antibodies testing showed no titer elevation.

HRCT of the chest was added for complementation of the initial diagnostic workup (Fig. 17.3 and 17.4). This revealed marked bilateral apical pleural fibrosis with marked involvement of the pulmonary fissures, with intraalveolar fibrotic reticulations of the subpleural lung parenchyma and patchy consolidations with upper lobe predominance. Traction bronchiectasis was noted, predominating in the upper lobes, together with a diverticulum of the distal trachea. Meanwhile, lower lobes showed subtle pleural thickening and volume loss. Moreover, a posteroanterior gradient of interstitial change was noted together with a deviation of the trachea. Ground-glass opacities documented in former CT scans of the patients were absent.

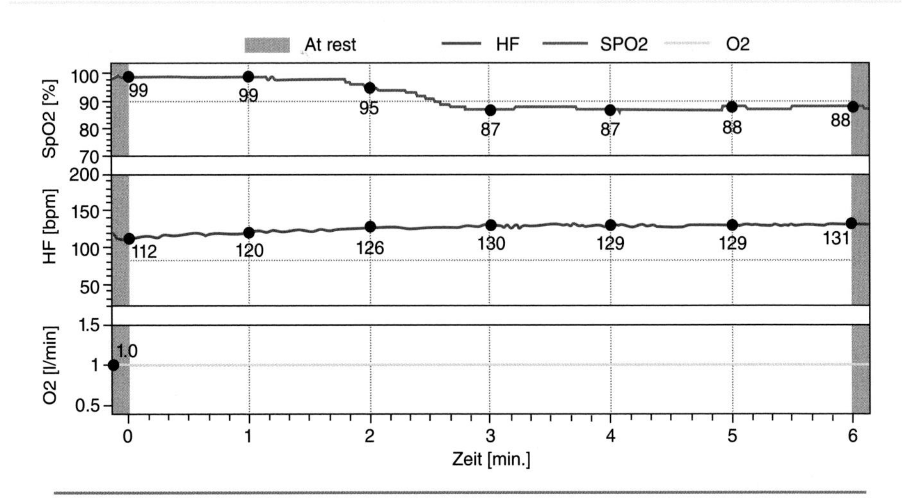

6-minute walk test

Oxygen	1L/Min
Shortness of breath at rest [BORG scale]	1
Shortness of breath at challenge [BORG scale]	3
Mean oxygen saturation at rest	99%
Mean oxygen saturation at challenge	91, 6% [–11%]
Minimum oxygen saturation at challenge	86%
6-min walking distance	457 m [79% expected]
Mean heart rate at rest	112 bpm
mean heart rate at challenge	126 bpm
Maximum heart rate at challenge	132 bpm

Fig. 17.2 Lung function and 6-minute walk test at presentation. HF, heart rate; SpO_2, oxygen saturation; VC, vital capacity; FEV_1, forced expiratory volume in 1 second; PEF, peak expiratory flow; MEF, mean expiratory flow; TLC, total lung capacity; TGV, thoracic gas volume; RAWtot, total airway resistance; DLCO, diffusion capacity of the lungs for carbon monoxide; KCO, alveolar gas transfer.

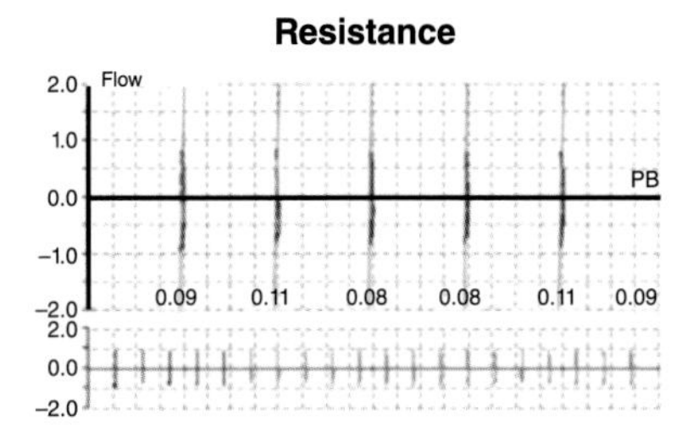

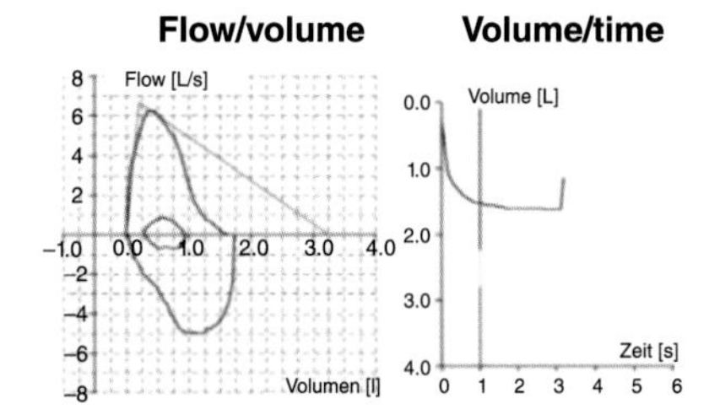

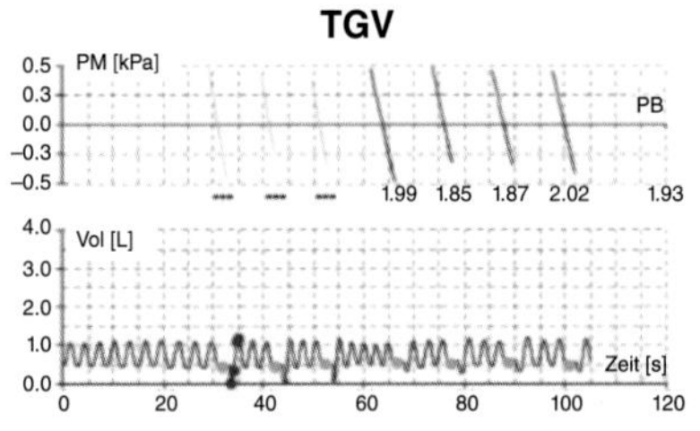

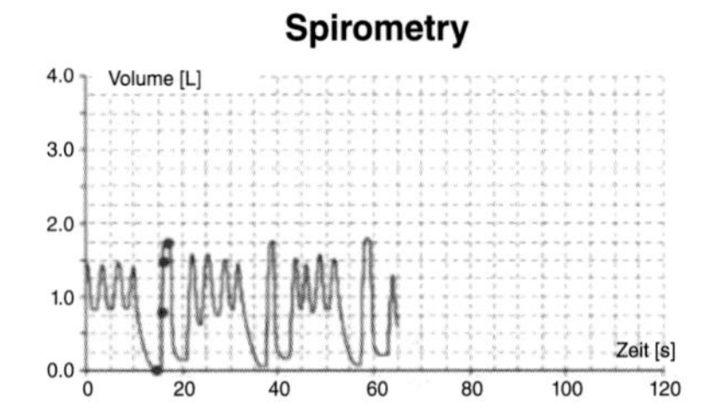

Lung function	Predicted	Actual	Actual/predicted
VC	3.37	1.74	51%
FEV1	2.79	1.52	54%
FEV1/VC	79	88	111%
PEF	6.67	6.29	94%
MEF25–75	3.25	2.98	92%
TLC	5.43	2.87	53%
TGV	2.87	1.93	67%
RAWtot	<0.35	0.09	26%
DLCO	8.97	4.49	50%
KCO	1.69	1.80	106%

Fig. 17.2, cont'd

TABLE 17.1 ■ **Laboratory Testing of Precipitins Against Various Frequently Detected Pulmonary Antigens Driving Development of Hypersensitivity Pneumonitis**

IgG CAP Antigen	Reference, mAg/L	Result, mAg/L	Interpretation
Pigeon	< 16	17.2	Borderline positive
Budgerigar	< 8	17.2	Weak positive
Saccharoplyspora rectivirgula	< 13	5.74	Negative
Aspergillus fumigatus	< 64	107	Intermediate positive
Penicillium chrysogenum	< 64	58.4	Negative
Aureobasidium pullulans	< 22	14.1	Negative
Cephalosporium acremonium	< 23	18.0	Negative
Fusarium proliferatum	< 46	14.4	Negative

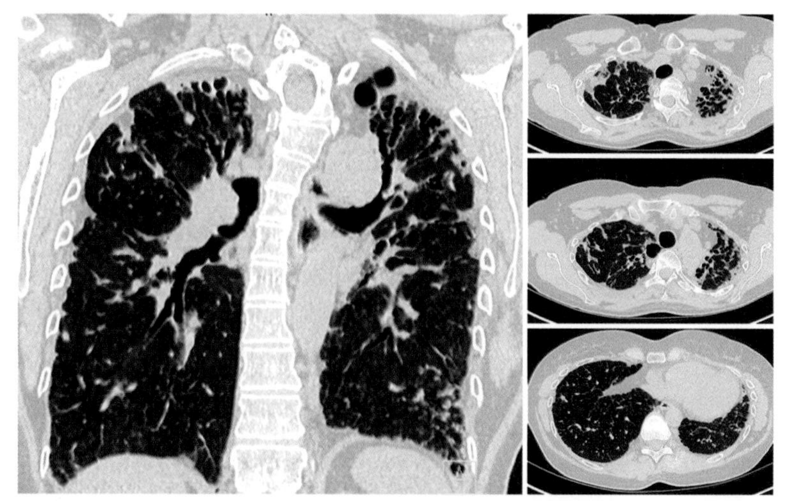

Fig. 17.3 High-resolution CT scan of the patient at initial presentation. The left panel depicts a reconstructed coronary view. Marked pleural thickening and subpleural consolidations are noted. Axial views emphasize a basal-to-apical gradient of the remodeling with relative sparing of the lower lobe. Volume loss of the upper lobes is underscored by the presence of pronounced tractions bronchiectasis.

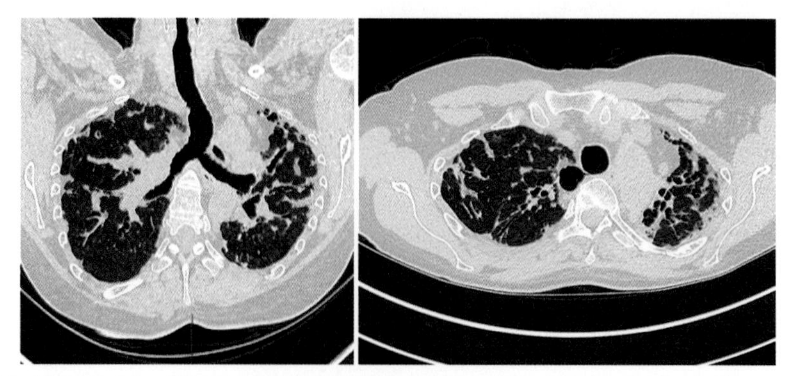

Fig. 17.4 High-resolution CT scan depicting hallmarks of pulmonary volume contraction in the upper lung. The left panel shows marked deviation of the trachea. The right panel shows a tracheal diverticulum, most likely resultant persistent tractional forces acting on the trachea.

Discussion Topic 2

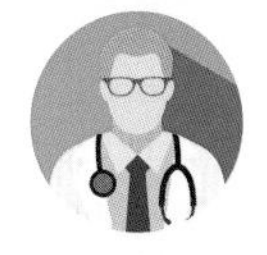

Pulmonologist A

On chest HRCT, there are no ground-glass opacities or signs of bronchiolitis. Overall, these findings do not seem indicative of sole fibrotic HP, do you agree?

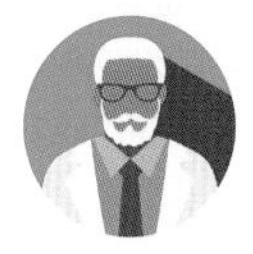

Radiologist

Yes, I do. Although fibrotic alterations in HP characteristically spare the lower lung lobes, signs of small airway disease are mandatory for the diagnosis, with ground-glass opacity, air entrapment, or centrilobular nodules.

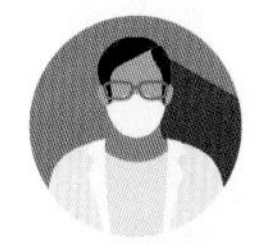

Pulmonologist B

Body plethysmography did not show signs of small airway disease either. Yet the patient's symptoms had been resolved under antigen eradication and immunosuppressive treatment with prednisolone. Furthermore, her history does not suggest persistent exposure to the antigen and subsequent fibrotic HP.

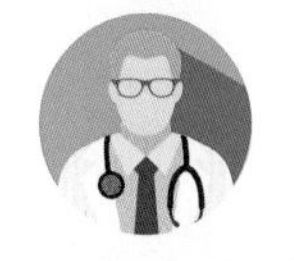

Pulmonologist A

I think so, too. She had no continued exposure to birds or other sources for avian antigens such as down-filled pillows; IgG titers decreased; and the ILD pattern on HRCT is indeterminate for HP. A chronic HP that turned into progressive fibrosis seems rather unlikely.

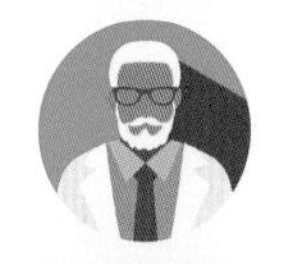

Radiologist

The diffuse pleural thickening and the predominant upper lobe involvement suggest a pleuroparenchymal fibroelastosis (PPFE).

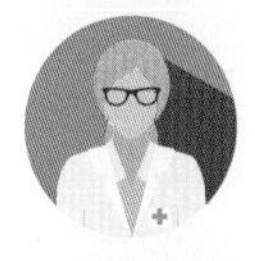

Pulmonologist C

HP may precede the development of chronic PPFE. However, the mild positivity of precipitins against birds and aspergillus still makes fibrosing HP a possible diagnosis.

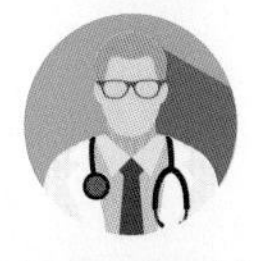

Pulmonologist A

Elevated precipitins for *Aspergillus fumigatus* have been repetitively reported in PPFE patients and are rather suggestive of pulmonary superinfection, aspergillosis, or allergic bronchopulmonary aspergillosis.

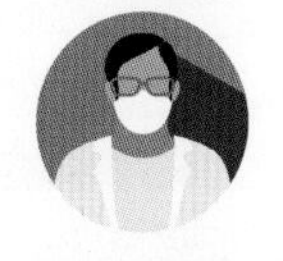

Pulmonologist B

It is important to distinguish between the two diseases given the lack of therapeutic options for patients with PPFE.
Histopathological examinations should be undertaken. I would suggest CT-guided pulmonary needle biopsies.

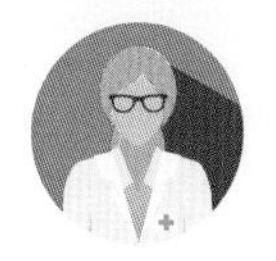

Pulmonologist C

However, an invasive diagnostic approach including lung biopsy carries an increased risk of pneumothorax. Spontaneous pneumothoraxes were also frequently observed in patients with PPFE at the time of diagnosis.

The patient was presented to the interdisciplinary ILD-board, which confirmed the diagnostic hypothesis of PPFE. She was referred to the radiologist to undergo CT-guided needle biopsy. The radiologist sampled a subpleural pulmonary abnormality that was accessible by dorsolateral puncture. Of note, immediate pneumothorax was found on follow-up CT imaging after the procedure was completed (Fig. 17.5). A small-bore chest tube was then placed. Further chest radiographs showed resolution of the pneumothorax, the drain was removed, and the patient was discharged after 1 week.

Histology revealed the pattern of alveolar fibroelastosis (Fig. 17.6) in the absence of inflammatory infiltrates or poorly formed granulomas. Although reminiscent HP cannot be fully ruled out by histopathological analysis of a single-sided biopsy, given its heterogenous nature, HP was considered to play a subordinate role in this case.

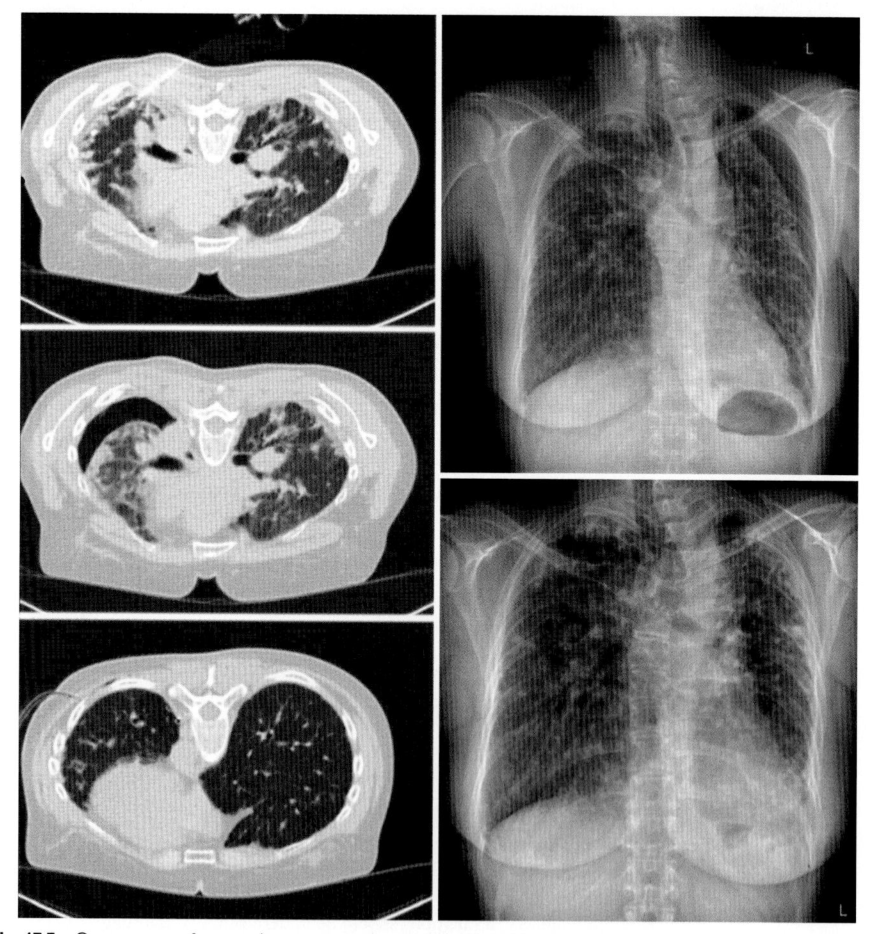

Fig. 17.5 Occurrence of secondary pneumothorax following CT-guided lung biopsy. Penetration of the fibrotic pleura by CT-guided lung biopsy (A) led to immediate formation of pneumothorax (B, C). PPFE patients are prone to develop either primary or secondary pneumothoraxes in the apical lung due to increased tractional forces acting on the stiff, fibrotic, and thickened pleura. The patient remained hemodynamically stable on pleural rupture but showed a rapid decline in oxygenation. Following insertion of drainage into the pleural space, the lung expanded (D, E) and the oxygenation status improved. The patient exhibited an uneventful recovery and was discharged 4 days after lung biopsy.

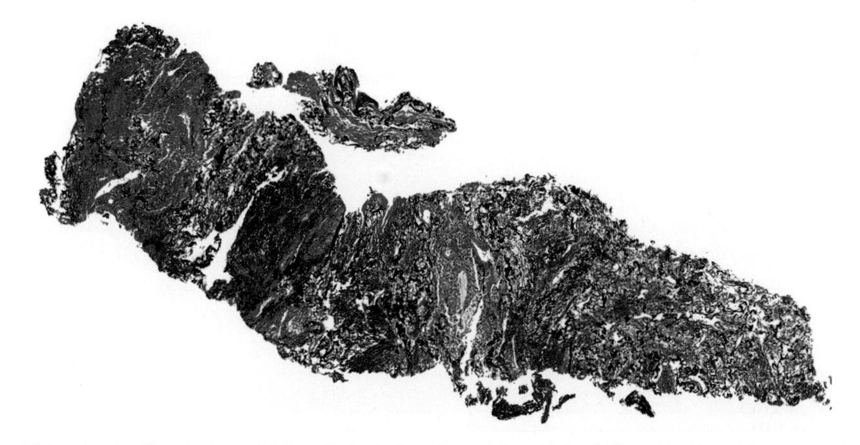

Fig. 17.6 Alveolar fibroelastosis. Histopathological workup of the obtained CT-guided lung biopsy specimen depicted zonal dense subpleural fibrosis in topographic proximity to elastotic remnants of obliterated airspaces drowning in coarse fibrils of collagen. The degree of parenchymal remodeling declines with increasing distance to the subpleural zone. Histopathological diagnosis of definite alveolar fibrelastosis (AFE) was made being in line with the radiographic findings.

Discussion Topic 3

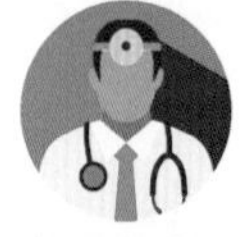

Interventional Radiologist

Unfortunately, pneumothorax occurred as complication on CT-guided fine needle biopsy. Thus, only a single biopsy specimen was obtained. Given the patchy spatial heterogeneity of consolidated PPFE lesions, quality of the biopsy sample cannot be taken for granted.

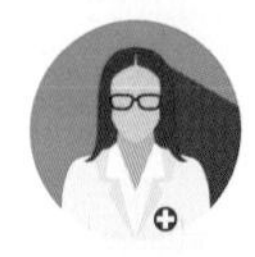

Pathologist

Luckily, lung biopsy of the subpleural regions of the right upper lobe was of sufficient quality. Marked alveolar fibroelastosis was noted consistent with the findings of subpleural fibrosis and alveolar fibrous obliteration with extensive collagen deposition in the airspaces adjacent to the pleura. Elastotic remnants of the former alveolar septa were noted in van Gieson elastin staining.

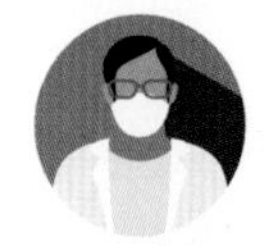

Pulmonologist B

A definite PPFE pattern on HRCT concomitant with manifest alveolar fibrelastosis (AFE) in histopathology leaves the patient with diagnosis of PPFE. Volume contraction in the upper lobes, platythorax, deepening of the suprasternal notch, and unspecific autoimmune features complete the typical clinical constellation.

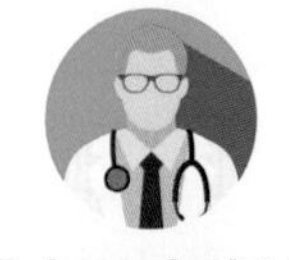

Pulmonologist A

What can we do for our patient?

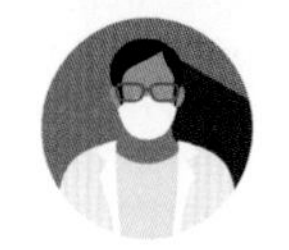

Pulmonologist B

Causative treatment options are, unfortunately, not available, leaving the treatment with the best supportive care. As the majority of PPFE cases depict a progressive course of the disease, the patient should be evaluated for lung transplantation in the near future.

Recommended Therapy and Further Indications

Prednisolone treatment had been already administered before referral to the ILD clinic, but shortness of breath, weight loss, and cough did not resolve since then. As neither chest HRCT nor laboratory workup depicted signs of ongoing pulmonary inflammation, steroids were carefully tapered down.

Given the lack of treatment options and the already manifest pulmonary functional impairment, the patient was referred to the lung transplantation unit to pursue further listing. The patient was instructed to keep her vaccination status updated (seasonal influenza, pneumococcal infection, and SARS-CoV-2), and the feasibility of pulmonary rehabilitation was evaluated.

Discussion Topic 4

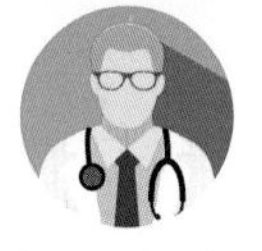

Pulmonologist A

I tapered the corticosteroid and finally stopped. Treatment with corticosteroids in idiopathic PPFE not secondary to autoimmune disease has solely shown subtle effects on inflammatory alterations on HRCT like ground-glass opacities but failed to improve or stabilize the decline in lung function or to reverse manifest fibrotic lesions.

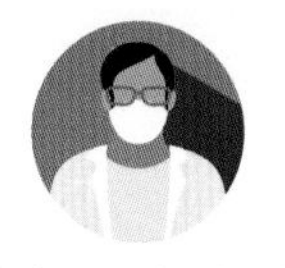

Pulmonologist B

I agree. Long-term immunosuppression increases the likelihood of infectious exacerbations. In addition, the patient had already tested positive for *A. fumigatus* antigen precipitins, raising the possibility of an overlying *Aspergillus* infection, as described in some PPFE case reports.

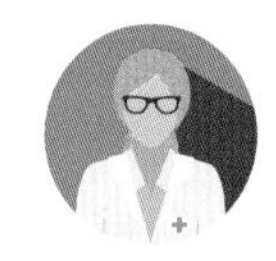

Pulmonologist C

Is there really no therapy that can help this patient?

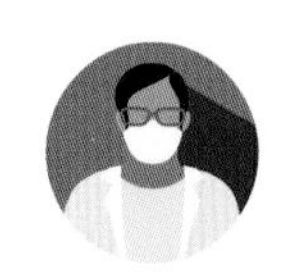

Pulmonologist B

Unfortunately, there are currently no causal treatment options available for patients with PPFE.
Available antifibrotic agents remain devoid of proven clinical benefit given the undeniable lack of prospective studies, although sustained pulmonary function has been reported during treatment with pirfenidone and nintedanib. Additionally, the effects of nintedanib are currently being studied in patients with chronic restrictive lung graft dysfunction.
I reiterate that the only option is to refer the patient to the lung transplant center.

Follow-Up and Outcomes

Approximately 6 months after diagnosis, the patient did pulmonary rehabilitation for 3 weeks but achieved only a slight improvement in exercise tolerance. She lost about 3 kg of weight and started taking dietary supplements of amino acids and proteins. Significant shortness of breath remained, PFTs showed further reduction in FVC, and oxygenation values were such that oxygen supplementation was required even at rest.

Focus on

Overview of PPFE

PPFE is listed among the idiopathic interstitial pneumonias (IIP) for more than two decades (Fig. 17.7). Epidemiological data are sparsely available, but one single-center study refers to up to 7.7% of PPFE cases among diagnosed IIP cases in one decade. Thereby, case reports are overrepresented among the Japanese literature. PPFE describes a fibroelastic lung disease initially described by Amitani as "pulmonary upper lobe fibrosis (PULF)," given its upper lobe predominance, and later coined as "idiopathic pleuroparenchymal fibroelastosis (PPFE)" by Frankel and coworkers in 2004. The disease has been stated to affect frequently nonsenile, female, never-smokers, but contradictive demographics are also available in the literature. A positive familial history is occasionally reported in patients with idiopathic PPFE. The histopathological counterpart is considered to be an alveolar fibroelastotic remodeling pattern termed alveolar fibroelastosis (AFE), which comprises alveolar obliteration due to marked intraalveolar collagen deposition in combination with reminiscent elastic fibers in the alveolar wall remnants. AFE predominates in the subpleural compartment but is also frequently localized in the parabronchial, paravascular, and interlobular parenchymal parts of the lung. Of note, subpleural thickening detectable in the HRCT usually co-locates with visceral pleura fibrosis.

ILDs with predominant upper lung lobe affection and sparing of the lower lung lobes are rarely seen in clinical practice. Differential diagnoses to be considered are idiopathic and secondary PPFE (iPPFE and sekPPFE, respectively), apical pleura caps, and certain pneumoconiosis such as asbestosis or aluminosis.

Diffuse pleural thickening including affection of the interlobar pleural fissures, upper lobe predominance of subpleural fibrosis, and relative sparing of the lower lobes resemble computed tomographic hallmarks of PPFE. Conversely, pronounced fibrotic, tractional distortion, and consecutive volume loss of the upper lung lobes as present in our patient is a characteristic finding in PPFE patients. Resultant clinical findings such as deepening of the suprasternal notch and plathythorax (shortened anteroposterior chest diameter) are early indicators of ongoing PPFE. These findings are usually explained by a disequilibrium of volume contraction and decreasing chest wall recoil forces driven by a characteristic permissive weight loss and sarcopenia.

Pneumothorax and pneumomediastinum are frequent complications in patients with PPFE, probably due to the pronounced tensile forces acting on the apical pleura. PPFE usually is a slowly progressive disease, and patients often have recurrent infections, increasing shortness of breath, and dry cough. Disease progression occurs in 60% of patients, and the prognosis is poor, with the large majority of patients dying of chronic respiratory failure, and a 5-year survival rate of 23.3% to 58.9%. Most of the literature reports the use of systemic corticosteroids, although there is no consistent evidence of efficacy, and lung transplantation remains an option for patients with end-stage lung disease.

Focus on

Pathogenetic Hypotheses of AFE and PPFE

A histopathological diagnosis of PPFE requires the demonstration of (intra)alveolar fibroelastosis (IAFE or AFE). This is defined by the presence of dense collagenous fibrosis filling alveolar spaces, with the residual alveolar walls highlighted by elastin deposition. Visceral pleural fibrosis further confirms the diagnosis, although it is not found in biopsies due to its patchy distribution. These features are prevalent in the upper lobes and are most easily detected by van Gieson elastin staining. The concurrent pathogenetic paradigm presumes AFE to be an aberrant wound repair mechanism secondary to a macrophage-driven lung injury. In this regard, pulmonary stem cell exhaustion may play a role in the formation of PPFE lesions as mutations in telomerase complex-associated genes (*TERT* and *TERC*) have been linked to progressive PPFE, similarly to the aberrant wound repair leading to the development of usual interstitial pneumonia in IPF. However, PPFE and UIP are distinct entities, although AFE was found to be spatially related to numerous histopathological patterns including UIP, nonspecific interstitial pneumonia, organizing pneumonia, bronchiolitis obliterans organizing pneumonia, and granulomas.

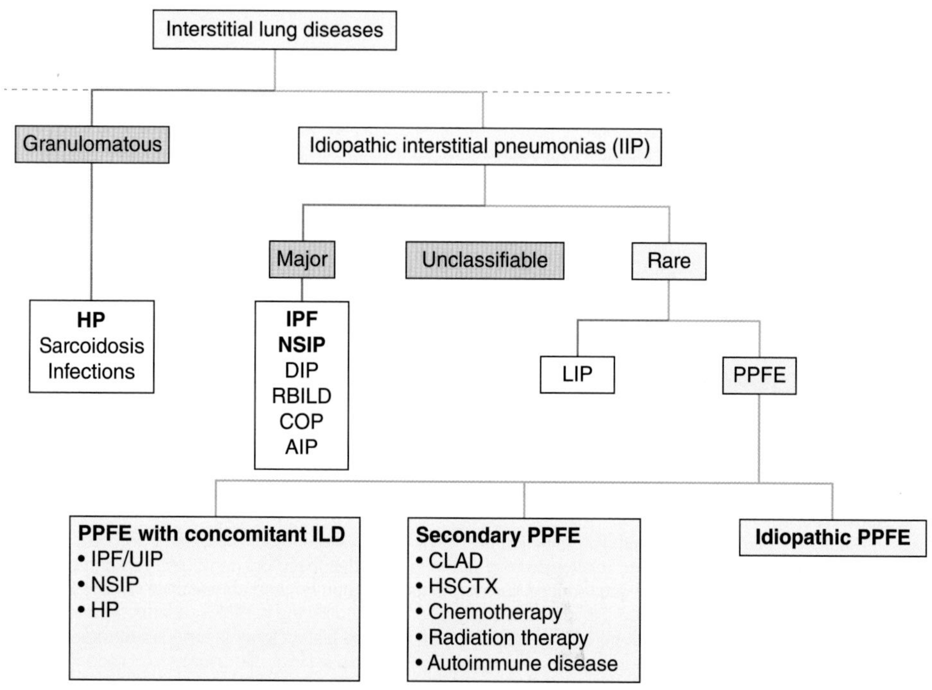

Fig. 17.7 Classification of pleuraparenchymal fibroelastosis (PPFE) within the interstitial lung diseases (outtake). PPFE is considered a rare idiopathic interstitial pneumonia (IIP). While it can occur in combination with other known interstitial entities (idiopathic pulmonary fibrosis [IPF], nonspecific interstitial pneumonia [NSIP], and organizing pneumonia [OP]), it has also been described in lung with chronic, fibrosing hypersensitivity pneumonitis (HP). Secondary PPFE can manifest following lung transplantation as chronic restrictive allograft syndrome (CLAD), hematopoetic stem cell transplantation (HSCTX), chemotherapy, radiation therapy, and autoimmune diseases, mainly systemic sclerosis and rheumatoid arthritis. Modified from Zibrak and Price, 2014.

Focus on

PPFE as a Possible Sequela in the Preinjured Lung

AFE can occur as an idiopathic entity in the context of PPFE on HRCT (idiopathic PPFE) but also with concomitant ILD and/or secondary to various exposures. In a well-conducted retrospective cohort analysis, 6 of 12 patients showed correlative features of an additional ILD on HRCT, of whom 3 patients depicted histopathological signs of UIP. Of note, PPFE concomitant with radiological, serological, and histopathological hallmarks of hypersensitivity pneumonitis, as in the current patient, was repeatedly noted throughout the literature. In this regard, AFE has been noted to occur with a prevalence of up to 23% in patients with HP. Likewise, secondary PPFE due to systemic sclerosis ILD or rheumatoid arthritis ILD was claimed to occur in approximately 10% of patients. Moreover, unspecific serologic abnormalities have been frequently noted in iPPFE patients. PPFE-like disease has also been reported secondary to exposure to chemotherapy, radiation, asbestos, and silicate as well as in patients who developed restrictive allograft syndrome after hematopoietic stem cell or lung transplantation, supporting the mechanism of aberrant wound repair following chronic alveolar injury in the development of PPFE. In contrast to UIP, only subtle involvement of the lower lung lobes and nono honeycombing is usually found in PPFE. Finally, coarse pleural fibrosis can occur as pulmonary apical cap (PAC), which has also been related to subtle AFE in the topographically proximate subpleural region. Differently from PPFE, PAC has been linked to a benign clinical course. Nevertheless, a transition of PAC into progressive PPFE has been suggested.

LEARNING POINTS

1. PPFE is a rare ILD characterized by predominant upper lobe fibrosis involving the pleura and subpleural lung parenchyma.
2. PPFE is an aberrant pulmonary wound repair with marked distinctive features from UIP/IPF.
3. PPFE is diagnosed by HRCT of the chest, but sometimes lung biopsy is required.
4. In most cases, PPFE is slowly progressive and has a poor prognosis.
5. Although most of the literature reports the use of corticosteroids, the appropriate treatment for PPFE is unknown, and lung transplantation is an option for patients with end-stage lung disease.

Further Reading

Amitani R, Niimi A, Kuse F. Idiopathic pulmonary upper lobe fibrosis (IPUF). *Kokyu* 1992;11:693-639.

Cheng SKH, Chuah KL. Pleuroparenchymal fibroelastosis of the lung: a review. *Arch Pathol Lab Med.* 2016;140(8):849-853.

Chua F, Desai SR, Nicholson AG, et al. Pleuroparenchymal fibroelastosis: a review of clinical, radiological, and pathological characteristics. *Ann Am Thorac Soc.* 2019;16(11):1351-1359.

Cottin V, Si-Mohamed S, Diesler R, Bonniaud P, Valenzuela C. Pleuroparenchymal fibroelastosis. *Curr Opin Pulm Med.* 2022;28(5):432-440.

Frankel SK, Cool CD, Lynch DA, Brown KK. Idiopathic pleuroparenchymal fibroelastosis: description of a novel clinicopathologic entity. *Chest.* 2004;126(6):2007-2013.

Harada T, Yoshida Y, Kitasato Y, et al. The thoracic cage becomes flattened in the progression of pleuroparenchymal fibroelastosis. *Eur Respir Rev.* 2014;23(132):263-266.

Kinoshita Y, Miyamura T, Ikeda T, et al. Limited efficacy of nintedanib for idiopathic pleuroparenchymal fibroelastosis. *Respir Investig.* 2022;60(4):562-569.

Nasser M, Si-Mohamed S, Turquier S, et al. Nintedanib in idiopathic and secondary pleuroparenchymal fibroelastosis. *Orphanet J Rare Dis.* 2021;16(1):419.

Newton CA, Batra K, Torrealba J, et al. Telomere-related lung fibrosis is diagnostically heterogeneous but uniformly progressive. *Eur Respir J.* 2016;48(6):1710-1720.

Piciucchi S, Tomassetti S, Casoni G, et al. High resolution CT and histological findings in idiopathic pleuroparenchymal fibroelastosis: features and differential diagnosis. *Respir Res.* 2011;12(1):111.

Raghu G, Collard HR, Egan JJ, et al. American Thoracic Society/European Respiratory Society International Multidisciplinary Consensus Classification of the Idiopathic Interstitial Pneumonias. *Am J Respir Crit Care Med.* 2002;165(2):277-304.

Reddy TL, Tominaga M, Hansell DM, et al. Pleuroparenchymal fibroelastosis: a spectrum of histopathological and imaging phenotypes. *Eur Respir J.* 2012;40(2):377-385.

Sato S, Hanibuchi M, Takahashi M, et al. A patient with idiopathic pleuroparenchymal fibroelastosis showing a sustained pulmonary function due to treatment with pirfenidone. *Intern Med (Tokyo, Japan).* 2016;55(5):497-501.

Shioya M, Otsuka M, Yamada G, et al. Poorer prognosis of idiopathic pleuroparenchymal fibroelastosis compared with idiopathic pulmonary fibrosis in advanced stage. *Can Respir J.* 2018.

Sugino K, Ono H, Saito M, et al. Immunoglobulin G4-positive interstitial pneumonia associated with pleuroparenchymal fibroelastosis. *Respir Case Rep.* 2022;10(4):e0925.

Tetikkurt C, Kubat B, Kulahci C, et al. Assessment score for the diagnosis of a case with pleuroparenchymal fibroelastosis. *Monaldi Arch Chest Dis.* 2021;91(3).

Watanabe S, Waseda Y, Takato H, et al. Pleuroparenchymal fibroelastosis: distinct pulmonary physiological features in nine patients. *Respir Investig.* 2015;3(4):149-155.

Xu L, Rassaei N, Caruso C. Pleuroparenchymal fibroelastosis with long history of asbestos and silicon exposure. *Int J Surg Pathol.* 2018;26(2):190-193.

Yoshida Y, Nagata N, Tsuruta N, et al. Heterogeneous clinical features in patients with pulmonary fibrosis showing histology of pleuroparenchymal fibroelastosis. *Respir Investig.* 2016;54(3):162-169.

Zibrak JD, Price D. Interstitial lung disease: raising the index of suspicion in primary care. *NPJ Prim Care Respir Med.* 2014;24:14054.

CHAPTER 18

IgG4-Related Disease as an Unexpected Cause of Hemoptysis

Lutz-Bernhard Jehn ■ Francesco Bonella

History of Present Illness

A 30-year-old never-smoker man was evaluated at the emergency department due to new onset of intermittent hemoptysis within a period of 4 weeks. Episodes increased in frequency, and the volume of expectorated fresh blood reached approximately 100 mL per day. The patient reported that a nonproductive cough had started 10 months before without any other systemic or thoracic symptoms. A chest radiograph in two planes revealed a hilo-mediastinal opacity with contact to the left upper lung lobe. A computed tomography (CT) scan of the chest with contrast material (Fig 18.1) showed a peribronchovascular mass compressing the left main bronchus and the left pulmonary artery. There was no evidence of pulmonary embolism, lymphadenopathy, bronchiectasis, pneumonia, or pleural effusions. For further evaluation, the patient was referred to the Center for Interstitial and Rare Lung Disease, a tertiary pulmonary care center that is located at the Ruhrlandklinik University Hospital Essen, Germany.

Past Medical History

The patient's medical history was unremarkable except for gastroesophageal reflux disease, which was well controlled under omeprazole therapy. He reported no other medications. He had no

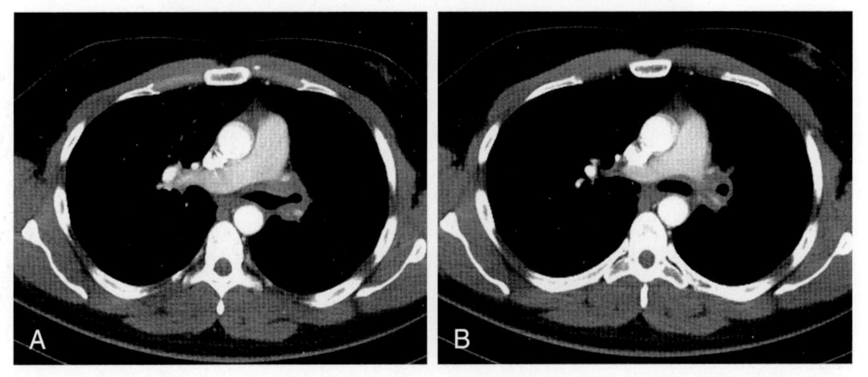

Fig 18.1 (A) Axial chest CT scan (mediastinal window) after the administration of intravenous contrast material showing a centrally located tumor formation surrounding the left main bronchus. (B) Reduced filling of the proximal left pulmonary artery with contrast material due to compression by the tumor is shown.

known drug allergies and did not consume alcohol or illicit drugs. He lived with his wife in an urban area of western Germany and worked as an office assistant. There were no known occupational or inhalational exposures. No familiarity for malignancies, autoimmune disorders, or pulmonary diseases was reported.

Physical Examination and Early Clinical Findings

At referral to the hospital, body temperature was 36.8°C (98.24°F), heart rate was 75 beats/min, blood pressure was 124/82 mmHg, respiratory rate was 16 breaths per minute, and oxygen saturation was 97% while the patient was breathing ambient air at rest. Auscultation of the chest revealed no abnormalities. No peripheral cyanosis or edema was present, and there were no ecchymoses or other signs of bleeding.

The laboratory tests showed normal counts of white blood cells, eosinophils, and platelets. Total serum protein concentration and electrophoresis were in the normal range.

Blood levels of immunoglobulin E (IgE), electrolytes, lipase, amylase, lactate dehydrogenase, and C-reactive protein were normal, as were the results of liver function, kidney function, and clotting tests.

Lung function tests were all in the normal range, and the diffusing capacity of the lungs for carbon monoxide (DLCO) was 90% of the predicted value when corrected for hemoglobin.

A cranial CT scan showed no cerebral metastases, paranasal sinus abnormalities, or other abnormal findings.

A total body positron emission tomography (PET)/CT scan (Fig 18.2) showed an increased ^{18}F-fluorodeoxyglucose (^{18}F-FDG) uptake of the peribronchovascular tumor (standardized uptake value [SUV] max. 12.3) but revealed no evidence of other ^{18}F-FDG–avid lesions.

Lung perfusion scintigraphy after the injection of technetium-99m (^{99m}Tc)-labeled macroaggregates of albumin revealed a pronounced left perfusion deficit with a mean activity distribution in the right lung of 92% compared to 8% in the left lung due to compression of the proximal left pulmonary artery by the tumor (Fig 18.3).

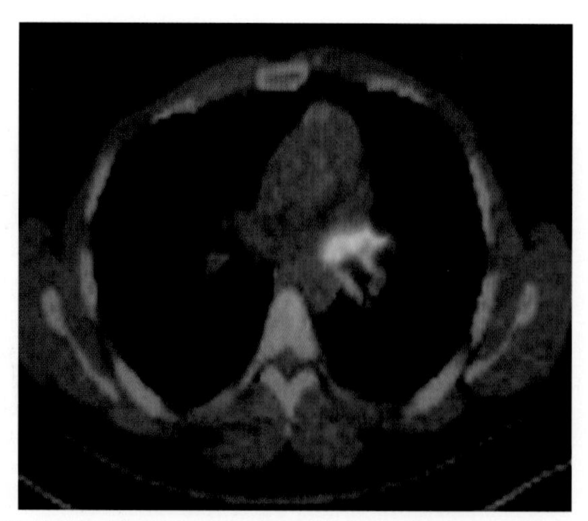

Fig 18.2 ^{18}F-FDG PET/CT showing a centrally located mass surrounding the left main bronchus with increased tracer uptake (standardized uptake value [SUV] max. 12.3) appearing as yellow-white mass.

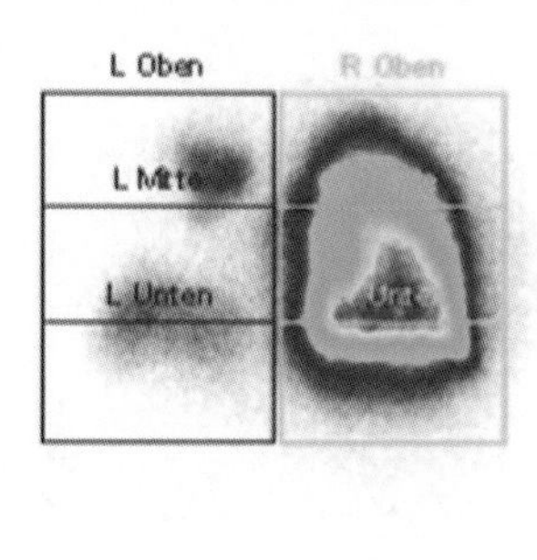

Fig 18.3 The technetium-99m (^{99m}Tc) activity distribution in the right lung is shown at three different levels (apical, intermediate, diaphragmatic) using tomographic gamma camera examination (single-photon emission computed tomography). A marked reduction of perfusion with predominance of the left apical and intermediate lung zones can be seen.

Discussion Topic 1 ■ Building a Differential Diagnosis

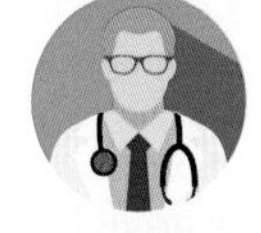

Pulmonologist A

The patient has a pulmonary mass surrounding the left main bronchus and the left pulmonary artery. Even uncommon in a 30-year-old, otherwise healthy, never-smoker man without familiarity for malignancies, we should consider the diagnosis of primary lung cancer.

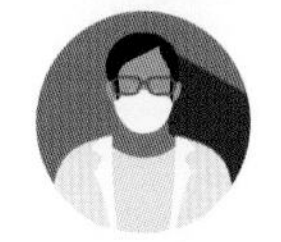

Pulmonologist B

Are there specific characteristics of primary lung cancer in the group of never-smokers?

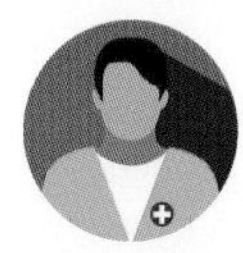

Oncologist

Adenocarcinoma is the predominant histological subtype of lung cancer in young never-smokers. There is a higher likelihood to detect targetable driver mutations, for example, activating *EGFR* or *ALK* gene mutations, in adenocarcinomas occurring in never-smokers compared to smokers. In contrast, small cell lung cancer in never-smokers is very rare.

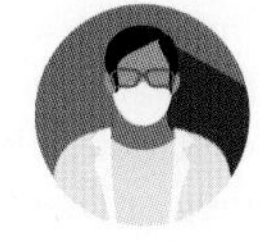

Pulmonologist B

What do you think about the possibility of metastatic cancer or pulmonary lymphoma?

Continued on following page

Discussion Topic 1 ■ Building a Differential Diagnosis (Continued)

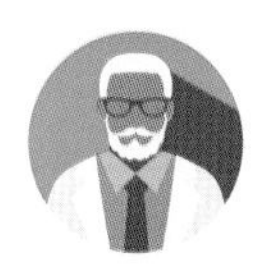

Radiologist

There is no evidence of mediastinal lymphadenopathy or other thoracic abnormalities on chest CT scan. Because total body FDG-PET/CT scan revealed no evidence of extrathoracic lesions, metastatic disease or secondary pulmonary lymphoma is unlikely.

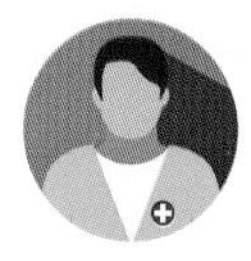

Oncologist

I agree. He doesn't have the typical "B-symptoms" that can be associated with lymphomas: no fever, no night sweats, and no unintentional weight loss. All these data further argue against secondary pulmonary lymphoma or systemic hematological diseases. Primary pulmonary lymphoma is extremely rare in young patients without underlying immunosuppression, although primary pulmonary lymphoma can occur with a peribronchovascular mass in isolation.

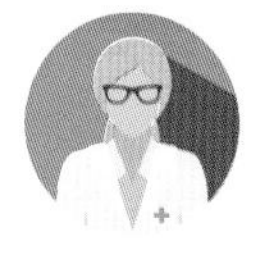

Pulmonologist C

Important immune-mediated disorders that should be considered in this case are sarcoidosis and antineutrophil cytoplasmic antibody (ANCA)-associated vasculitis, especially eosinophilic granulomatosis with polyangiitis (EGPA) and granulomatosis with polyangiitis (GPA). Additional laboratory tests should therefore include tests for antinuclear antibodies (ANAs) and ANCAs. Serum levels of angiotensin-converting enzyme (ACE) and the soluble interleukin 2 receptor (sIL-2R) should also be determined.

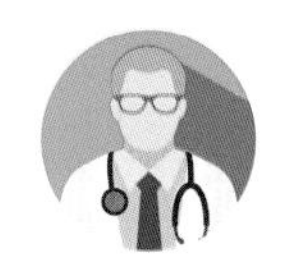

Pulmonologist A

Let´s perform transbronchial core needle biopsies to obtain tissue specimens directly from the tumor, endobronchial ultrasound-guided transbronchial needle aspirations (EBUS-TBNAs) for cytological analysis of selected lymph node stations, and mucosal forceps biopsies from the involved bronchial mucosa. Bronchoalveolar lavage (BAL) with differential cytology might be helpful to detect inflammatory alveolar processes or underlying infections; in particular, we should look for mycobacteria (tuberculosis as well atypical), fungi, and bacteria.

Clinical Course

ANA and ANCA tests were negative and there were normal serum levels of ACE (< 12 U/L, normal range 8–62 U/L) and sIL-2R (300 U/L, normal range 223–710 U/L).

A rigid diagnostic bronchoscopy with BAL, transbronchial core needle biopsies from the mass, and EBUS-TBNAs from suspicious lymph node stations was performed. Rigid bronchoscopy was chosen to facilitate the removal of preexisting blood clots and to optimize the management of potential bleeding complications in comparison to the use of a flexible bronchoscope. The left main bronchus was compressed by the surrounding tumor formation. Macroscopically, edema and hypervascularization of the mucosa, also involving the proximal left upper lobe bronchus, were seen. Forceps biopsy specimens were obtained from the visually altered mucosa of the left main bronchus and the left upper lobe bronchus. The mucosa was extremely vulnerable to manipulation with the bronchoscope and reacted with easy bleeding. There were no signs of active bleeding or endobronchial tumor growth. The remaining examination of the bronchial system was normal.

The recovered BAL fluid (BALF), obtained from the lingula, was clear, and the BALF differential cytology was normal. Perls Prussian blue staining revealed an increased number of hemosiderin-laden macrophages.

BALF staining for acid-fast bacilli was negative, and sputum polymerase chain reaction tests for tuberculous and nontuberculous mycobacteria were negative. An interferon-γ release assay revealed no prior immunization against mycobacterium tuberculosis.

Histological analysis of the tissue specimens obtained from the peribronchovascular mass showed a dense lymphoplasmacytic infiltrate, tissue fibrosis, and obliterative phlebitis accompanied by a mild granulocytic infiltrate. Lymph node TBNAs revealed unspecific inflammatory changes. Mucosal biopsy specimens of the left main and upper lobe bronchus showed signs of chronic bronchitis.

Because neoplastic cells in masses with extended inflammation or marked fibrosis can be missed by transbronchial core needle biopsy due to sampling bias, a surgical biopsy approach was recommended by the institutional tumor board to rule out malignancy with a higher negative predictive value.

Minimal thoracotomy was performed after placement of a double-lumen endotracheal tube for selective ventilation of the right lung. During palpation of the collapsed left lung, a centrally located solid mass was detectable and biopsy specimens were directly obtained from the tumor. The histological findings were compatible with the prior findings; again, there was no evidence of malignancy (Fig 18.4).

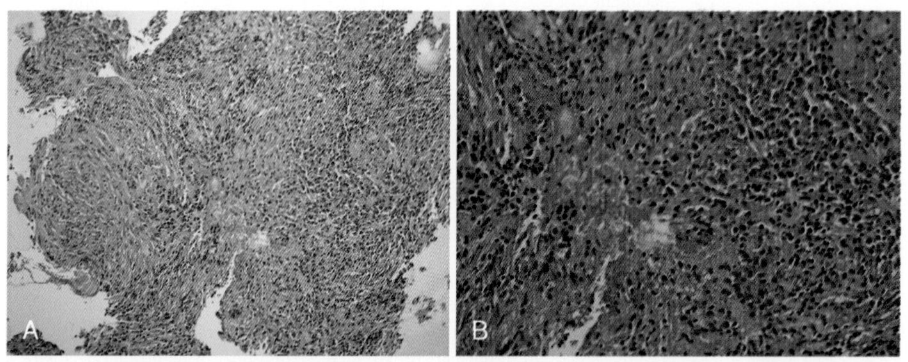

Fig 18.4 (A) Hematoxylin and eosin staining of specimens obtained from the surgical biopsy show evidence of fibrosis and a lymphoplasmacytic infiltrate of mixed density (×100 original magnification). (B) The same specimen with a dense lymphoplasmacytic infiltrate. There is no evidence of giant cells, granulomas, or necrosis (×200 original magnification).

Discussion Topic 2 ■ Narrowing the Differential Diagnosis and Evaluation of Further Diagnostic Tests

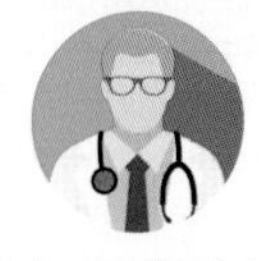

Pulmonologist A

Do you think we can exclude malignancy or infections on the basis of the findings we have obtained so far?

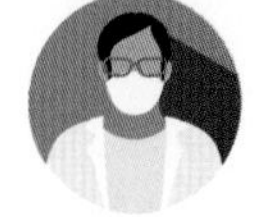

Pulmonologist B

On CT imaging, primary lung cancer commonly presents as ground-glass opacification or discrete nodules or masses with a spiculated margin frequently accompanied by lymphadenopathy. The noninvasive character of this peribronchovascular process on CT scans without lymphadenopathy and several negative biopsy results strongly argue against lung cancer in this case.

Continued on following page

Discussion Topic 2 ■ Narrowing the Differential Diagnosis and Evaluation of Further Diagnostic Tests (Continued)

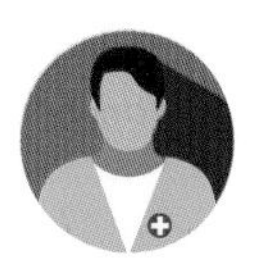

Oncologist

The most frequent types of primary pulmonary lymphoma are marginal zone B-cell lymphoma (MZL) of the mucosa-associated lymphatic tissue (MALT) and diffuse large B-cell lymphoma (DLBCL). Both typically occur between 50 and 70 years of age and are commonly associated with immunosuppression. Lymphomatoid granulomatosis, usually presenting in middle-aged adults and associated with immunosuppression, is an Epstein-Barr virus (EBV)-associated lymphoproliferative disorder. Hodgkin lymphoma or multicentric Castleman disease can present as a peribronchovascular mass in younger patients even without underlying immunosuppression. However, the absence of lymphadenopathy, the lack of B-symptoms, and the histopathological findings are not suggestive of any of these entities.

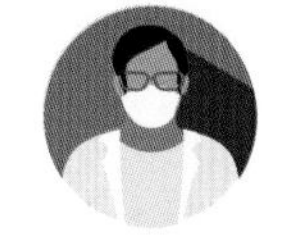

Pulmonologist B

Further, numerous microbiological analyses were unremarkable, and tissue specimens did not show evidence of necrotizing granulomatous inflammation. Thus, we can rule out an infectious process with a very high likelihood.

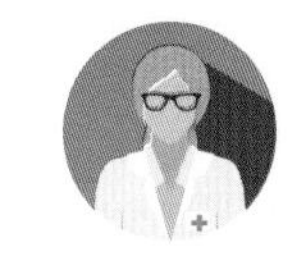

Pulmonologist C

I think we should focus on immune-mediated disorders. What are your ideas in this case?

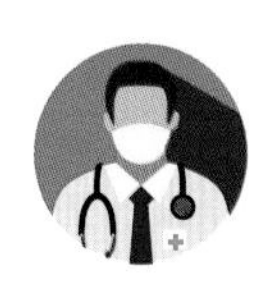

Rheumatologist

In this case, negative ANA/ANCA test results make a diagnosis of GPA unlikely. Conversely, ANCA-negative EGPA is quite common. Granulomas, necrosis, and giant cells are typical histological findings in EGPA and GPA but are also absent in our patient. An increased number of hemosiderin-laden macrophages in the BALF is common in alveolar hemorrhage syndromes, which can occur in a broad range of diseases including pulmonary ANCA-associated vasculitis. However, increased numbers of hemosiderin-laden macrophages can be the result of chronic endobronchial blood loss with consecutive phagocytosis of red blood cells in the alveolar spaces. Normal ACE and sIL-2R serum levels, combined with the absence of BALF lymphocytosis, missing noncaseating granulomas, and no additional organ involvement, are associated with a very low likelihood of sarcoidosis.

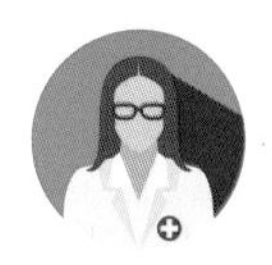

Pathologist

A dense lymphoplasmacytic infiltrate, a varying degree of tissue fibrosis, and obliterative phlebitis are the main histological findings of IgG4-Related Disease (IgG4-RD), which are all present in our case. Tissue staining for $IgG4^{+}$ plasma cells is required for a definite diagnosis of thoracic involvement in IgG4-RD. Additional laboratory tests should include serum concentrations of IgG4. Circulating plasmablasts are frequently expanded in peripheral blood irrespective of serum IgG4-levels in patients with IgG4-RD and could be determined with flow cytometry.

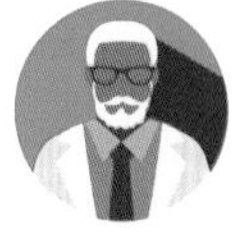

Radiologist

The most frequent HRCT patterns of thoracic IgG4-RD are peribronchovascular involvement and lymph node enlargement. Thus, the radiographic findings also support a diagnosis of IgG4-RD in this case.

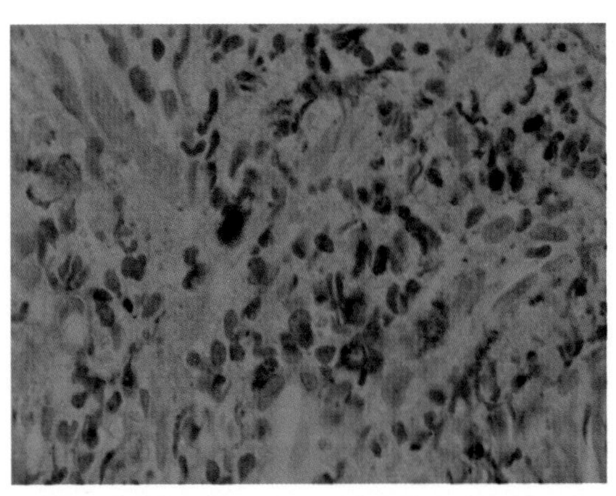

Fig 18.5 A marked increase in IgG4-positive plasma cells among the inflammatory infiltrates is shown (×600 original magnification).

Staining for IgG4 performed on tissue samples obtained from surgical biopsy specimens showed an increased number of IgG4$^+$ plasma cells with an IgG4$^+$/IgG$^+$ plasma cell ratio of 50% (Fig 18.5). However, serum IgG4 concentration was in the normal range (0.276 g/L, with a suggested cut-off of 1.35 g/L).

Integrating all clinical, serological, radiological, and pathological findings, a diagnosis of IgG4-RD was finally made in accordance with the 2019 American College of Rheumatology/ European Alliance of Associations for Rheumatology (ACR/EULAR) classification criteria for IgG4-RD.

Recommended Therapy

Steroid induction therapy was initiated for IgG4-RD with 40 mg prednisone/day. At the first follow-up after 3 months, cough and hemoptysis had resolved completely, and the mass had decreased in size on CT scan (Fig 18.6).

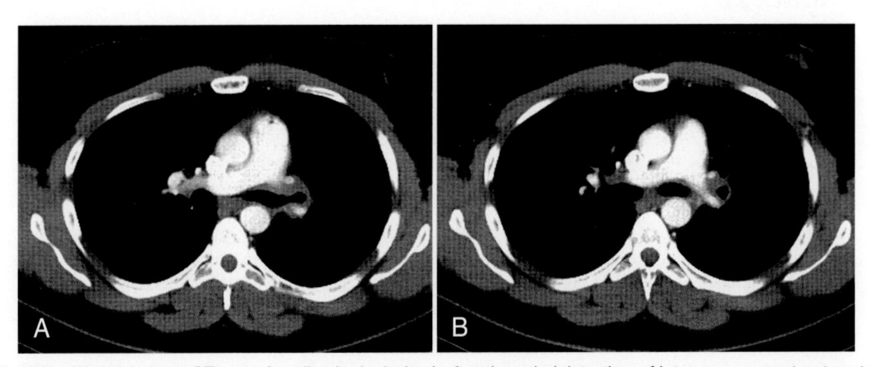

Fig 18.6 (A) Axial chest CT scan (mediastinal window) after the administration of intravenous contrast material showing a decreased size of the mass around the left main bronchus. (B) The filling of the proximal left pulmonary artery with contrast material seemed to be increased 3 months after steroid induction therapy compared to the initial findings (shown in Fig. 1).

Follow-Up and Outcomes

Steroids were gradually tapered down 4 weeks after initiation, and a sustained clinical remission was achieved with a maintenance dose of 15 mg/day. Because low-dose steroid maintenance was associated with an unintended weight gain of 11 kg, steroid treatment was completely discontinued. At 18 months after steroid initiation, relapse occurred with the new onset of severe hemoptysis.

Steroid therapy was restarted with 40 mg prednisone/day achieving a good and rapid clinical response. Due to stable clinical course, steroids were gradually reduced, but hemoptysis reoccurred at a maintenance dose of 5 mg prednisone/day. Second-line treatment with rituximab was initiated at the rheumatological department of our hospital and a complete clinical remission was achieved.

Discussion Topic 4 ■ Therapeutic Approaches and Biomarkers to Predict Disease Activity and Treatment Response in IgG4-RD

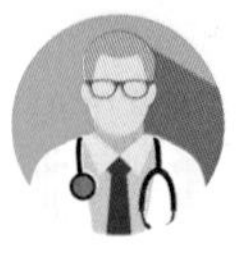

Pulmonologist A

There was a good clinical response to steroids, but the mass decreased only a little in size. What is your opinion about this finding?

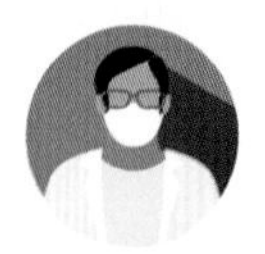

Pulmonologist B

Steroids are considered as first-line treatment for remission induction in all patients with active, untreated IgG4-RD disease. Thoracic manifestations of IgG4-RD typically are also associated with high response rates to steroids. The lack of a significant size reduction on imaging analyses might be due to a high degree of fibrosis, which cannot be addressed by any pharmacological agent.

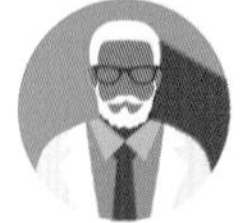

Radiologist

After complete tapering of steroids, disease relapse occurred. Are steroids appropriate for reinduction in IgG4-RD?

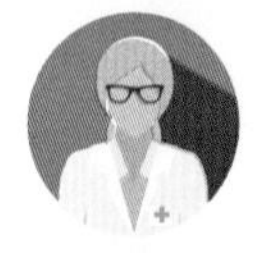

Pulmonologist C

If remission is achieved with steroid induction therapy, patients can benefit from low-dose steroid maintenance. Relapse is common when steroids have been tapered, but reinduction with steroids is usually effective. The induction dosage of steroids should be continued for 2 to 4 weeks, after which steroids can be gradually tapered down.

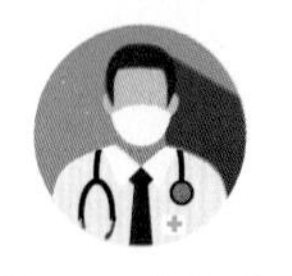

Rheumatologist

Because of the high rate of treatment failure with low-dose steroids and the substantial long-term side effects, steroid-sparing agents should be considered as maintenance therapy. One highly effective option in IgG4-RD is B-cell depletion with rituximab, which is also associated with high response rates in thoracic IgG4-RD.

Discussion Topic 4 ■ Therapeutic Approaches and Biomarkers to Predict Disease Activity and Treatment Response in IgG4-RD (Continued)

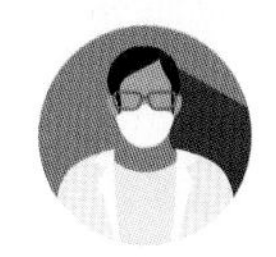

Pulmonologist B

Are there any specific biomarkers to determine the optimal time to initiate B-cell–depleting therapy after steroid-induced remission, to predict treatment responses to steroids or rituximab and to identify optimal dose intervals for rituximab maintenance?

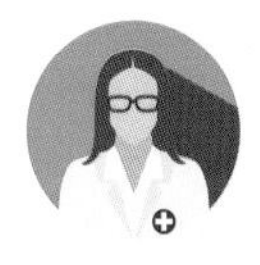

Pathologist

The number of circulating $CD20^{+}$ memory B-cells rises before IgG4-RD relapses after steroid-induced remission, and these cells can be targeted with rituximab. Also, the number of circulating plasmablasts and serum IgG4 levels seem to correlate with disease activity; both were shown to decrease after response to steroids or rituximab and can increase at disease flare.

Focus on

Overview of Thoracic IgG4-Related Disease

IgG4-RD is a rare systemic fibroinflammatory disease of unknown etiology that can affect virtually any organ. Investigations from Japan report a disease prevalence of about 100 cases per million. The disease has a male predominance and is usually diagnosed in patients > 50 years of age. An association has been described between various disease manifestations of the respiratory system, including chronic rhinosinusitis, asthma, bronchiectasis, pulmonary fibrosis, emphysema, pleuritis, and mediastinal fibrosis with increased tissue or serum levels of IgG4. Thoracic involvement of IgG4-RD seems to be underestimated and may be found in up to 30% of patients diagnosed with IgG4-RD in association with other organ disease or in isolation in about 10% of cases. The exposition to tobacco use or other occupational or environmental agents is not a known risk factor for thoracic IgG4-RD, and the role of genetic risk factors contributing to thoracic manifestations of IgG4-RD is unclear. The male predilection of IgG4-RD and the common occurrence in elderly adults are reflected by a predominance of the male gender with a mean age at diagnosis of about 60 years in retrospective case series of patients with thoracic IgG4-RD. Because IgG4-RD was described as a unique disease only two decades ago, there is a lack of prospective long-term data on the mortality of patients with IgG4-RD. Based on retrospective case series, no differences in mortality between patients with and without thoracic involvement of IgG4-RD were observed. While early studies reported a mortality rate of 60% with a median survival of 3 years, in the newest case series a 5-year survival rate > 80% has been described. Thoracic IgG4-RD can cause a variety of unspecific symptoms, including chronic cough, hemoptysis, and dyspnea. Acute or fulminant symptoms like acute hypoxemic respiratory failure are typically absent and rather would be the result of progressive local organ damage due to the fibroinflammatory process.

Focus on

Diagnostic Issues of Thoracic IgG4-Related Disease

Differential diagnoses of suspected thoracic IgG4-RD mainly include immune-mediated disorders such as sarcoidosis and ANCA-associated vasculitis, neoplasms comprising primary lung cancer, and lymphoproliferative disorders, as well as bacterial, fungal, and viral infections. A diagnosis of thoracic IgG4-RD can be classified as definite, highly probable, probable, possible, and alternative to IgG4-RD. For a diagnosis of definite thoracic IgG4-RD, histological confirmation is mandatory.

Continued on following page

Focus on (Continued)

Diagnostic Issues of Thoracic IgG4-Related Disease

However, the newest ACR/EULAR IgG4-RD classification criteria 2019 do not strictly require a positive biopsy nor elevated serum IgG4 concentration for confirmation of IgG4-RD, when the diagnosis of IgG4-RD is straightforward on the basis of clinical, serological, and radiological findings. This is clinically relevant, because up to 10% of patients with biopsy-proven IgG4-RD reveal normal serum levels of IgG4. Based on HRCT findings, pulmonary IgG4-RD can be categorized into nodular, round-shaped ground-glass opacity, interstitial disease, or peribronchovascular patterns, but a pathognomonic pattern does not exist. Lymph node enlargement, retromediastinal fibrosis, and pleural disease are further ancillary HRCT patterns associated with thoracic IgG4-RD. ^{18}F-FDG PET/CT is a useful tool to detect thoracic manifestations of IgG4-RD, to select the optimal biopsy side, and to assess disease activity and treatment response. BALF cytology is not specific for pulmonary IgG4-RD, but moderate lymphocytosis has been described. For histological confirmation, transbronchial core needle or cryobiopsies for lung parenchymal involvement, transbronchial needle aspirations for mediastinal lymph node sampling, percutaneous core needle biopsies for pleural involvement, or surgical procedures can be performed. Surgical biopsy specimens usually reveal higher numbers of IgG4$^+$ plasma cells than nonsurgical biopsies (consensus threshold of $>$ 50 IgG4$^+$ plasma cells per high-power field for surgical biopsies vs. $>$ 20 IgG4$^+$ plasma cells per high-power field for nonsurgical biopsies). Independent of the sample type and size an IgG4$^+$/IgG$^+$ plasma cell ratio $>$ 40% strongly supports a diagnosis of IgG4-RD. Storiform fibrosis and obliterative phlebitis are distinguishing features of IgG4-RD but can be absent in lung tissue. Additional findings include neutrophilic aggregates and obliterative arteritis in the lung interstitium and alveolar spaces, uncommon in other organs.

Focus on

Treatment of Thoracic IgG4-Related Disease

Treatment aims to prevent or control organ damage, which can be life-threatening, and relieve symptoms. Because spontaneous remissions in thoracic IgG4-RD have been reported, patients do not always require treatment and a "watchful waiting" strategy might be appropriate, such as in case of asymptomatic nonprogressive lymphadenopathy. Thoracic IgG4-RD is associated with a high clinical and radiological response to steroids, comparable to the extrathoracic form. The tendency to relapse after remission under steroids seems to be a common feature of both intrathoracic and extrathoracic forms. It is unclear if the response to treatment or the risk of relapse could vary according to the underlying HRCT patterns. Steroids are generally used as first-line treatment (prednisone or equivalent, 30–40 mg/day), and an inadequate response to these agents is considered an excluding IgG4-RD diagnostic criterion by the 2019 ACR/EULAR guideline. After induction over 2 to 4 weeks, steroids can be gradually tapered down, generally over months. Because of a high treatment failure rate after steroid discontinuation and even under low-dose steroid maintenance treatment, steroid-sparing agents like azathioprine, mycophenolate, methotrexate, and cyclophosphamide have been used. Their value in thoracic IgG4-RD is still unclear. B-cell–depleting therapy with rituximab has been shown to be highly effective in IgG4-RD and may be considered when treatment to steroids fails or is not tolerated. Promising treatment approaches are represented by monoclonal antibodies against B-cell and T-cell surface molecules including CD19 (inebilizumab), CD38 (daratumumab), and SLAMF-7 (elotuzumab) or small molecules targeting the proteasome (bortezomib), Bruton tyrosine kinase (rilzabrutinib), or CTLA4 (abatacept). Their role in the treatment of IgG4-RD needs to be further investigated.

LEARNING POINTS

- IgG4-RD is a systemic fibroinflammatory disease that can affect airways, lung parenchyma, pleura, and mediastinum.
- Diagnosis of pulmonary IgG4-RD relies on all clinical, radiological, and histopathological findings because symptoms and radiological findings are not specific. Moreover, elevated serum IgG4-levels and increased concentration of IgG4-positive plasma cells in tissue can be found in several malignant, inflammatory, and infectious processes of the lung.
- BALF findings in pulmonary IgG4-RD are not specific, and the diagnostic utility of BALF cellular analysis or BALF IgG4-levels in pulmonary IgG4-RD needs to be clarified.
- Cytology and histology with special staining can confirm the diagnosis of pulmonary IgG4-RD. The optimal sampling technique depends on the type, site, and distribution of the lesions, including EBUS–guided TBNA, transbronchial biopsies, and surgical biopsies.
- Steroids are recommended as first-line treatment for remission induction in IgG4-RD independent of the sides of manifestation and show high response rates although relapses are common when they are tapered.
- B-cell–depleting therapy with rituximab is a highly effective alternative treatment of IgG4-RD in case of steroid intolerance or disease relapse after their tapering.
- Acute or fulminant presentation, B-symptoms, and the initial failure of response to an adequate course of steroids (0.6 mg/kg per day of prednisone or equivalent) should question the diagnosis of thoracic IgG4-RD.

Further Readings

Carruthers MN, Khosroshahi A, Augustin T, et al. The diagnostic utility of serum IgG4 concentrations in IgG4-related disease. *Ann Rheum Dis.* 2015;74(1):14-18.

Carruthers MN, Topazian MD, Khosroshahi A, et al. Rituximab for IgG4-related disease: a prospective, open-label trial. *Ann Rheum Dis.* 2015;74(6):1171-1177.

Corcoran JP, Culver EL, Anstey RM, et al. Thoracic involvement in IgG4-related disease in a UK-based patient cohort. *Respir Med.* 2017;132:117-121.

Deshpande V, Zen Y, Chan JK, et al. Consensus statement on the pathology of IgG4-related disease. *Mod Pathol.* 2012;25(9):1181-1192.

Ebbo M, Grados A, Guedj E, et al. Usefulness of 2-[18F]-fluoro-2-deoxy-D-glucose-positron emission tomography/computed tomography for staging and evaluation of treatment response in IgG4-related disease: a retrospective multicenter study. *Arthritis Care Res.* 2014;66:86-96.

Kamisawa T, Funata N, Hayashi Y, et al. A new clinicopathological entity of IgG4-related autoimmune disease. *J Gastroenterol.* 2003;38(10):982-984.

Khosroshahi A, Wallace ZS, Crowe JL, et al. International Consensus Guidance Statement on the management and treatment of IgG4-related disease. *Arthritis Rheumatol.* 2015;67(7):1688-1699.

Lanzillotta M, Della-Torre E, Milani R, et al. Increase of circulating memory B cells after glucocorticoid-induced remission identifies patients at risk of IgG4-related disease relapse. *Arthritis Res Ther.* 2018;20(1):222.

Mattoo H, Mahajan VS, Della-Torre E, et al. De novo oligoclonal expansions of circulating plasmablasts in active and relapsing IgG4-related disease. *J Allergy Clin Immunol.* 2014;134(3):679-687.

Muller R, Habert P, Ebbo M, et al. Thoracic involvement and imaging patterns in IgG4-related disease. *Eur Respir Rev*. 2021;30(162):210078.

Ryu JH, Sekiguchi H, Yi ES. Pulmonary manifestations of immunoglobulin G4-related sclerosing disease. *Eur Respir J*. 2012;39(1):180-186.

Strehl JD, Hartmann A, Agaimy A. Numerous IgG4-positive plasma cells are ubiquitous in diverse localised non-specific chronic inflammatory conditions and need to be distinguished from IgG4-related systemic disorders. *J Clin Pathol*. 2011;64(3):237-243.

Wallace ZS, Khosroshahi A, Carruthers MD, et al. An International Multispecialty Validation Study of the IgG4-related disease responder index. *Arthritis Care Res (Hoboken)*. 2018;70(11):1671-1678.

Wallace ZS, Mattoo H, Mahajan VS, et al. Predictors of disease relapse in IgG4-related disease following rituximab. *Rheumatology*. 2016;55(6):1000-1008.

Wallace ZS, Naden RP, Chari S, et al. The 2019 American College of Rheumatology/European League Against Rheumatism classification criteria for IgG4-related disease. *Ann Rheum Dis*. 2020;79(1):7-87.

PART VI

Miscellanea

CHAPTER 19

Amyloid-Associated Cystic Lung Disease in a Woman With Sjögren Syndrome

Claudio Tirelli ■ Claudia Cigala ■ Silvia Terraneo ■ Giovanni Palladini ■ Michele Mondoni

History of Present Illness

A 68-year-old Caucasian female was admitted to the emergency department after a traumatic accident and a consequent transient loss of consciousness. A total body computed tomography (CT) scan was immediately performed. Brain CT scan showed an occipital subarachnoid hemorrhage and bilateral subdural hematoma, while chest CT scan revealed multiple bilateral cysts (from a few millimeters to 2 cm in size) with a well-defined wall. Bilateral, partly calcified nodules with regular margins (the largest with 21-mm long-axis CT diameter) were also evident (Fig 19.1).

Blood tests showed only a mild lymphocytosis (white blood cell [WBC] count 12,000 cells/μL, normal values: 4,300 cells μL; neutrophils 80%) and a very slight increase in the indices of inflammation (C-reactive protein [CRP] 18 mg/L, normal values <5 mg/L).

Blood pressure was 115/70 mmHg, heart rate was 85 beats/min, body temperature was 36.4°C, and peripheral oxygen saturation (SpO_2) was 98% on room air. The patient was then admitted to the neurology unit and showed rapid clinical improvement.

Past Medical History

The patient was a former mild smoker (smoking history of 5 pack-years) who had quit smoking more than 30 years ago. In her past medical history, she had gastroesophageal reflux disease secondary to a hiatal hernia and a diagnosis of osteoporosis, treated with α-calcifediol and alendronate.

She denied any familiar history of respiratory diseases or occupational exposures to irritant agents. She only had two lower tract respiratory infections during the past 10 years.

Physical Examination and Early Clinical Findings

During the pulmonology consultation, she was eupneic and denied any respiratory symptoms. SpO_2 values continued to be normal on room air. At chest examination, the respiratory sound was bilaterally present, without pathological sounds. Heart and abdomen examinations were unremarkable. No digital fissures or clubbing were detectable.

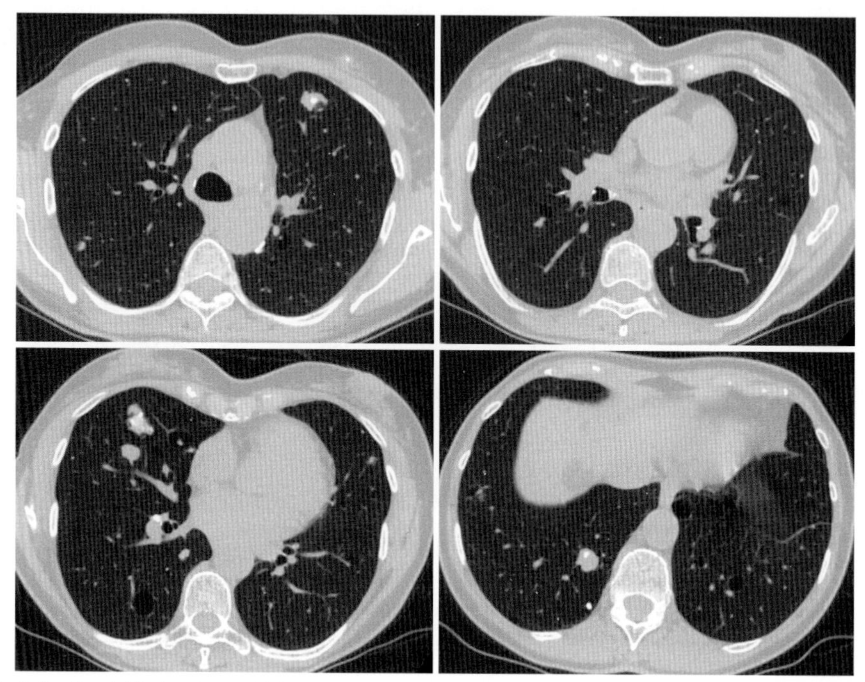

Fig 19.1 Chest CT showing multiple bilateral nodules, partly calcified, and cysts of various diameters (from few millimeters to 2 cm). Cysts present a defined but irregular wall.

Discussion Topic 1

Neurologist

There are bilateral lung nodules at the chest CT scan, and the blood tests show neutrophilia. Could the patient have a pulmonary infection? Do you think these findings are compatible with primary or secondary lung neoplasm?

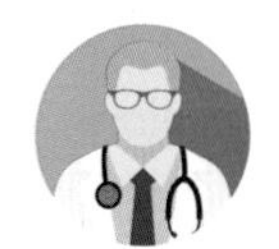

Pulmonologist A

It doesn't seem like it. The indices of inflammation are quite low for a lung infection. On the other side, calcifying pulmonary metastases are rare and can occur mainly in tumors of osteoid origin.

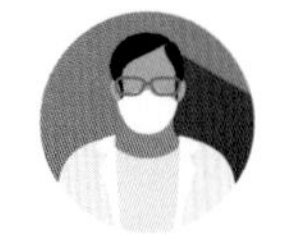

Pulmonologist B

The CT shows both nodules and cysts. Moreover, sparse calcifications are present. In my opinion, diffuse lung disease should also be considered.

Discussion Topic 1 (Continued)

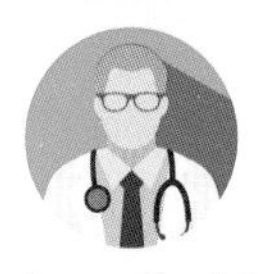

Pulmonologist A

I agree. These findings deserve further investigation. A transthoracic needle aspiration or a surgical biopsy should be considered.

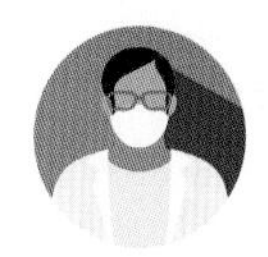

Pulmonologist B

We should wait until the patient is neurologically stable.

Thoracic Surgeon

It would be useful to perform a positron emission tomography (PET)/CT scan before a biopsy to detect other possible distant metastasis and mediastinal lymph nodes involvement.

The patient referred mild xerophthalmia without xerostomia or Raynaud phenomenon. She denied morning stiffness or inflammatory joint pains.

To exclude the presence of a connective tissue disease (CTD), a complete serum autoimmunity screening was requested, including antinuclear antibodies (ANA), extractable nuclear antigens (ENA), anti–neutrophil cytoplasmic antibodies (ANCAs), anti–cyclic citrullinated peptide (ACCP), and anti–double-stranded DNA (ds-DNA). Positivities for ANA (titer 1:640 with speckled pattern) and ENA (anti-SSA/Ro-52) were detected.

Discussion Topic 2

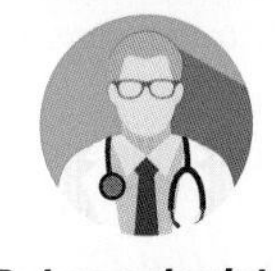

Pulmonologist A

A rheumatology consultation is needed. The patient complains of mild xerophthalmia. She might have Sjögren syndrome.

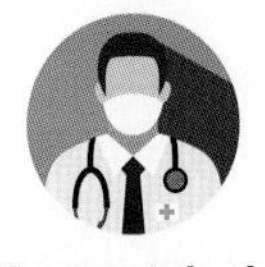

Rheumatologist

The autoantibody panel was positive for ANA and anti-SSA/Ro-52; Sjögren syndrome is possible. I suggest performing the Schirmer test, sialometry, and ultrasonography of the salivary glands.

Continued on following page

Discussion Topic 2 (Continued)

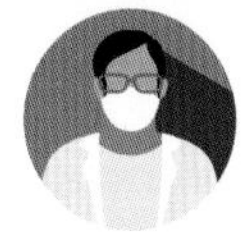

Pulmonologist B The patient doesn't seem to have a sicca syndrome, and CT scan shows many lung cysts. I think we should measure serum vascular endothelial growth factor D (VEGF-D) and check for the presence of abdominal angiomyolipomas to exclude lymphangioleiomyomatosis (LAM).

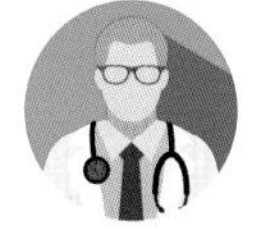

Pulmonologist A Chest CT scan pattern doesn't seem characteristic of LAM because of the concomitant presence of nodules. Abdomen CT scan does not show renal angiomyolipomas. The patient has a positivity for anti-SSA/Ro-52. While waiting for ultrasonography and the other tests, I suggest extending the autoantibody panel with the myositis- and scleroderma-specific immunoblots.

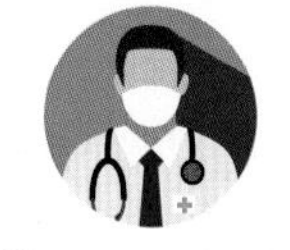

Rheumatologist This is a good observation. Anti-SSA/Ro-52 positivity can be associated with Sjögren syndrome, but they may also hide myositis and antisynthetase syndrome, although the patient did not show any other clinical or instrumental signs of these diseases.

The patient was evaluated by a rheumatologist who detected chronic sialadenitis with fibrotic evolution on ultrasonography of the salivary glands. Schirmer test and sialometry were positive. The myositis- and scleroderma-specific immunoblots confirmed the isolate positivity for anti-SSA/Ro-52. A diagnosis of Sjögren syndrome was made but no specific rheumatologic treatment was retained to be started at the time of diagnosis.

A PET/CT scan revealed a low glycolytic activity (standardized uptake value [SUV] max 1.3) of all the nodules.

Clinical Course

Once neurologically recovered and discharged from the hospital, the patient underwent a complete clinical and functional evaluation in our pulmonology clinic.

The spirometry was normal (forced vital capacity [FVC] was 92%, forced expiratory volume in 1 second [FEV_1] was 95% of the predicted value, and Tiffenau Index was 81.3), and a moderate reduction in diffusing capacity for carbon monoxide (DLCO) was detected (DLCO 57% of the predicted value). A lung surgical biopsy was proposed, but the patient refused. Strict clinical and radiological follow-up was then recommended.

A chest CT scan performed 1 year after the baseline assessment confirmed the stability of the number and size of the cysts and the nodules. The patient was asymptomatic, and pulmonary function tests were within the normal limits.

A new CT scan performed 1 year later revealed a slight increase in the size of a para-aortic nodule of the right upper lobe (Fig 19.2). Significant ^{18}F-fluorodeoxyglucose (FDG) uptake of the nodule was then detected with a new PET/CT scan (Fig 19.3).

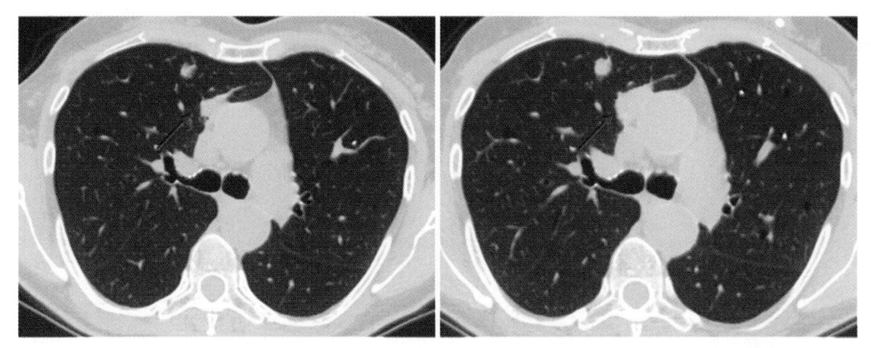

Fig 19.2 Chest CT scan at the first assessment (left) and after 1 year (right), showing a dimensional increase of the para-aortic nodule located in the right superior lobe

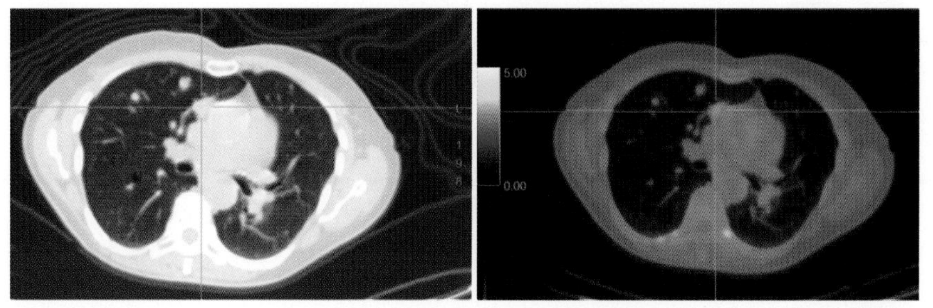

Fig 19.3 PET/CT scan showing a significant FDG uptake of the right para-aortic nodule, which was dimensionally increased after 2 years of follow-up.

Discussion Topic 3

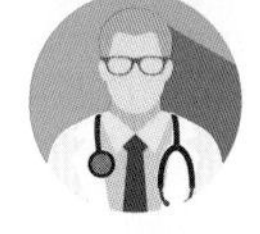

Pulmonologist A

The presence of cysts and nodules together with calcifications might be the expression of pulmonary nodular amyloidosis, a rare condition that may be associated with Sjögren syndrome. Moreover, one nodule slightly increased.

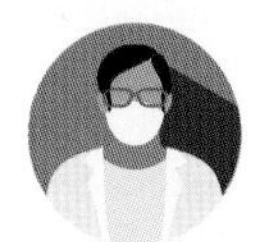

Pulmonologist B

We could perform an abdominal fat biopsy. It's a minimally invasive and safe procedure that can lead to the histological confirmation and typing of amyloid deposits.

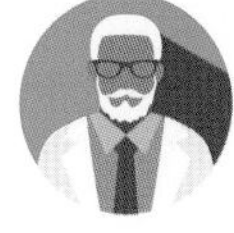

Radiologist

I think the diagnosis of amyloidosis may be possible, but a mucosa-associated lymphoid tissue (MALT) lymphoma and lung cancer should be excluded. A lung biopsy with a histopathological evaluation is needed.

Continued on following page

Discussion Topic 3 (Continued)

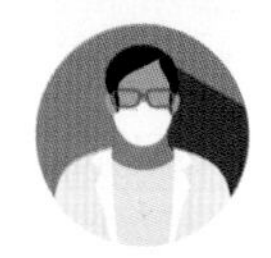

Pulmonologist B

Can a CT-guided percutaneous fine needle aspiration biopsy be performed?

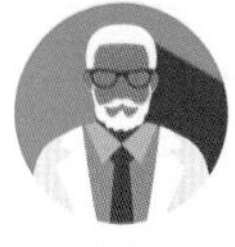

Radiologist

In my opinion, due to the complexity of the case with many types of lesions in the lung parenchyma, a surgical biopsy might be more useful.

Thoracic Surgeon

I fully agree. A video-assisted thoracoscopic biopsy could help obtaining adequate tissue for a precise histopathological diagnosis.

In the suspicion of a lung malignancy associated with a cystic disease, a surgical video-assisted thoracoscopic biopsy of the nodule of the superior right lobe was performed. Histopathological evaluation revealed the presence of eosinophilic material with a Congo red–staining positivity, associated with an apple-green birefringence on polarized microscopy. The findings were consistent with the diagnosis of amyloidosis (Fig 19.4).

The case and the biopsy specimens were then evaluated at the National Amyloidosis Centre.

Amyloid typing with electron microscopy immunohistochemistry (immunogold post-embedding) showed immunoreactivity for anti-κ light chain polyclonal antibodies. The biopsy of the periumbilical fat was negative after Congo red staining under polarized light, while the levels of serum N terminal pro–brain natriuretic peptide, cardiac troponin I, creatinine, and alkaline phosphatase were normal, and there was no relevant albuminuria. The echocardiogram did not show any findings compatible with cardiac amyloidosis. Serum and urine immunofixation did not show monoclonal components, and the circulating free light chain ratio was normal.

Since no clinical or instrumental signs of systemic amyloidosis were found, a diagnosis of pulmonary nodular AL κ amyloidosis, in the context of a Sjögren syndrome, was made.

Recommended Therapy and Further Indications

Based on review by the Pavia Amyloidosis Research and Treatment Center, no specific treatment was started. The rheumatologist also did not suggest starting any immunosuppressive drugs.

Follow-Up and Outcomes

The patient did not develop any new symptoms during the clinical and radiological follow-up.

Chest CT scan and pulmonary function tests were stable at 12 and 24 months after the diagnosis. No signs of systemic amyloidosis have been detected to date.

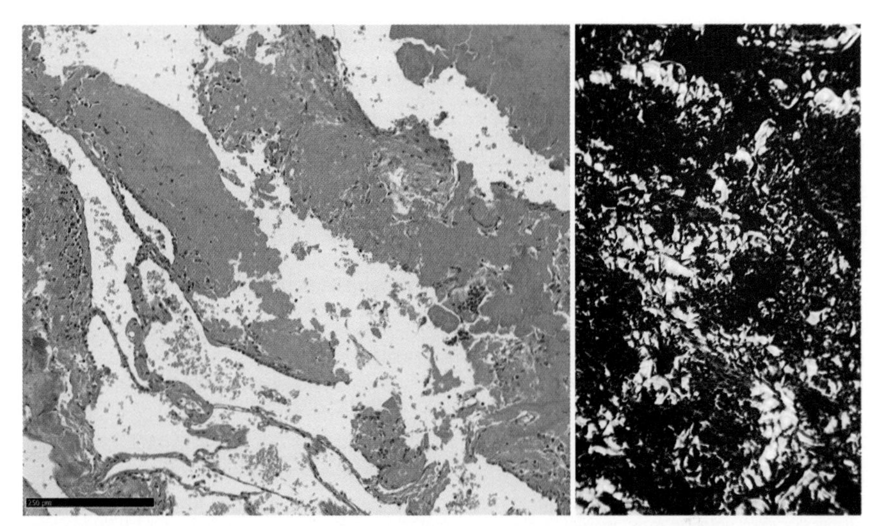

Fig 19.4 Histopathological evaluation of the resected nodule of the right upper lobe showing homogeneous aggregates of eosinophilic material (hematoxylin-eosin staining, on the left). Congo-red staining positivity with typical green birefringence under polarized light, confirming the presence of amyloid (on the right).

Focus on

Sjögren Syndrome Associated Interstitial Lung Disease (SS-ILD)

Sjögren syndrome (SS) is a systemic autoimmune disease characterized by an impairment of exocrine glands that may involve multiple organs, with interstitial lung disease (ILD) being the most frequent respiratory system involvement (SS-ILD). Symptoms of SS-ILD include cough and exertional dyspnea, and chest examination can detect inspiratory Velcro-like crackles. Spirometry can be normal at diagnosis or detect a restrictive ventilatory pattern. Reduction of DLCO may be an early sign of the disease. Chest CT usually shows nonspecific interstitial pneumonia (NSIP), although lymphoid interstitial pneumonia (LIP) and, less frequently, usual interstitial pneumonia (UIP) patterns may be detected. Isolated lung nodules and cysts may also be present in a minority of the patients. SS may be associated with pulmonary amyloidosis, which radiologically may show the presence of solid nodules, often large, irregular, and with bizarre calcifications. The occurrence of LIP and amyloidosis in SS patients should be carefully investigated, since it could be associated with an increased risk of pulmonary MALT lymphoma.

Progression of the disease can be monitored by clinical, functional, and radiological (i.e., with CT scan) evaluation. In case of progressive or symptomatic disease, therapy with glucocorticoids alone or in combination with other, steroid-sparing, immunosuppressive agents (e.g., cyclophosphamide and/or mycophenolate mofetil) should be started.

Focus on

Pulmonary Amyloidosis

Amyloidosis is a rare disease, caused by an extracellular deposition of misfolded autologous proteins as fibrils. Different molecular mechanisms have been found to contribute to fibril formation and deposition. The International Society of Amyloidosis classifies the disease on the basis of the different fibrillar proteins.

Pulmonary amyloidosis may be both localized and part of a systemic disease. Three forms of pulmonary amyloidosis have been described: nodular pulmonary amyloidosis, diffuse alveolar-septal amyloidosis, and tracheobronchial amyloidosis.

Nodular pulmonary amyloidosis is characterized by the presence of one or more amyloid nodules, typically peripheral, subpleural, and, often, bilateral. Nodular pulmonary amyloidosis is usually a benign

Continued on following page

Focus on (Continued)

Pulmonary Amyloidosis

form of localized immunoglobulin amyloid light chain (AL) amyloidosis, although cases of systemic AL amyloidosis or other rarer forms of amyloidosis have been reported. Immunoglobulin light chains are more frequently γ than κ in nodular pulmonary amyloidosis. Nodules usually remain stable, and the prognosis is good without the need of systemic therapy. A mucosa-associated lymphoid tissue (MALT) lymphoma, a lymphoproliferative disorder in the spectrum of extranodal marginal zone lymphoma, may be associated with pulmonary nodular amyloidosis, particularly in patients with an underlying systemic disorder like SS.

Diffuse alveolar-septal amyloidosis is a form of systemic amyloidosis characterized by the amyloid deposition in the small vessel walls, interstitium, and alveolar septa. Diffuse interlobular septal thickenings, reticular opacities, small nodules, and ground-glass opacifications can be detected at CT. If the visceral pleura is affected, pleural effusion can be found. Immunoglobulin light chains are more frequently in this subset of disease. Pulmonary function tests typically show a restrictive pattern with decreased diffusion capacity of carbon monoxide (DLCO). Exertional dyspnea is the most frequent symptom. Treatment is based on chemotherapy regimens for systemic amyloidosis.

Tracheobronchial amyloidosis is a form of localized AL amyloidosis. Amyloid deposits in the trachea and large bronchi as multifocal submucosal plaques may cause airway stenosis, thus inducing symptoms and respiratory failure. Atelectasis and pneumonia may be present. The treatment is based on bronchoscopic ablation (e.g., with laser therapy). Systemic chemotherapy and external beam radiation have also been successfully reported.

Focus on

Amyloid-Associated Cystic Lung Disease

Amyloid-associated cystic lung disease is a rare entity, usually associated with AL amyloidosis (λ or κ). Cysts are typically multiple, thin walled, round, or lobulated, of small to moderate size. Cysts can be either predominantly distributed in the lower lung zones or sparse and are typically accompanied by nodules, partly calcific. Amyloid-associated cystic lung disease can be found in association with connective tissue diseases, particularly Sjögren syndrome. Several cystic lung diseases should be considered in the differential diagnosis. In lymphocytic interstitial pneumonia, ground-glass, centrilobular, not calcific nodules are usually detected. Pulmonary light chain deposition disease can show thin-walled cystic lesions and nodules, which are less commonly calcified. In these cases, the histopathological evaluation is necessary for a correct etiological diagnosis, with only amyloidosis staining positive for Congo red.

Birt-Hogg-Dubè syndrome and lymphangioleiomyomatosis can be differentiated from amyloid-associated cystic lung disease by the absence of the nodules on the CT scan. Pulmonary Langerhans cell histiocytosis shows the typical upper lung predominance of bizarre-shaped cysts, with noncalcified cavitary nodules. It usually presents in young male smokers. Cystic pulmonary metastatic lesions should also be excluded in the diagnostic pathway of patients with cystic lung disease.

LEARNING POINTS

- Sjögren syndrome is a systemic autoimmune disease with impairment of exocrine glands and involvement of multiple organs, particularly the respiratory system. Interstitial lung disease is the most frequent type of lung involvement.
- The occurrence of LIP and amyloidosis in patients with Sjögren syndrome must be carefully investigated, since it could be associated with an increased risk of pulmonary MALT lymphoma.
- Amyloidosis is a rare disease, caused by extracellular deposition of misfolded autologous proteins as fibrils. Three forms of pulmonary amyloidosis have been described: nodular pulmonary amyloidosis, diffuse alveolar-septal amyloidosis, and tracheobronchial amyloidosis.
- Amyloid-associated cystic lung disease is a rare form of amyloidosis.

Further Readings

Cha SI, Fessler MB, Cool CD, et al. Lymphoid interstitial pneumonia: clinical features, associations and prognosis. *Eur Respir J.* 2006;28:364-369.

Flament T, Bigot A, Chaigne B, et al. Pulmonary manifestations of Sjögren's syndrome. *Eur Respir Rev.* 2016;25:110-123.

Gupta N, Vassallo R, Wikenheiser-Brokamp KA, et al. Diffuse cystic lung disease. Part II. *Am J Respir Crit Care Med.* 2015;192(1):17-29.

Luppi F, Sebastiani M, Silva M, et al. Interstitial lung disease in Sjögren's syndrome: a clinical review. *Clin Exp Rheumatol.* 2020;38(suppl 126):S291-S300.

Milani P, Basset M, Russo F, et al. The lung in amyloidosis. *Eur Respir Rev.* 2017;26:170046.

Raoof S, Bondalapati P, Vydyula R, et al. Cystic lung diseases. Algorithmic approach. *Chest.* 2016;150(4): 945-965.

Swigris JJ, Berry GJ, Raffin TA, et al. Lymphoid interstitial pneumonia: a narrative review. *Chest.* 2002;122:2150-2164.

Tirelli C, Morandi V, Valentini A, et al. Multidisciplinary approach in the early detection of undiagnosed connective tissue diseases in patients with interstitial lung disease: a retrospective cohort study. *Front Med.* 2020;7:11.

Tirelli C, Zanframundo G, Valentini A, et al. CT-guided biopsy in the differential diagnosis of Sjögren syndrome associated cystic lung disease: a case of lung nodular AL-κ amyloidosis. *Radiol Case Rep.* 2020;15:2331-2334.

Zamora AC, White DB, Sykes AG, et al. Amyloid-associated cystic lung disease. *Chest.* 2016;149(5): 1223-1233.

CHAPTER 20

Sporadic Lymphangioleiomyomatosis in a Woman Previously Diagnosed With Asthma

SilviaTerraneo ■ OlgaTorre ■ Fausta Alfano ■ Claudio Sorino ■
Stefano Centanni ■ Michele Mondoni

History of Present Illness

A 49-year-old Caucasian woman was referred to the pulmonary clinic complaining of 2-year worsening dyspnea and sporadic dry cough despite treatment with inhaled bronchodilators and corticosteroids due to atopic asthma. Chest radiograph revealed a diffuse reticular pattern without pleural effusion.

Past Medical History

The patient was a steelworker with minimal exposure to mineral oil. She never smoked, had never been pregnant, and had no familial history of pulmonary diseases. She had arterial hypertension and several years earlier was diagnosed with atopic asthma. Skin prick testing revealed sensitization to grass pollen, olive pollen, and dust mites. Previous spirometry showed a partially reversible airflow obstruction.

Her daily medical treatment included inhaled β_2-agonists and corticosteroids and oral 5 mg amlodipine. She sometimes used oral antihistamines and had taken a birth control pill for 3 years in the past. Drug allergies were not reported.

Physical Examination and Early Clinical Findings

The patient was in good general condition. Oxygen saturation measured by pulse oximetry (SpO_2) was 95% on room air, heart rate was 80 beats/min, respiratory rate was 14 breaths/min, and blood pressure was 120/75 mmHg. Chest examination revealed a diffuse reduction of *vesicular murmur* without additional breath sounds. No pallor, clubbing, or peripheral edema was apparent.

Discussion Topic 1

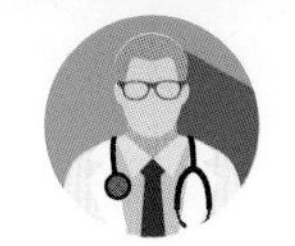

Pulmonologist A

The patient appears to have difficult-to-treat asthma.

Continued on following page

Discussion Topic 1 (Continued)

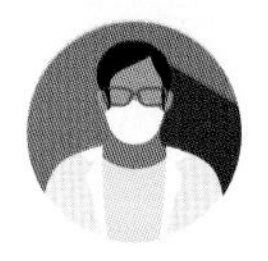

Pulmonologist B

Are we sure that she is taking the inhalation therapy correctly?

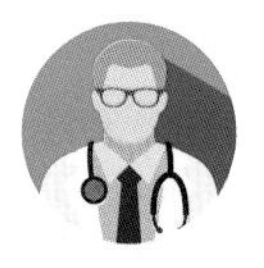

Pulmonologist A

Yes, I checked both the adherence and the inhalation technique.

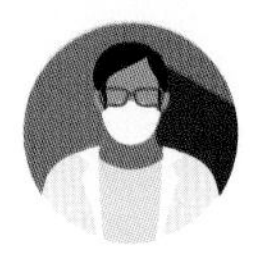

Pulmonologist B

She had spirometry 3 years ago for the last time. I suggest repeating the lung function tests, including a lung diffusion test.

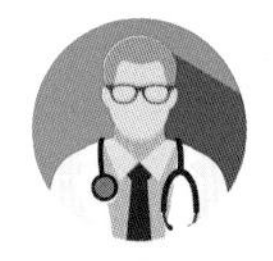

Pulmonologist A

I would also do a chest CT scan. She has an interstitial reticular pattern on chest radiography; it is important to rule out other lung diseases.

Clinical Course

Spirometry revealed a severe airflow obstruction with forced expiratory volume in 1 second (FEV_1) 47.1% of predicted value and forced vital capacity (FVC) 71% of predicted. Bronchodilator reversibility testing was negative. Diffusing capacity of the lungs for carbon monoxide (DLCO) was severely impaired (31.2% of predicted value) (Fig. 20.1).

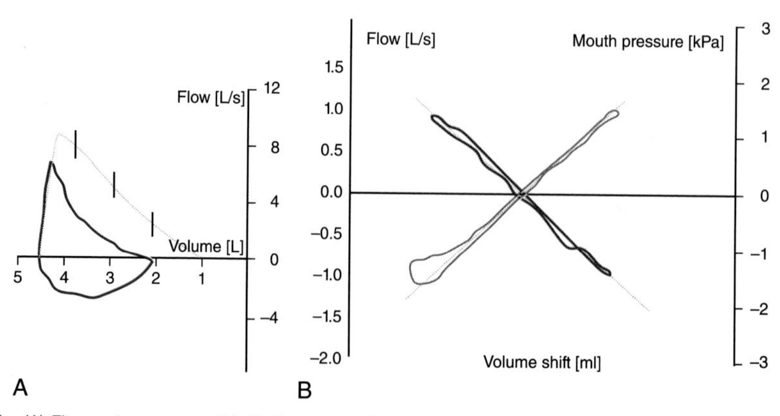

Fig 20.1 (A) Flow-volume curve. (B) Plethysmography.

Continued on following page

ID: ****** ******		Gender: Female		Height: 161 cm
Age: 49 years		Race: Caucasian		Weight: 64 Kg
	Observed	Predicted	LLN	% Observed/Predicted
FEV_1 (Lit)	1.29	2.73	2.14	47.1
FVC (Lit)	2.42	3.40	2.67	71.0
FEV_1/FVC	0.53	0.81	0.70	65.9
Raw (TkPa*s/L)	0.65	0.30	-	216
RV (Lit)	1.56	1.44	0.85	108.1
TLC (Lit)	4.83	5.10	4.17	94.9
DLCO (mL/min/mmHg)	2.12	6.82	5.34	31.2

C

Fig 20.1, cont'd (C) Measured parameters. Pulmonary function tests. The reduction of FEV_1/VC below the LLN indicates an obstructive pattern. Note the marked increase in airway resistance (Raw). FEV_1, forced expiratory volume in 1 second; LLN, lower limit of normal; VC, vital capacity; RV, residual volume; TLC, total lung capacity. DLCO, diffusing capacity of the lungs for carbon monoxide.

A high-resolution computed tomography (HRCT) scan of the chest revealed multiple and diffuse radiolucent areas together with interstitial thickening and parenchymal destruction. These findings deserved a differential diagnosis between cysts and emphysematous blebs/bullae (Fig. 20.2).

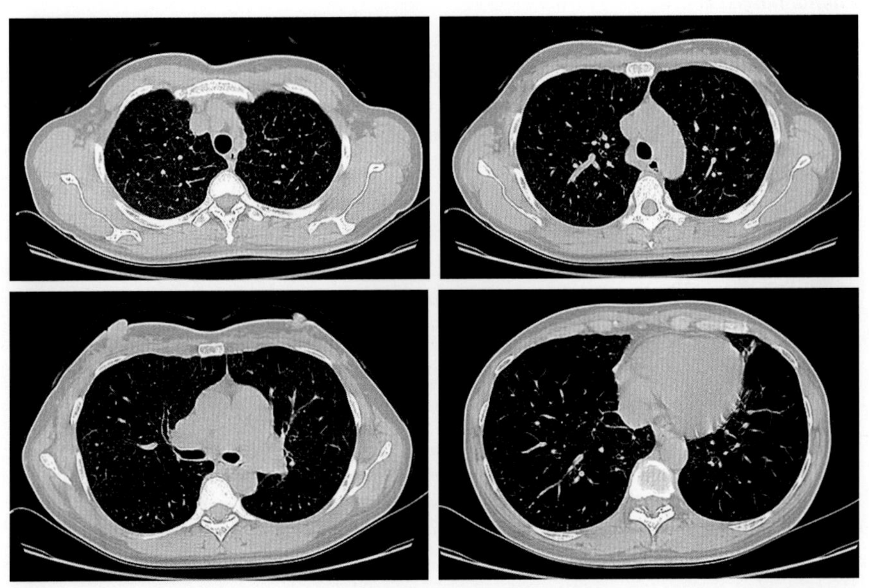

Fig 20.2 Axial chest HRCT in the lung window showing multiple, diffused, small cysts without nodular evidence and areas of merged cysts and destroyed parenchyma that mimics emphysema.

Discussion Topic 2

Pulmonologist A

This appears to be a case of severe emphysema. As the patient is a young, never-smoker woman, we should measure serum levels of α_1-antitrypsin (AAT) and perform gene sequencing to evaluate mutations that cause AAT deficiency or malfunction.

Continued on following page

Discussion Topic 2 (Continued)

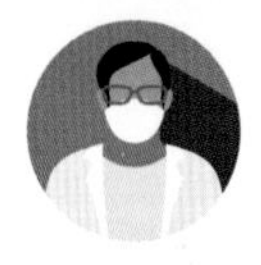

Pulmonologist B

I think this may not be emphysema but rather a highly evolved diffuse cystic lung disease.

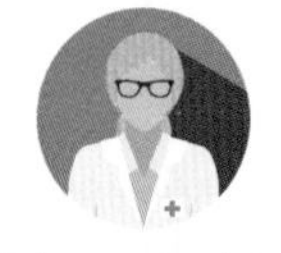

Pulmonologist C

Yes, this seems a severe advanced cystic lung disease with some area of destroyed parenchyma that mimics emphysema.

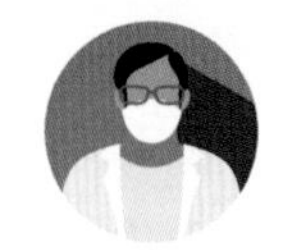

Pulmonologist B

We should ask for other tests to explore different diagnoses. HRCT alone is not usually enough to make a definite diagnosis.

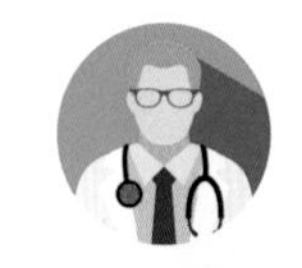

Pulmonologist A

How about consulting a thoracic surgeon to perform a lung biopsy?

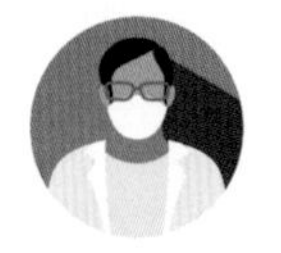

Pulmonologist B

Before invasive diagnostic tests, we should explore possible differential diagnoses using noninvasive tests.

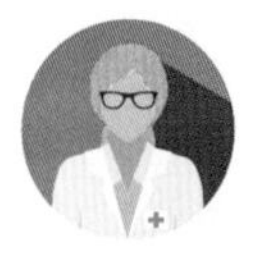

Pulmonologist C

I agree. Serum vascular endothelial growth factor D (VEGF-D) can be measured to explore the hypothesis of lymphangioleiomyomatosis (LAM). We should also evaluate autoantibodies to rule out lymphocytic interstitial pneumonia related to an autoimmune disease such as Sjögren syndrome.

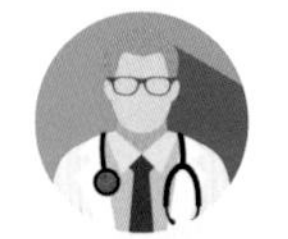

Pulmonologist A

Protein electrophoresis and free light chains dosage will be useful to rule out a light chain deposition disease.

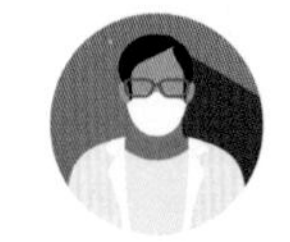

Pulmonologist B

I will also ask a complete blood count and HIV antibodies to explore acquired immunodeficiencies. Moreover, abdominal magnetic resonance should be performed to detect angiomyolipomas or lymphangioleiomyomas related to LAM, or kidney tumors, frequent in Birt-Hogg-Dubè syndrome.

The chest CT scan was revised by an experienced radiologist, and multiple, round, well-circumscribed cysts diffusely distributed throughout the lung parenchyma were identified. There was no evidence of nodules or other interstitial abnormalities (Video 20.1) .

Laboratory exams were then requested. Hemoglobin was 16.7 g/dL (normal values 12–16 g/dL), hematocrit was 49.1%, and leukocytes and renal and hepatic function indexes were within the normal range. Antinuclear antibodies (ANAs), antibodies against extractable nuclear antigen (ENA), as well as perinuclear and cytoplasmic anti–neutrophil cytoplasmic antibodies (pANCAs and c ANCAs) were absent. Protein electrophoresis and free light chains dosage were in the normality range. Human immunodeficiency virus (HIV) types 1 and 2 autoantibodies were negative. Serum α_1-Antitrypsin level was 134 mg/dL (normal value > 80 mg/dL; genetic sequencing was taking much longer to get ready), and C-reactive protein was 0.3 mg/dL (normal value < 0.5 mg/dL). Serum vascular endothelial growth factor (VEGF) D was 1387.6 pg/mL. Abdominal magnetic resonance imaging (MRI) revealed bilateral renal angiomyolipomas, abdominal tubular structures with irregular development with internal septa, and pseudo-cystic dilatations along iliac vessel in periaortic region. The findings were compatible with lymphangioleiomyomas (Fig 20.3).

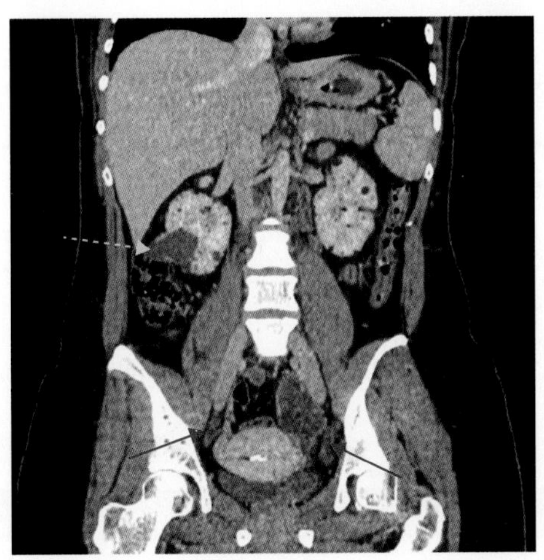

Fig 20.3 Abdominal MRI showing renal angiomyolipomas of the right kidney (blue arrow) and abdominal lymphangioleiomyomas along iliac vessels (red arrows).

Discussion Topic 3

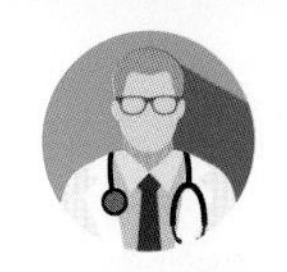

Pulmonologist A

We need an experienced thoracic radiologist consultation to detect radiological findings compatible with LAM or with other cystic lung diseases.

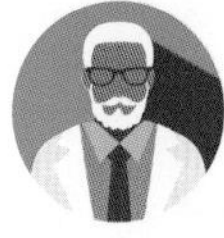

Radiologist

I reviewed HRCT images. I confirm that there are multiple rounded, thin-walled and air-filled parenchymal cysts, without internal septa or vessels. Cysts are randomly distributed throughout pulmonary parenchyma. There is no evidence of zonal predominance and no evidence of ground-glass opacity, consolidation, nodules, reticulation, or honeycombing. Cysts are > 10. Hence, all the HRCT features are typical of LAM.

Continued on following page

Discussion Topic 3 (Continued)

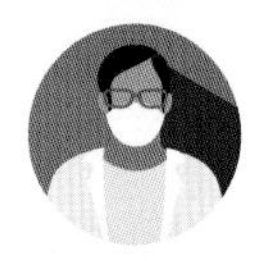

Pulmonologist B

Are the abdominal findings compatible with LAM?

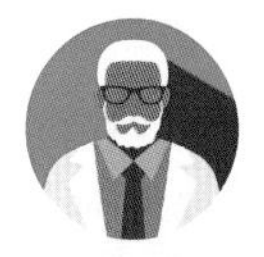

Radiologist

Abdominal MRI shows bilateral angiomyolipomas (AMLs). MRI also reveals tubular structures with irregular development, internal slight septa, and some pseudo-cystic dilatations along iliac vessel and in periaortic region. They are compatible with lymphangioleiomyomas. Both AMLs and lymphangioleiomyomas could represent extrathoracic involvement of LAM.

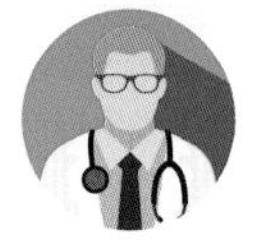

Pulmonologist A

Because of the combination of HRCT features typical of LAM, the presence of AMLs, abdominal lymphangioleiomyoma, and VEGF-D serum level > 800 pg/mL, we can conclude for a *definite* diagnosis of LAM.

A final diagnosis of LAM was made. A 6-minute walk test in room air was interrupted after 3 minutes because of severe desaturation (nadir SpO_2 82%) associated with exertional dyspnea. Arterial blood gas analysis revealed mild hypoxemia with PaO_2 66.5 mmHg, $PaCO_2$ 33 mmHg, pH 7.44, and HCO_3^- 23.4 mmol/L. Overnight oximetry reveals severe nocturnal respiratory (mean SpO_2 86%, nadir SpO_2 83%). Oxygen supplementation was prescribed during night and exertion.

Discussion Topic 4

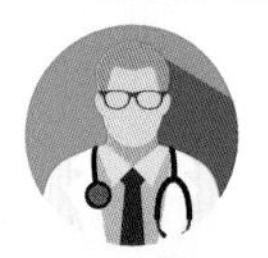

Pulmonologist A

The patient is a young woman, and there is a wide parenchymal involvement. Do you think we should consider a medical treatment with sirolimus?

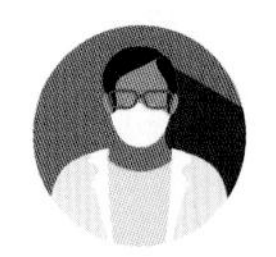

Pulmonologist B

Yes, guidelines recommend starting a pharmacological treatment when functional impairment is present at diagnosis or a functional worsening develops during the follow-up.

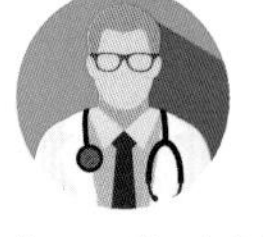

Pulmonologist A

We already performed a 6-minute walk test before starting treatment. Together with spirometric findings, this will be useful to monitor the disease evolution.

Discussion Topic 4 (Continued)

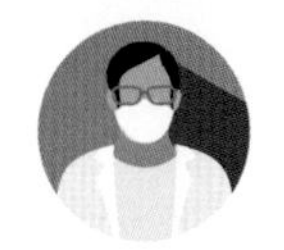

Pulmonologist B

It is also necessary to evaluate the presence of tuberous sclerosis complex (TSC). Dermatological evaluation, brain CT, and fundus oculi must be performed in order to individuate the clinical signs of the disease. *TSC1* and *TSC2* gene mutations must also be investigated.

To explore the hypothesis of a tuberous sclerosis complex associated with LAM (TSC-LAM) further, clinical evaluations were performed. TSC findings were not found during the dermatological examination, in the brain CT scan, or during eye fundus examination. Echocardiography resulted in regular with normal ejection fraction (55%), systolic pulmonary artery pressure (PAPs) of 31 mmHg, and no signs of rhabdomyomas. Since the evidence of bilateral angiomyolipomas, mutations in *TSC1* and *TSC2* genes were also searched in peripheral blood through denaturing high-performance liquid chromatography (DHPLC) and with multiple ligation-dependent probe amplification (MLPA). No mutations were identified.

Discussion Topic 5

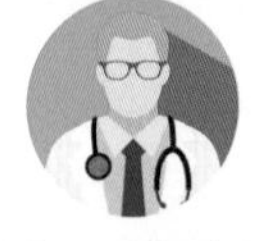

Pulmonologist A

In addition to drug therapy, we should recommend vaccinations against the most common causes of lower respiratory tract infections. Also, estrogens should be avoided as they may accelerate the deterioration of respiratory function in patients with LAM.

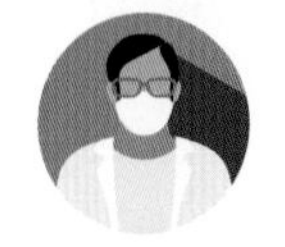

Pulmonologist B

What do you think of inhalation therapies? Can they be useful? The patient has breathlessness and evidence of airflow obstruction.

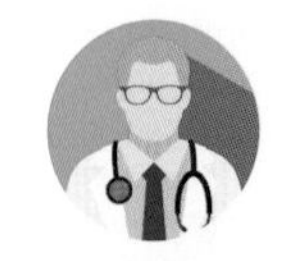

Pulmonologist A

Not sure if she really had asthma. Probably the onset of LAM was misdiagnosed. However, she is allergic and initially the airflow obstruction was partially reversible. I should recommend inhaled therapy with β_2-agonists and corticosteroids.

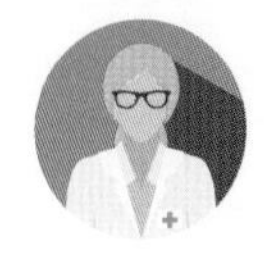

Pulmonologist C

Despite the medical treatment, this is an advanced disease with latent respiratory failure. The patient should be referred to a lung transplant center.

Recommended Therapy and Further Indications

Yearly immunization against influenza and *Streptococcus pneumoniae* was recommended, and avoidance of estrogen-based therapy was advised. The patient was notified about the most common LAM acute complications (e.g., pneumothorax).

Because of her asthma history and obstructive pattern on pulmonary function tests, therapy with inhaled β_2-agonist, antimuscarinic, and corticosteroids was prescribed.

Due to impaired lung function and latent respiratory failure, treatment with a mammalian target of rapamycin (mTOR) inhibitor was also prescribed (2 mg/day of oral sirolimus). Before starting therapy, testing for HIV antibodies and screening for hepatitis infections were both negative. Liver and renal functions were normal, and a mild hypercholesterolemia was observed (total cholesterol 202 mg/dL; normal value ≤ 115 mg/dL). Outpatient follow-up visits in the pulmonary clinic were scheduled with clinical and functional evaluation.

Follow-Up and Outcomes

The exertional dyspnea improved with supplemental oxygen during physical activity, and the 6-minute walk test was successfully completed without oxygen desaturation (oxygen flow used 2 liters/minute). Hemoglobin and hematocrit levels lowered to 14.7 g/dL and 43.6%, respectively. Sirolimus serum level, complete blood count, hepatic and renal function, and cholesterol levels were monitored 15 and 30 days after starting therapy and then every 4 months. During the follow-up, the patient developed worsening hypercholesterolemia, unresponsive to a low-fat diet and requiring a low-dose statin therapy. She also experienced diarrhea, which was easily controlled with dietary indications and symptomatic drugs. Consequently, sirolimus dosage reduction was not required.

Given the presence of respiratory failure and functional impairment, the patient was quickly referred to a transplant center.

Two years after the diagnosis, a thoracic CT scan and echocardiography were repeated. There was no evidence of worsening in parenchymal cystic involvement, but an increased pulmonary pressure (PAPs of 41 mmHg) was detected.

The patient is currently undergoing a clinical and functional follow-up, with overall stability of the course of the disease.

Focus on

Diagnosis of Lymphangioleiomyomatosis (LAM)

LAM is a rare, progressive, cystic lung disease with systemic involvement, affecting almost exclusively women of childbearing age. Thoracic involvement includes mediastinal lymphadenopathy and chylous pleural effusion. Extrathoracic manifestations consist of abdominal chylous effusion, renal angiomyolipomas (AMLs), cystic lymphatic masses (lymphangioleiomyomas), chylous ascites, and abdominal lymphadenopathy. LAM can occur sporadically (sporadic LAM; S-LAM) or as part of tuberous sclerosis complex (TSC; TSC-LAM). The latter is a rare autosomal dominant syndrome with multiorgan involvement due to germline mutations in *TSC1* and *TSC2* genes. Up to 60% of women with TSC have radiological evidence of LAM, while the disease is very rare in males with TSC and anecdotal in males without TSC.

The natural history of LAM is quite variable. At the beginning of the disease, patients may be asymptomatic or experience mild and insidious symptoms (usually progressive dyspnea). In some cases, the diagnosis is reached after an acute complication of the disease (i.e., pneumothorax, chylothorax, or rupture of renal AMLs). The suspicion of LAM arises when parenchymal cysts are detected at a chest HRCT scan. As pulmonary cysts can express the normal consequence of aging, a minimum of four cysts has been suggested as the threshold for considering them pathological. The typical LAM pulmonary cysts are rounded, thin-walled, air-containing, well-circumscribed, and scattered bilaterally in the lung parenchyma. Cyst size and number range from a few to up to 30 mm and from four cysts to the

Focus on (Continued)

Diagnosis of Lymphangioleiomyomatosis (LAM)

entire replacement of the lung parenchyma. Cysts are typically round, but in severe disease they could merge, becoming polygonal or atypically shaped. The thickness of cyst walls ranges from barely perceptible to 2 mm. HRCT showing at least 10 parenchymal cysts with the above-mentioned features may be considered *characteristic* of LAM. In patients with TSC, the presence of at least four cysts is considered *diagnostic* for LAM without the need for other elements. However, except for patients with TSC, HRCT alone is not enough for a definite diagnosis of LAM, and additional clinical and laboratory data are needed. A definite diagnosis of LAM is reached with lung biopsy with histological evidence of LAM cells or through a combination of radiological and clinical elements (i.e., renal angiomyolipoma, abdominal or thoracic chylous effusion, identification of thoracic or abdominal lymphangioleiomyomas). In the case of a radiological suspicion of LAM, abdominal MRI or CT scan should be performed. Last, in the presence of a *characteristic* chest CT scan, a serum VEGF-D value > 800 pg/mL may be considered diagnostic. Fig 20.4 shows a possible algorithm for the diagnosis of LAM.

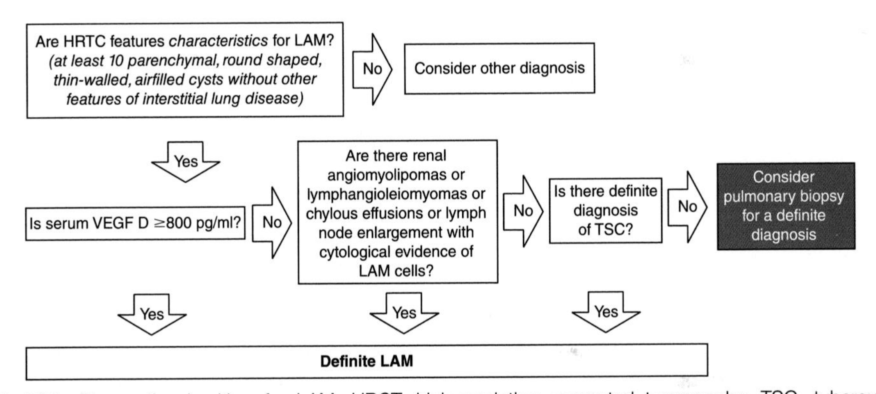

Fig 20.4 Diagnostic algorithm for LAM. HRCT, high-resolution computed tomography; TSC, tuberous sclerosis complex; LAM, lymphangioleiomyomatosis; VEGF-D, vascular endothelial growth factor.

Focus on

Cystic Lung Diseases, Differential Diagnosis

Other cystic lung diseases can mimic LAM. Emphysema, Birt-Hogg-Dubé syndrome, follicular bronchiolitis or lymphoid interstitial pneumonia (LIP), light-chain deposition disease, pulmonary amyloidosis, and pulmonary Langerhans cell histiocytosis (PLCH) are the main differential diagnosis. Because chest HRCT findings alone are not diagnostic, the identification of specific patterns can orientate the differential diagnosis (Table 20.1). Parenchymal cysts in Birt-Hogg-Dubé syndrome have round to lentiform shape, and lung involvement is limited compared to LAM; nodules are rarely described. In the early phase of PLCH, centrilobular or peribronchial nodules are usually detected; nodules tend to cavitate with consequent irregular cystic lesions development with thick-wall and upper-middle pulmonary distribution. In the end stage of the disease, cysts tend to coalesce, and nodules disappear. In LIP, few large cystic lesions are associated with ground-glass opacities and centrilobular nodules, sometimes with interlobular septal and bronchovascular bundle thickening. LIP may be idiopathic or associated with autoimmune diseases or immunodeficiency states. α_1-Antitrypsin serum level, autoantibodies (rheumatoid factor, antinuclear antibodies, anti-Ro, and anti-La), serum free light chains, and serum and urine protein electrophoresis should be tested. Dermatologic evaluation is needed to investigate signs of TSC (i.e., facial angiofibromas, forehead plaques, hypomelanotic macules, shagreen patches, and ungual fibroma) or the presence of fibrofolliculomas. The latter, most commonly located in the head and neck, are characteristic for Birt-Hogg-Dubè syndrome.

Continued on following page

Focus on (Continued)

Cystic Lung Diseases, Differential Diagnosis

Once the diagnosis of LAM is established, a TSC-associated form should be investigated. Brain CT scan for encephalic manifestations (i.e., cortical tubers, subependymal nodules, and subependymal giant cell astrocytoma), fundus oculi for retinal involvement, and echocardiography for rhabdomyoma should be performed. Finally, an abdomen CT scan or MRI for renal or hepatic angiomyolipomas and dermatological evaluation is needed.

TABLE 20.1 ■ **Differential Diagnoses of Cystic Lung Diseases**

	Parenchymal cysts appearance (HRCT)	Cystic lung involvement	Other parenchymal features	Diagnostic evaluation
Lymphangioleiomyomatosis	Round Thin-walled Well- circumscribed No internal septa or vessels	No zonal predominance Diffusely distributed	Nodules absent except in TSC-LAM	HRCT characteristics VEGF-D Abdominal involvement Pulmonary biopsy
Birt-Hogg-Dubè syndrome	Thin-walled Variable size Irregular shape	Limited Predominantly in medial lung bases	Nodules rarely described	Dermatologist evaluation* Abdominal MRI† Folliculin (*FLNC*) gene mutation
Pulmonary Langerhans cell histiocytosis	Thick-wall Irregular shape In end stage cysts tend to coalesce	Upper-middle distribution	Centrilobular or peribronchial nodules in the early phase of disease Nodules rarely described in end stage disease	HRCT is evocative Bronchoalveolar lavage‡ Improvement after smoke cessation
Lymphocytic interstitial pneumonia	Thin-walled cysts Variable in shape	Lower lung predominant and perivascular or randomly distributed	GGOs Centrilobular nodules Interlobular septal and bronchovascular thickening	Evaluation of underlying conditions*
Light chain deposition disease	Thin-wall Multiple Round up to 2 cm in size	Diffuse or a lower lung predominance	Nodules, GGOs, interlobular septal thickening, lymph node enlargement	Serum free light chains, and serum and urine protein electrophoresis

TABLE 20.1 ■ **Differential Diagnoses of Cystic Lung Diseases** (Continued)

	Parenchymal cysts appearance (HRCT)	Cystic lung involvement	Other parenchymal features	Diagnostic evaluation
Amyloidosis	Irregular shape	Subpleural	Nodules and calcifications Superimposed ground glass is possible	Evaluation of underlying conditions*
Other: metastases (usually squamous cell carcinoma or sarcoma) Infections (usually *Pneumocystis jirovecii* pneumonia)	Variable in shape and size	Bilateral, upper lobes	Nodules (may cavitate)	Immunocompromised patients Bronchoscopy diagnosis

HRCT, high-resolution computed tomography; TSC, tuberous sclerosis complex; LAM, lymphangioleiomyomatosis; VEGF-D, vascular endothelial growth factor D; MRI, magnetic resonance imaging; GGO, ground-glass opacity.

*To search for follicular tumors of the skin.

†To investigate renal neoplasms.

‡Cytology with immunostaining for CD1a > 5% and CD207 strongly support the diagnosis.

Focus on

Management of LAM and Relevant Complications

All patients diagnosed with LAM should undergo annual influenza vaccination with inactivated vaccine, as well as pneumococcal vaccination with PCV13 and PPSV23. Patients > 50 years old and patients treated with mechanistic target of rapamycin (mTOR) inhibitors should undergo Herpes zoster vaccination. Spirometry, body plethysmography, and lung diffusion tests should be performed to evaluate the affect of the disease on respiratory function. Airway obstruction, often reversible, associated with a reduced diffusing capacity of the lungs for carbon monoxide is typical for LAM. Inhaled bronchodilators should be prescribed to patients with airflow limitations. Estrogens have been shown to accelerate the loss of function of the respiratory system in patients with LAM. Estrogen-based therapy (i.e., contraceptive therapy or hormonal replacement therapy) in these patients must therefore be avoided. In women of childbearing age, counseling about the possible accelerated disease progression and increased risk of spontaneous pneumothorax related to pregnancy is mandatory. Treatment with mTOR inhibitors is indicated in 1) patients with LAM with abnormal lung function at diagnosis or with an estimated annual loss of FEV_1 of ≥ 90 mL/year or greater; 2) patients with significant disease burden (i.e., elevated residual volume, reduced diffusing capacity, desaturation on exercise, or resting hypoxemia); and 3) patients with relapsing chylothorax. Sirolimus is usually administered orally at 2 mg/day to obtain trough serum values between 5 and 15 ng/mL. Sirolimus can stabilize or improve lung function (monitored with FEV_1 and FVC), functional performance, and health-related quality of life. It can also reduce the volume of angiomyolipomas, lymphangioleiomyomas, and chylothorax or chylous ascites.

The most common adverse events of the drug are mucositis, diarrhea, nausea, hypercholesterolemia, acneiform rash, and swelling in the lower extremities. Additional toxicities that are encountered

Continued on following page

Focus on (Continued)

Management of LAM and Relevant Complications

with sirolimus include ovarian cyst formation, dysmenorrhea, proteinuria, elevated liver function tests, drug-induced pneumonitis, and the risk of infections due to immunosuppression.

The most frequent thoracic complication of LAM is pneumothorax, often relapsing. The first episode must be approached with video-assisted thoracoscopic surgery-guided mechanical pleurodesis. For recurrent pneumothorax, further chemical pleurodesis, talc pleurodesis, or pleurectomy must be considered. Pleurodesis, both unilateral and/or bilateral, should not be considered a contraindication to lung transplant.

In patients with chylothorax, mTOR inhibitors are recommended as first-line treatment; pleural drainage must be considered in severe cases with large effusions. In recurrent or refractory cases, lymphatic imaging and thoracic duct embolization could be considered.

Angiomyolipomas < 3 cm in diameter must be radiologically followed every 12 to 24 months. For larger, multiple, bilateral or growing angiomyolipomas, mTOR inhibitors are indicated. Embolization should be considered for single large lesions or for lesions that are refractory to mTOR inhibitors. Surgical resection is to be considered for large, complex lesions refractory to mTOR inhibitors.

The last stage of the disease is characterized by the development of respiratory failure. Patients refractory to mTOR inhibitors in whom FEV_1% predicted is $\leq 30\%$, who experience resting hypoxemia, progressive lung function decline, or dyspnea of New York Heart Association (NYHA) functional class 4, must be urgently referred to a lung transplant center.

LEARNING POINTS

- Lymphangioleiomyomatosis (LAM) is a rare, progressive, cystic lung disease affecting almost exclusively women of childbearing age.
- LAM may occur with renal angiomyolipomas, thoracic and abdominal lymphadenopathies, chylous effusion, and cystic lymphatic masses (lymphangioleiomyomas).
- Two subtypes of LAM are described: sporadic (S-LAM) and associated with tuberous sclerosis complex (TSC-LAM), a rare neurocutaneous disorder secondary to mutations in the *TSC1* or *TSC2* tumor suppressor genes.
- A definite diagnosis of LAM is based on a combination of radiological with clinical and laboratory findings. A lung biopsy is required when a noninvasive diagnosis cannot be reached.
- LAM usually causes airflow obstruction, often reversible, and impairment of gas exchange.
- A pharmacological treatment with the mTOR inhibitor sirolimus should be considered in the case of abnormal lung function at diagnosis or functional impairment during follow-up.

Further Readings

Crivelli P, Ledda RE, Terraneo S, et al. Role of thoracic imaging in the management of lymphangioleiomyomatosis. *Respir Med.* 2019;157:14-20.

Di Marco F, Terraneo S, Dias OM, et al. Natural history of incidental sporadic and tuberous sclerosis complex associated lymphangioleiomyomatosis. *Respir Med.* 2020;168:105993.

Johnson SR, Cordier JF, Lazor R, et al; Review Panel of the ERS LAM Task Force. European Respiratory Society guidelines for the diagnosis and management of lymphangioleiomyomatosis. *Eur Respir J.* 2010;35(1):14-26.

McCarthy C, Gupta N, Johnson SR, Yu JJ, McCormack FX. Lymphangioleiomyomatosis: pathogenesis, clinical features, diagnosis, and management. *Lancet Respir Med.* 2021;9(11):1313-1327.

McCormack FX, Gupta N, Finlay GR, et al; ATS/JRS Committee on Lymphangioleiomyomatosis. Official American Thoracic Society/Japanese Respiratory Society Clinical Practice Guidelines: lymphangioleiomyomatosis diagnosis and management. *Am J Respir Crit Care Med.* 2016;194(6):748-761.

Northrup H, Aronow ME, Bebin EM, et al; International Tuberous Sclerosis Complex Consensus Group. Updated international tuberous sclerosis complex diagnostic criteria and surveillance and management recommendations. *Pediatr Neurol.* 2021;123:50-66.

Raoof S, Bondalapati P, Vydyula R, et al. Cystic lung diseases: algorithmic approach. *Chest.* 2016;150(4): 945-965.

CHAPTER 21

Acute Respiratory Failure in a Patient With Diffuse Ground-Glass Opacities During the COVID-19 Pandemic

Claudio Sorino ■ Daniela Ceriani ■ Sergio Agati

History of Present Illness

A 78-year-old woman arrived in the emergency department (ED) due to a dry cough, worsening dyspnea, and fever. Before that ED visit, the general practitioner placed her on oral azithromycin 500 mg once daily, oral acetylcysteine 600 mg once daily, and paracetamol as needed. However, she had no improvement in the symptoms after 3 days of treatment.

Past Medical History

The patient had been a heavy smoker from the age of 18 to 60 years (42 pack-years). She had a history of arterial hypertension and gastroesophageal reflux disease. About 6 months before the current presentation, she was hospitalized for obstructive jaundice from gallstones, and her gallbladder was removed. On that occasion, atrial fibrillation was found and she underwent pharmacological cardioversion with amiodarone. She received an intravenous loading dose of 300 mg diluted in 250 mL of 5% glucose over 60 minutes, followed by 450 mg in 250 mL of 5% glucose at 21 mL/hr for 8 hours, when restoration of sinus rhythm was documented. The patient then continued maintenance treatment with oral amiodarone.

Her home medication list included pantoprazole 20 mg/day, ramipril 5 mg/day, amiodarone 200 mg/day Monday through Friday, and rivaroxaban 20 mg once daily.

No vaccine for the novel coronavirus (severe acute respiratory syndrome coronavirus 2 [SARS-CoV-2]) was available at the time of clinical presentation.

Physical Examination and Early Clinical Findings

On presentation in ED, the patient was dyspneic, tachycardic, and feverish with a body temperature of 37.9°C (100.2°F). Peripheral oxygen saturation at the pulse oximeter (SpO_2) was 86% while the patient was breathing room air. Respiratory rate was about 30 breaths per minute, and blood pressure was 135/85 mm Hg. On auscultation, the breath sounds were slightly reduced and expiratory wheezing was heard in the middle and lower lung fields. Supplemental oxygen was promptly administered. However, a 50% fraction of inspired oxygen (FiO_2) via Venturi mask was required to obtain sufficient oxygen levels (SpO_2 92%). Arterial blood gas analysis (ABGA) with such oxygen supplement showed respiratory alkalosis with pH 7.48, partial pressure of oxygen (pO_2) 68 mm Hg, and partial pressure of carbon dioxide (pCO_2) 31 mmHg.

Blood tests showed leukocytosis (white blood cell count 11.820/mm^3), raised D-dimer (1560 μg/L FEU; normal value for patients > 50 years: age × 10 μg/L FEU), and a marked increase in C-reactive protein (CRP: 226 mg/L; normal values < 5 mg/L), whereas procalcitonin (PCT) was slightly raised (0.45 ng/mL; normal values < 0.1 ng/mL). No anemia or alteration of electrolytes or liver and kidney function was found.

Bedside ultrasound showed interstitial syndrome with several abnormal vertical artifacts (B-lines) bilaterally (Fig. 21.1).

The chest radiograph demonstrated a diffuse reduction of lung transparency and multiple patchy ground-glass opacities (Fig. 21.2).

Reverse transcriptase–polymerase chain reaction (RT-PCR) for SARS-CoV-2 on nasopharyngeal swab was negative.

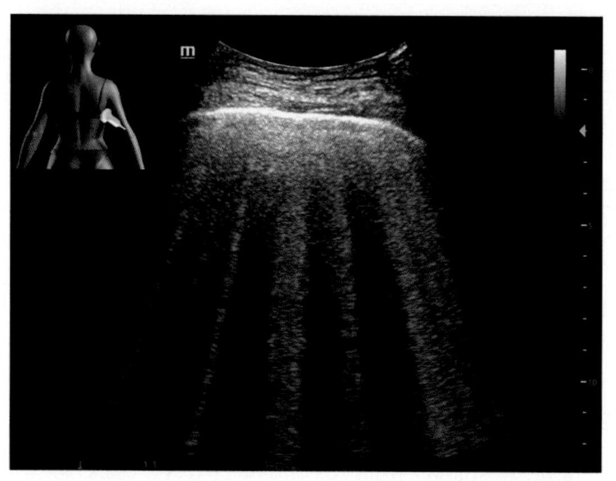

Fig. 21.1 Chest ultrasound (convex probe) demonstrating interstitial syndrome with multiple vertical pulmonary artifacts (B-lines).

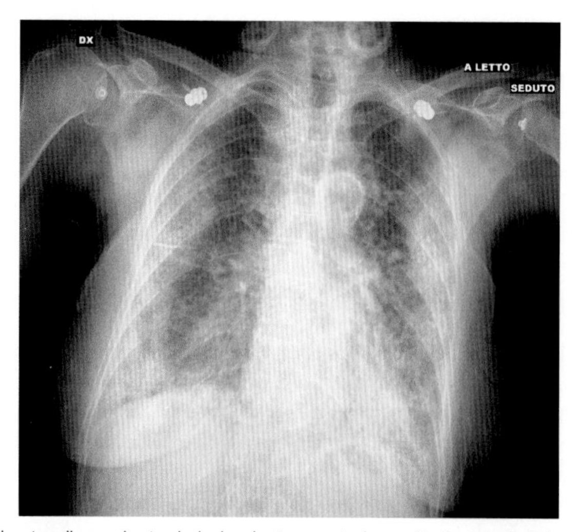

Fig. 21.2 Portable chest radiograph at admission (anteroposterior projection, patient in a semi-sitting position in bed). A diffuse reduction of lung transparency and multiple patchy areas of ground-glass opacities are evident.

Discussion Topic 1

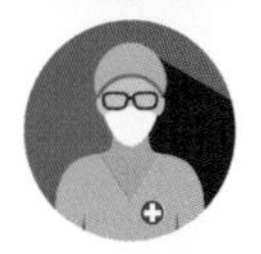

ER doctor A

This woman has a severe acute hypoxemic respiratory failure. The PaO_2:FiO_2 ratio is 136.

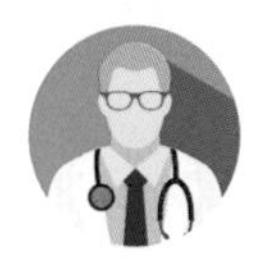

Pulmonologist A

With these oxygen values, she risks tracheal intubation.

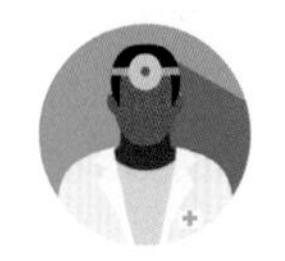

Resuscitator

We should see if she benefits from noninvasive respiratory support such as a high-flow nasal cannula (HFNC), continuous positive airway pressure (CPAP), or bilevel noninvasive ventilation (NIV). They could prevent intubation.

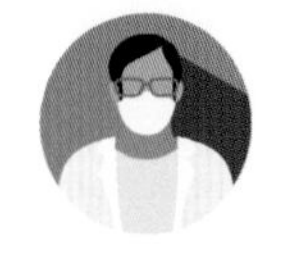

Pulmonologist B

I agree. Let's prepare a CPAP with the helmet! In my opinion, it's better tolerated than the bilevel NIV with a facial mask.
Furthermore, she does not require bilevel ventilation or guaranteed tidal volume because she is not hypercapnic.

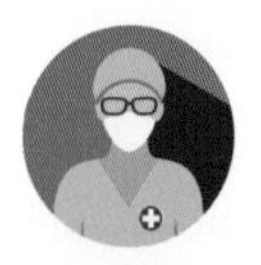

ER doctor A

We should also understand the cause of her respiratory failure.
I already asked for a CT pulmonary angiography as the patient has an increased D-dimer. So we will be able to evaluate the lung parenchyma and whether she has a pulmonary embolism.

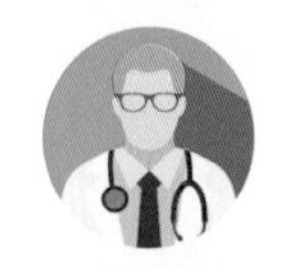

Pulmonologist A

Okay, even if the embolic risk is reduced, as the patient is already on oral anticoagulant therapy from when she had her episode of atrial fibrillation.

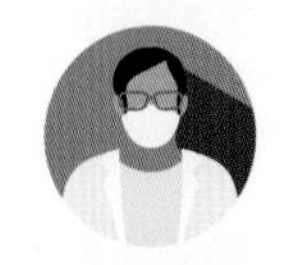

Pulmonologist B

Chest ultrasound and radiograph suggest an interstitial syndrome. As she has no clinical signs of pulmonary edema, the most likely diagnoses, in my opinion, are interstitial pneumonia or pulmonary fibrosis.

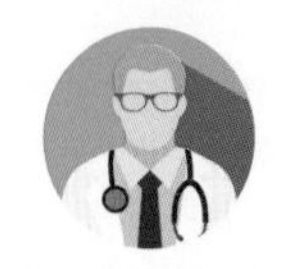

Pulmonologist A

The latter commonly doesn't have an acute onset. Moreover, the patient has a fever; therefore, I would suspect coronavirus disease 2019 (COVID-19).

Continued on following page

Discussion Topic 1 (Continued)

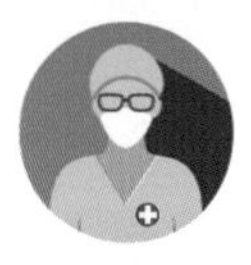

ER doctor A

Yet the nasopharyngeal swab for SARS-COV-2 is negative.

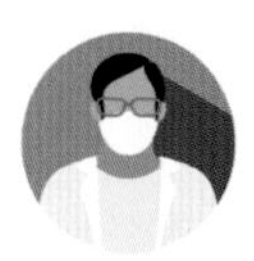

Pulmonologist B

I think it's preferable to repeat it. False-negative swabs are possible.

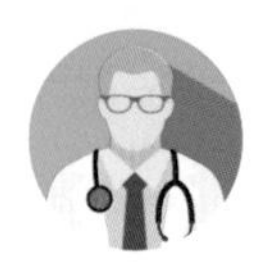

Pulmonologist A

We can also test for H1N1 influenza and the main causative pathogens of community-acquired pneumonia.

Clinical Course

The patient started helmet CPAP treatment with positive end-expiratory pressure (PEEP) of 7.5 cmH_2O and FiO_2 of 50%; then she was admitted to the pulmonology department. She obtained an improvement in oxygen parameters (SpO_2 97%, pO_2 88 mmHg), and the respiratory rate decreased to approximately 22 breaths/minute. Therefore, the use of CPAP was confirmed. Empiric administration of intravenous corticosteroids and antibiotics was initiated (dexamethasone 6 mg/day, ceftriaxone 2 mg/day), and the current anticoagulant (rivaroxaban) was continued.

Due to the evidence of breath sounds suggesting bronchospasm and the significant exposure to smoke, inhaled bronchodilators were added, assuming the patient had unrecognized COPD. In particular, the doctors chose the combination of a long-acting β_2-agonist (LABA) and a long-acting muscarinic agent (LAMA).

The computed tomography pulmonary angiography (CTPA) was negative for pulmonary embolism but showed diffuse ground-glass opacities in all pulmonary lobes, with a slight prevalence in the subpleural regions compared to the central ones. There were also focal lucencies due to preexisting emphysema, and no pleural effusion nor mediastinal lymphadenopathies were observed (Fig. 21.3).

For the first 72 hours of hospitalization, the patient maintained SpO_2 between 97% and 99% when using CPAP. During the short meal breaks, she was using a Venturi mask with the same FiO_2 of 50%, and the SpO_2 diminished to about 91%.

As a precaution, the patient was kept in airborne infection isolation. However, three molecular tests on nasopharyngeal swabs for SARS-CoV-2, repeated for 3 consecutive days, were all negative. Throat swabs for the H1N1 virus and *Mycoplasma pneumoniae* were negative as well as urinary antigen testing for *Streptococcus pneumoniae* and *Legionella pneumophila*. The search for IgM antibodies anti–*Chlamydia pneumoniae* in serum was negative, too.

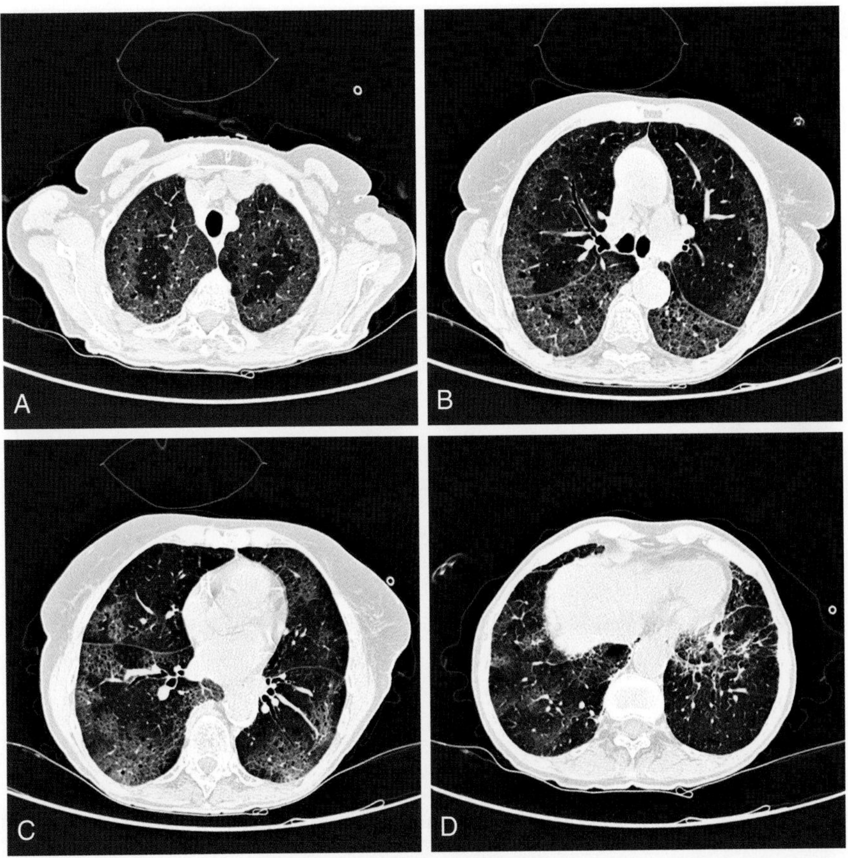

Fig. 21.3 Axial chest CT scan showing bilateral patchy areas of ground-glass opacities, involving all lung lobes, with a mainly peripheral distribution. Small focal lucencies due to emphysematous spaces (< 10 mm in size) are also visible.

Discussion Topic 2

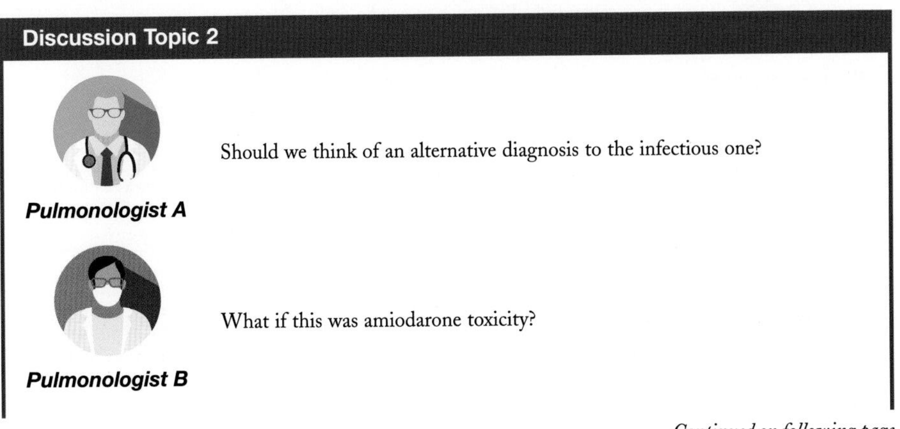

Pulmonologist A

Should we think of an alternative diagnosis to the infectious one?

Pulmonologist B

What if this was amiodarone toxicity?

Continued on following page

Discussion Topic 2 (Continued)

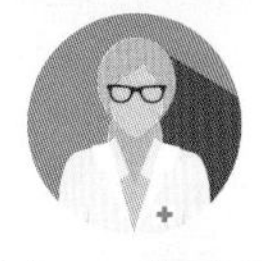

Pulmonologist C

Amiodarone can cause interstitial pneumonitis. It usually occurs after > 2 months of therapy, as in the case of our patient.

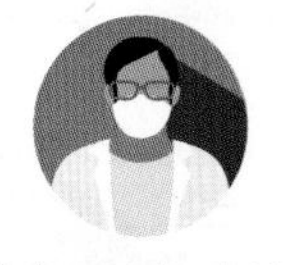

Pulmonologist B

The onset of toxicity after such a short time occurs more frequently when the daily dose of amiodarone exceeds 400 mg. In any case, we suspended its administration due to respiratory failure.

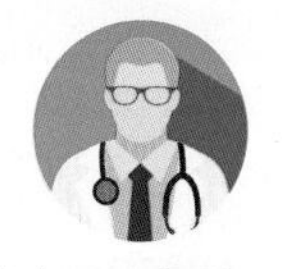

Pulmonologist A

In this period of the COVID-19 pandemic, a patient with acute respiratory failure and widespread ground-glass opacities on chest CT deserves further investigation.

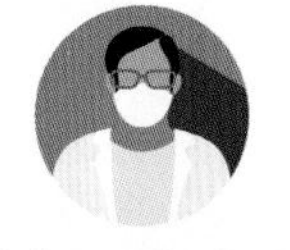

Pulmonologist B

Bronchoscopy with bronchial aspiration or bronchoalveolar lavage (BAL) could be the best way to obtain lower respiratory tract specimens and to try to settle the diagnosis.

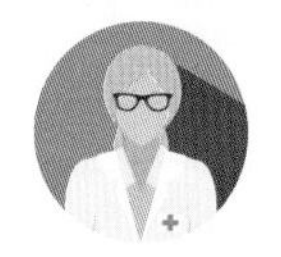

Pulmonologist C

Bronchoscopy is an aerosol-generating procedure. Don't you think it exposes operators to a high risk of transmission if the patient is infected with SARS-CoV-2?

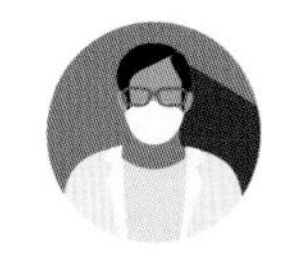

Pulmonologist B

If necessary, and I believe so, it can be done with appropriate personal protective equipment and precautions.

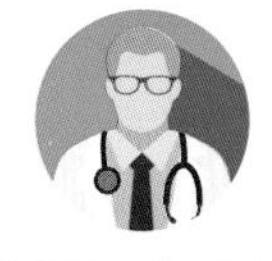

Pulmonologist A

How dangerous would that be for the patient, given that she has a severe respiratory failure?

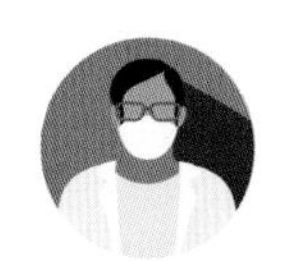

Pulmonologist B

Respiratory failure certainly exposes the patient to a greater risk of complications. We may ask for assistance from the anesthetist during the procedure. We should also limit the amount of saline instilled in the airways to a minimum.

Discussion Topic 2 (Continued)

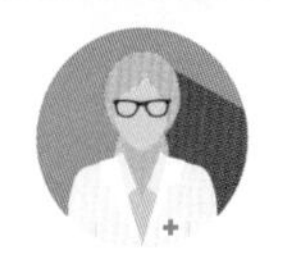

Pulmonologist C

I think the risk:benefit ratio is favorable. However, we should make the patient aware that a deteriorating condition related to the procedure may require intubation.

The patient underwent bronchoscopy using precautions intended for people infected with coronavirus, although there was still no positivity for COVID-19. The procedure was performed under the supervision of an anesthetist, using intravenous propofol and midazolam as sedation. To reduce the impact of bronchoscopy on the patient's clinical conditions, doctors performed just a small bronchial lavage by instilling a limited amount of saline solution (20 mL in this case), which allowed the collection of an adequate lower respiratory specimen for analysis.

RT–PCR for SARS-CoV-2 in bronchial lavage fluid turned positive and the patient continued her hospitalization in the ward dedicated to COVID-19 patients. Instead, bacterial cultures were negative.

After the bronchoscopy, the patient had a worsening gas exchange. SpO_2 dropped to 94% during CPAP with PEEP of 7.5 cmH_2O and FiO_2 of 50%, while ABGA showed mild hypercapnia and respiratory acidosis: pH 7.33, pO_2 70 mmHg, and pCO_2 49 mmHg.

Discussion Topic 3

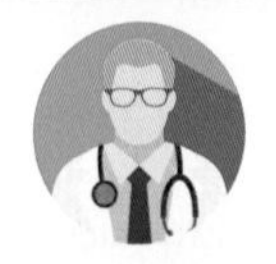

Pulmonologist A

The patient developed respiratory acidosis. Could this be related to a high supplement of oxygen during bronchoscopy?

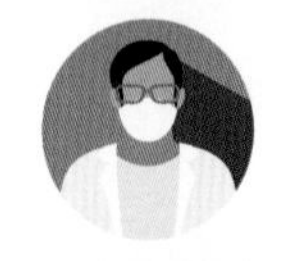

Pulmonologist B

Partially yes, excessive oxygen supplementation in a patient with chronic obstructive pulmonary disease (COPD) can depress the respiratory centers. Moreover, she received sedation.

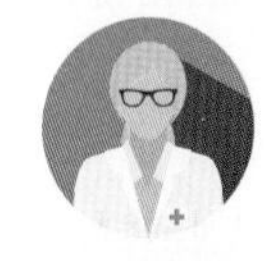

Pulmonologist C

We could keep the FiO_2 to lower levels. In patients with COPD and hypercapnia, it's sufficient to reach a saturation of just 90%.

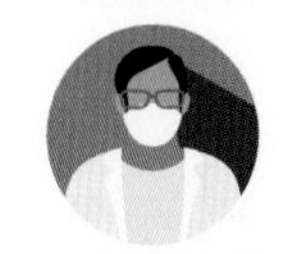

Pulmonologist B

It's also likely that her respiratory muscles are wearing out. I would switch to bilevel ventilation.

Continued on following page

Discussion Topic 3 (Continued)

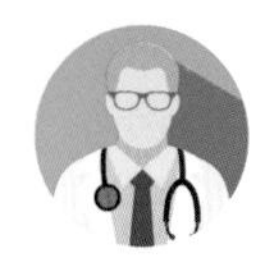

Pulmonologist A

We could also evaluate whether she benefits from pronation. It can enhance perfusion to less damaged areas of the lungs and improve ventilation-perfusion matching.

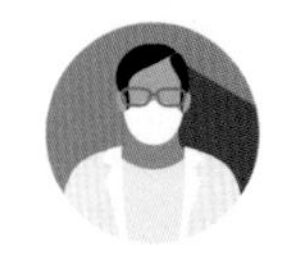

Pulmonologist B

If the patient does not tolerate pronation, we could ask her to stay in the "tripod position," sitting with the chest resting forward on a flat surface.

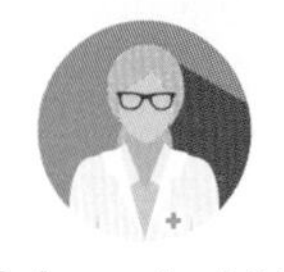

Pulmonologist C

In other patients, I also have used this position with success.
It is also known as "Rodin's position," as it resembles the famous sculpture *The Thinker* by Auguste Rodin.

In the following days, the patient showed a progressive clinical improvement with the resolution of wheezing, improvement of oxygenation parameters, and reduction of inflammation indices. Arterial pH and pCO_2 values normalized. Doctors reduced the use of noninvasive respiratory support and FiO_2. When ABGA with FiO_2 40% via Venturi mask revealed a PaO_2:FiO_2 > 200 (pO_2 86 mmHg), they stopped the mechanical ventilation. After 10 days, the systemic corticosteroid was tapered and shifted to oral administration. However, it took > 2 weeks for SpO_2 to be stably sufficient without supplemental oxygen.

Several electrocardiograms showed that the patient maintained sinus, slightly tachycardic rhythm.

Recommended Therapy and Further Indications at Discharge

The patient was discharged home after a total of 18 days of hospitalization, with the diagnosis of acute respiratory failure due to COVID-19 pneumonia and possible acute exacerbation of COPD.

Amiodarone was reintroduced in therapy (200 mg/day from Monday to Friday). A low dose of oral prednisone was recommended with further tapering (12.5 mg/day for 3 days, then 6.25 mg/day for an additional 3 days).

Pulmonary function tests after 3 months and chest high-resolution (HR) CT after 6 months were scheduled.

Follow-up and Outcomes

Three months after the acute episode, the patient regained clinical conditions and quality of life similar to those she had before admission. Pulmonary function tests revealed a moderate airway obstruction, without significant reversibility at the bronchodilation test (postbronchodilator FEV_1/VC 64%, FEV_1 72% of predicted). Diffusing capacity of the lungs for carbon monoxide (DLCO) was reduced to 74% of predicted. Thus, the diagnosis of COPD was confirmed and the use of inhaled LABA/LAMA was continued.

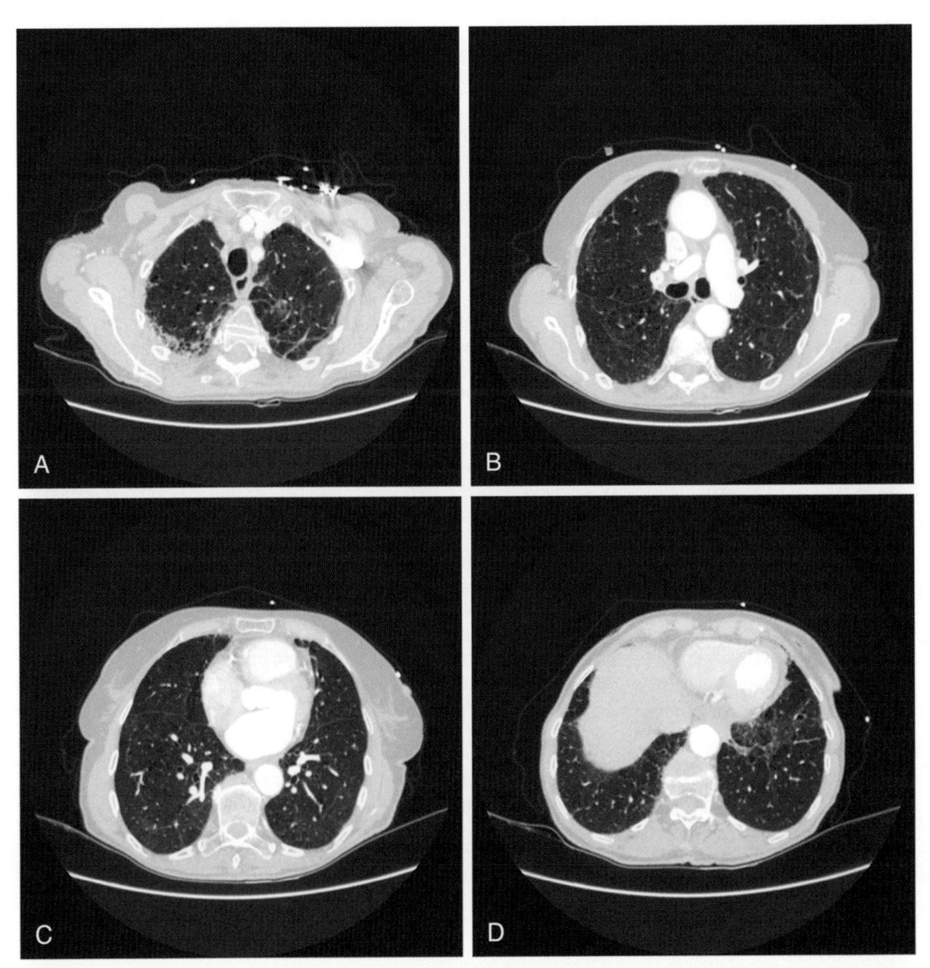

Fig. 21.4 Chest CT scan with contrast media (lung window) performed 6 months postdischarge. Pulmonary emphysema and the residual aspects of COVID-19 bilateral pneumonia are evident.

A chest HRCT scan performed 6 months after discharge showed residual peripheral opacities referable to scarring fibrotic outcomes, in addition to the previously noted pulmonary emphysema. The ground-glass areas had disappeared from all lobes (Fig. 21.4).

Focus on

Pulmonary Ground-Glass Opacities

Ground-glass opacity (GGO) is a radiological finding on chest CT scan consisting of an increased density that does not obscure the underlying bronchial structures or pulmonary vessels. Indeed, this appearance resembles glass in which the surface is artificially roughened.

The term is sometimes used in chest radiography to indicate an area of hazy lung opacity, often fairly diffuse, where pulmonary vessels are difficult to appreciate.

GGO is a nonspecific finding and may correspond to interstitial thickening, partial filling or collapse of the alveoli, or even increased blood supply. Therefore, this tomographic pattern should be always

Continued on following page

Focus on (Continued)

Pulmonary Ground-Glass Opacities

correlated with the patient's clinical presentation, laboratory tests, and associated radiology findings. Moreover, it is important to exclude false GGO, which may be due to an expiratory scan or mosaic perfusion.

GGO can be diffuse, patchy, or nodular and recognize acute (arising within 7–10 days), subacute (occurring in 10–30 days), or chronic (present for > 1 month) causes (Table. 21.1).

Acute causes of GGO include infections (mainly due to atypical bacteria and viruses), alveolar hemorrhage, pulmonary edema, diffuse alveolar damage, and pulmonary embolism.

Bilateral GGO, with or without consolidations, preferably with peripheral distribution and in the posterior segments, is the main hallmark of COVID-19 pneumonia.

Pulmonary edema is caused by the accumulation of fluid in the extravascular compartments and usually appears with GGO associated with bilateral and symmetric smooth septal thickening, sparing the periphery of the lungs (the batwing sign). Asymmetric distribution of the edema can be related to mitral valve regurgitation or chronic obstructive pulmonary disease. In such circumstances, GGO prevails in the right upper lobe and the areas least affected by emphysema, respectively. In cardiogenic pulmonary edema, pleural effusion may be present.

A wide spectrum of chronic conditions may occur with GGO, and radiological evaluation is based also on the presence of typical parenchymal signs of disease (e.g., fibrosis, honeycombing, and architectural distortion).

Nonspecific interstitial pneumonia and desquamative interstitial pneumonia are the most frequent ILD, presenting with diffuse GGO, typically peripheral, in the lower lobes and without honeycombing.

GGO may be also present (although generally not the main finding) in idiopathic pulmonary fibrosis, hypersensitivity pneumonitis, respiratory-bronchiolitis ILD, organizing pneumonia, pulmonary sarcoidosis, lung involvement in drug toxicities, alveolar proteinosis, and aspiration pneumonia.

Adenocarcinoma is the most common histology among patients with pure GGO nodules.

TABLE 21.1 ■ **Main Conditions in Which the Chest CT Scan Can Reveal GGO and Correlation With the Most Frequent Clinical Presentations and Distribution**

It should be noted that in some pathologies (eg, IPF) the GGO may be present in association with other findings, but it is not a typical element, nor is it usually the most represented.

	Onset	
Distribution	**Acute**	**Subacute/chronic**
Nodular	HP Hemorrhage	HP Adenocarcinoma DIP
Peripheral/patchy	Infections* NSIP Hemorrhage	Fibrosing HP OP DIP
Diffuse	Infections Pulmonary edema DAD ARDS Hemorrhage Eosinophilic pneumonia	Sarcoidosis Fibrosing HP NSIP Alveolar proteinosis Drug toxicity**

ARDS, acute respiratory distress syndrome; DAD, diffuse alveolar damage; DIP, desquamative interstitial pneumonia; HP, hypersensitivity pneumonitis; NSIP, nonspecific interstitial pneumonia; OP, organizing pneumonia.

*For example, coronavirus (severe acute respiratory syndrome [SARS], Middle East respiratory syndrome [MERS], COVID-19), influenza A (H1N1) virus, *Mycoplasma pneumoniae, Chlamydia pneumoniae, Pneumocystis jiroveci*, cytomegalovirus.

**For example, cyclophosphamide, bleomycin, amiodarone, tumor necrosis factor (TNF)-α blockers.

Focus on

Bronchoscopy in COVID-19

During the COVID-19 pandemic, bronchoscopy has proved to be a valuable tool for confirming the diagnosis in subjects with symptoms and imaging strongly suggestive of an ongoing infection but negative molecular nasopharyngeal swabs for SARS-CoV-2.

Bronchoscopy is also useful for differentiating COVID-19 infection from other viral interstitial pneumonias (e.g., H1N1 influenza, cytomegalovirus, *Pneumocystis jiroveci*), particularly in immunocompromised subjects. Similarly, lower airways sampling can identify superadded bacterial and/or fungal infections such as *Aspergillus* and *Candida* spp. Additionally, bronchoscopy enables the operator to perform therapeutic interventions, which can be lifesaving. For instance, in mechanically ventilated patients, it could be required for mucus plug removal, hemoptysis, and tracheostomy management.

Bronchoscopy carries a high risk of virus transmission to the bronchoscopist and other involved health care workers due to the stimulation of cough and consequent aerosol dispersion. For this reason, some precautions are required, such as:

- execution when strictly necessary, e.g., in the presence of well-founded suspicion of COVID-19 pneumonia and at least two negative molecular tests on nasopharyngeal swabs;
- provision of adequate personal protective equipment (PPE: FFP3 mask, water-repellent coat, gloves, and eye protection devices);
- dedicated room with adequate air changes (at least six per hour); and
- anesthesiological assistance, especially in the case of severe impairment of gas exchange, requiring invasive ventilatory support, curarization, and cough inhibition.

The use of disposable bronchoscopes can be convenient but not mandatory.

Focus on

Post–COVID-19 Pulmonary Fibrosis (PCPF)

Studies of previous coronavirus outbreaks have shown that pulmonary fibrosis occurred in more than half of patients after SARS-CoV infection and in one-third of those who had MERS. Similarly, COVID-19 can lead to postviral fibrosis (PCPF), characterized by an architectural distortion of the lung parenchyma, and overall impairment of lung function, with consequent physiological impairment and decreased quality of life.

The severity of COVID-19 is one of the main risk factors for PCPF development, although its exact prevalence is still unknown. This can be indicated by the need for invasive mechanical ventilation or noninvasive respiratory support, intensive care unit admission, and long hospitalization.

Fibrosis is considered to be due to the abnormal healing of the injured lung parenchyma. In COVID-19 patients, possible sources of injury include the cytokine storm caused by an improper inflammatory response, bacterial coinfections, and thromboembolic events producing microvascular damage and endothelial dysfunction. The renin-angiotensin system is also believed to be involved due to the high affinity of the SARS-CoV-2 viral spike protein to the angiotensin-converting enzyme-2 (ACE2) receptor.

The most frequent chest HRCT findings in patients with PCPF include parenchymal bands, interlobular septal thickening, and coarse reticulations. Less frequently, ground-glass opacities and consolidations are found (most often within 6–8 weeks of discharge, when an organized pneumonia-like pattern may be present).

Impaired lung diffusion capacity is the most common abnormality on pulmonary function tests (30–40%) and often persists after 6 to 12 months of follow-up, while restrictive pulmonary dysfunction is less frequent (about 10%).

To date, there is no proven treatment for PCPF, although a short postdischarge course of corticosteroids has been shown to improve symptoms and physiological parameters in patients with persistent inflammatory ILD following SARS-CoV-2 infection.

Moreover, antifibrotic drugs could have a potential role to decrease pulmonary injury in individuals with severe COVID-19.

Close follow-up of patients after SARS-CoV-2 pneumonia is essential.

LEARNING POINTS

- Lung infections from viruses and atypical bacteria can cause GGO. Clinical presentation, laboratory tests, distribution of lesions, and associated radiological findings aid in the differential diagnosis.
- Diagnostic bronchoscopy can be indicated in patients with clinical and radiological features of COVID-19 but nondiagnostic nasopharyngeal swabs.
- The risks of patient complications and transmission of SARS-CoV-2 to health care workers during bronchoscopy are low if adequate safety measures are followed.
- Pulmonary fibrosis is one of the major sequelae of COVID-19 pneumonia and deserves proper follow-up.
- Impaired lung diffusion capacity can persist beyond 1 year after COVID-19 pneumonia.

Further Reading

Guarnera A, Podda P, Santini E, Paolantonio P, Laghi A. Differential diagnoses of COVID-19 pneumonia: the current challenge for the radiologist: a pictorial essay. *Insights Imaging*. 2021;12(1):34.

Hama Amin BJ, Kakamad FH, Ahmed GS, et al. Post COVID-19 pulmonary fibrosis: a meta-analysis study. *Ann Med Surg (Lond)*. 2022;77:103590.

Lee JH, Yim JJ, Park J. Pulmonary function and chest computed tomography abnormalities 6-12 months after recovery from COVID-19: a systematic review and meta-analysis. *Respir Res*. 2022;23(1):233.

Mohammadi A, Balan I, Yadav S, et al. Post-COVID-19 pulmonary fibrosis. *Cureus*. 2022;14(3):e22770.

Mondoni M, Sferrazza Papa GF, Rinaldo R, et al. Utility and safety of bronchoscopy during the SARS-CoV-2 outbreak in Italy: a retrospective, multicentre study. *Eur Respir J*. 2020;56(4):2002767.

Myall KJ, Mukherjee B, Castanheira AM, et al. Persistent post-COVID-19 interstitial lung disease. An observational study of corticosteroid treatment. *Ann Am Thorac Soc*. 2021;18(5):799-806.

Saha BK, Chaudhary R, Saha S, et al. Bronchoscopy during coronavirus disease 2019 pandemic: a bronchoscopist's perspective. *Crit Care Explor*. 2021;3(9):e0522.

Wahidi MM, Shojaee S, Lamb CR, et al. The use of bronchoscopy during the coronavirus disease 2019 pandemic: CHEST/AABIP guideline and expert panel report. *Chest*. 2020;158(3):1268-1281.

INDEX

A

D

E

I

Q

R